Communication Disorders
Educational and
Medical Settings

*An Introduction for Speech-Language Pathologists,
Educators, and Health Professionals*

WILLIAM O. HAYNES, PHD
Professor Emeritus
Department of Communication Disorders
Auburn University

MICHAEL J. MORAN, PHD
Professor
Department of Communication Disorders
Auburn University

REBEKAH H. PINDZOLA, PHD
Professor and Chair
Department of Communication Disorders
Auburn University

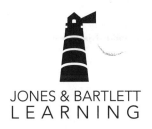

JONES & BARTLETT
LEARNING

World Headquarters

Jones & Bartlett Learning
40 Tall Pine Drive
Sudbury, MA 01776
978-443-5000
info@jblearning.com
www.jblearning.com

Jones & Bartlett Learning
Canada
6339 Ormindale Way
Mississauga, Ontario L5V 1J2
Canada

Jones & Bartlett Learning
International
Barb House, Barb Mews
London W6 7PA
United Kingdom

Jones & Bartlett Learning books and products are available through most bookstores and online booksellers. To contact Jones & Bartlett Learning directly, call 800-832-0034, fax 978-443-8000, or visit our website, www.jblearning.com.

Substantial discounts on bulk quantities of Jones & Bartlett Learning publications are available to corporations, professional associations, and other qualified organizations. For details and specific discount information, contact the special sales department at Jones & Bartlett Learning via the above contact information or send an email to specialsales@jblearning.com.

Production Credits

Publisher: David Cella
Associate Editor: Maro Gartside
Production Manager: Julie Champagne Bolduc
Production Editor: Jessica Steele Newfell
Marketing Manager: Grace Richards
Manufacturing and Inventory Control
  Supervisor: Amy Bacus

Composition: Glyph International
Cover Design: Scott Moden
Photo Research and Permissions Manager:
  Kimberly Potvin
Printing and Binding: Malloy, Inc.
Cover Printing: Malloy, Inc.

Library of Congress Cataloging-in-Publication Data
Haynes, William O.
  Communication disorders in educational and medical settings : an introduction for speech-language pathologists, educators, and health professionals / William O. Haynes, Michael J. Moran, Rebekah H. Pindzola.
    p. ; cm.
  Includes bibliographical references and index.
  ISBN 978-0-7637-7648-0 (pbk. : alk. paper)
  1. Communicative disorders. 2. Communicative disorders in children. I. Moran, Michael J., Ph. D. II. Pindzola, Rebekah H. (Rebekah Hand) III. Title.
  [DNLM: 1. Communication Disorders. WL 340.2 H424c 2010]
  RC423.H38256 2010
  362.196'855—dc22
                              2010025904
6048

Printed in the United States of America
14 13 12 11 10   10 9 8 7 6 5 4 3 2 1

CONTENTS

PREFACE

CONCEPTS UNDERLYING THE PRESENT TEXT AND TARGET AUDIENCES

The discipline of communication disorders involves the two professions of audiology and speech-language pathology. Audiologists are involved in the assessment and rehabilitation of people who have hearing loss. Speech-language pathologists (SLPs) focus on the assessment and treatment of disorders affecting speech, language, voice, and swallowing. Both audiologists and SLPs serve as primary interventionists for communication disorders that affect children, adolescents, and adults.

Most introductory texts on communication disorders place heavy emphasis on speech-language pathology and devote only a single chapter to audiology. One reason for this is because training programs typically require students to take another course titled "Introduction to Audiology" in which hearing is the sole topic of consideration. This text is designed to be an introductory text for communication disorders as well as a text that could be used in the training of educational and health professionals. It is designed in the traditional way, with a single chapter on hearing disorders that provides treatment implications for speech-language pathologists, educators, and health professionals. Students interested in audiology as a potential career can find a general introduction in the present text that can then be elaborated in additional coursework on hearing disorders.

The two most common environments in which audiologists and SLPs provide services are educational settings (school systems) and medical settings (hospitals, rehabilitation centers, long-term care facilities, medical clinics). Educational professionals (classroom teachers, special educators, school psychologists, teaching assistants) in the school setting and health professionals (physicians, nurses, occupational therapists, physical therapists, nurses' aides) in the medical/clinical environment frequently encounter communication disorders. As speech-language pathologists perform assessment and treatment activities in educational and medical settings, they typically make an effort to collaborate with setting-specific professionals in providing services. These relationships are depicted in **Figure 1**. For example, classroom teachers and special educators can play a vital role in providing assessment information to the SLP and can also become involved in the treatment program to promote generalization of communication skills to the natural environment. Similarly, in medical settings, health professionals are in a position to provide critical

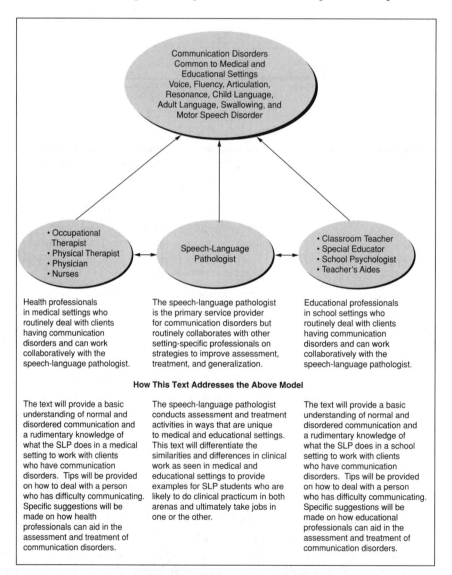

FIGURE 1   **Relationships among health professionals, speech-language pathologists, and educators in medical and educational settings.**

help in generalizing communication goals while the patient is receiving nursing care, physical therapy, or occupational therapy.

To collaborate in treatment or assessment activities, health and educational professionals must have a basic knowledge of the nature of various communication disorders and awareness of how they might play a role in the treatment process. Likewise, students in training to become speech-language pathologists must gain an appreciation of how their role is similar and different as they move from educational to medical settings and how to work with educational and health professionals. Thus, there are several important uses of this text:

1. The primary use of the book is as an introductory text in communication disorders that illustrates not only normal and disordered communication in children and adults but also how professionals deal with these disorders in school and medical settings.
2. Educators and health professionals can also use the text in training or in coursework on various disorders encountered in school and medical settings. Communication disorders are among the most frequently encountered problems in both school and medical environments. The text provides an introduction to normal and disordered communication in medical and educational settings. We make specific suggestions for health and educational professionals in terms of how to deal with clients with communication disorders and how to collaborate with the SLP in assessment and treatment.
3. The book is useful as a guide for the SLP in working with other professionals in school and medical environments because it includes practical suggestions for involvement of other professionals in the assessment and remediation processes.

Table 1 shows an example of how the disorders of communication are both similar and different across medical/clinical and educational settings. The various chapters covering communication disorders are listed in the left column and the work settings and client populations are included in the next two columns. Chapters 1, 2, 3, and 7 address normal aspects of the field and the communication processes that are applicable to medical/clinical and educational work settings.

OUR APPROACH TO PEDAGOGY

The field of communication disorders, similar to many other disciplines, has undergone an information explosion in the past 25 years. Both the fields of speech-language pathology and audiology have experienced quantum leaps in technology and empirical research since the turn of the new century. These fields have embraced evidence-based practice that combines use of relevant research with clinical skills and the unique needs of patients. Now, more than ever before, training programs are straining to provide adequate coverage of all dimensions of communication sciences and disorders. Master's programs in speech-language pathology have been lengthened, and now a clinical doctorate is the required credential in the field of audiology. Students often report that it is a struggle to process all of the classroom information and learn the diverse clinical skills necessary for certification as a professional.

TABLE I An Example of How the Various Disorders of Communication Are Seen in Educational and Medical Settings

Disorder	Educational Setting	Medical/Clinical Setting
Voice disorders Chapter 9	Disorders of vocal fold mass and approximation, intensity, quality, pitch, and so forth in children and adolescents.	Disorders of vocal fold mass and approximation, intensity, quality, pitch, and so forth in adults. Adult disorders such as laryngectomy, vocal cord paralysis, spasmodic dysphonia, and hysterical aphonia are often seen in medical settings.
Articulation disorders Chapter 4	Developmental phonology disorders, articulation disorders.	Glossectomy, jaw and oral cancer.
Motor speech disorders Chapter 13	Dysarthrias seen in children with cerebral palsy and other conditions, developmental apraxia, apraxia of speech in brain-injured adolescents.	Dysarthrias and apraxia seen in postcerebrovascular accident (CVA) patients and in some degenerative diseases.
Early child language disorders Chapter 5	Disorders of syntax, semantics, morphology in preschool children. Autism and cognitive limitations in young children.	Working with neonatal ICU and families of high-risk children during the infant/toddler period.
School-age, adolescent, and adult language disorders Chapter 6 Chapter 12 Chapter 13 Chapter 14	Disorders of syntax, semantics, morphology, and pragmatics in older children/adolescents; literacy-based problems in school settings. Adolescents with traumatic brain injury and other brain injury exhibit problems with word retrieval, memory, executive function, and other difficulties seen in adults with brain injury.	Adults with aphasia, dementia, TBI, and degenerative neurologic conditions, and so forth.
Fluency disorders Chapter 8	Stuttering, cluttering seen in children and adolescents.	Fluency problems in adults associated with motor speech disorders, word finding difficulties, and language processing load. Adult stuttering.
Swallowing disorders Chapter 13	Children/adolescents with dysphagia as a product of neurologic conditions.	Adults with dysphagia as a result of neurologic insult are seen in acute care and rehabilitation medical settings.
Hearing impairments Chapter 10	Children/adolescents with hearing impairment that is either congenital or acquired.	Adults with hearing impairment.
Resonance disorders Chapters 9 and 11	Children with clefts and other velopharyngeal problems.	Children with clefts seen by cleft palate teams. Adults with resonance disorders secondary to brain injury, surgery, or degenerative conditions.

In most training programs, students are initially exposed to the field of communication disorders in an introductory course. The goal of such a course is to provide an overview of basic processes of speech, hearing, and language and discuss common disorders that professionals deal with in communication disorders. After or concurrently with the introductory course, students take courses in the normal processes of speech, hearing, and language such as phonetics, speech and hearing science, anatomy and physiology, and introduction to audiology. The next step is completion of courses focusing on disorders of speech, hearing, and language that discuss in considerable detail the nature of each type of impairment and assessment and treatment approaches used in remediation. Then, on the graduate level, students also take even more advanced courses in all of the communication disorders and participate in extensive clinical practicum experiences.

As veteran instructors who have many years of experience introducing students to the field of communication disorders, we have observed several recurring issues:

- When students begin taking more focused courses in the field, we have found that they most often do not remember the specific terms they "learned" in the introductory course, mainly because concepts were introduced too quickly and superficially to facilitate recall. Our task in these later courses, then, becomes reintroducing the specifics of each disorder in earnest.
- We have noticed that colleagues teaching the introductory courses and using a very complex text often have to omit certain information to cover all relevant areas in a given semester. Thus, some students have the experience of being required to "know" certain information from the text for test purposes and are not responsible for other facts in preparation for an examination.
- The average semester has only about 40 class days of approximately one hour in which to cover material. If an instructor administers four 1-hour examinations during a semester, that reduces the number of teaching days to 36. Especially in introductory courses, instructors tend to show DVD presentations of the various disorders, and many of these videos are not specifically designed to be compatible with the introductory textbook. Thus, when you remove teaching time lost as a result of video presentations, there are precious few hours left to cover normal aspects of speech, hearing, and language plus all of the disorder areas. It is not unusual for instructors to have only two or three days to address a particular area of interest such as fluency disorders, articulation, anatomy, language disorders, or vocal disorders. The bottom line is that teaching opportunities are limited and the broad base of an introductory overview course makes it important that instructors cover material at a consistent depth that allows for understanding but that does not overload the student.

As a result of the preceding points, we saw the need to create an introductory textbook that covers all relevant areas, but that does so in a way so as not to overwhelm students. It is axiomatic that an introductory text should cover the *breadth* of a discipline to give students a sampling of its relevant components and a flavor for the duties of professional practitioners. In a field as vast as communication disorders, it is a challenge to do justice even to the breadth of the field. And the real challenge concerns the *depth* at which each area is considered. Our solution is to attempt to control the depth in each section by limiting inclusion of more technical information that will be covered in later courses. We also make a conscious effort to minimize the use of references to the research literature that students will study in more specific coursework. We use references to support major points in the text without overwhelming students with a large bibliography.

This, of course, is a judgment call on the part of the present authors, but our goal is to have each chapter be similar in depth, creating an evenness of content throughout the book. Instructors can always add information if they deem it important for introductory students. This, in many ways, is more workable than telling students to ignore sections of a text that have provided too much depth for beginning students. We carefully considered the selection of information that is critical to an overview of the profession with the goals of keeping the text readable and not overwhelming students and instructors. Even this approach results in ample detail in all the areas of normal processes and disorders; students will find learning the material challenging but doable. Students can use the general foundation they develop in their introductory courses to build more in-depth knowledge in later courses in the training program.

No matter what a student's major or a reader's profession, he or she is still in the position of learning about communication sciences and disorders for the first time. We intend this text primarily for speech-language pathologists in training, and we also make the information accessible to professionals in education and allied health and anyone unfamiliar with this field. Whether you are an educator, health professional, or speech-language pathologist in training, we are certain that you will find this introduction to the field of communication disorders exciting, interesting, and relevant to your future work.

COMMUNICATION DISORDERS IN EDUCATIONAL AND MEDICAL SETTINGS: BACKGROUND, LEGAL/ ADMINISTRATIVE ISSUES, PROFESSIONAL ROLES, AND SERVICE DELIVERY MODELS

Whether you are reading this textbook as a communication disorders major or are a student majoring in education or allied health professions (e.g., physical therapy, nursing, occupational therapy), you are starting out at the same place as many other students. You probably know little about communication sciences and disorders and are taking this course to gain an overview of the field. We cover the breadth of the profession while controlling the depth to which we go in each chapter so the information is not overwhelming. We also keep the references and technical terms to a minimum so you can focus on the big picture while still learning some detail.

BACKGROUND INFORMATION: THE COMMUNICATION DISORDERS PROFESSIONAL

Communication takes many forms, some verbal and some nonverbal. **Language** is a major part of the human communication system because it includes words and rules for organizing them. **Speech** is the process by which sound is shaped into meaningful units, such as words, whereas **audition** is the process of hearing what is said. A multitude of genetic, prenatal and perinatal (at birth) factors can interfere with a child's normal development of speech, language, and audition. Acquired damage, as from traumatic injuries and diseases, also can affect a child's or adult's ability to use speech and language or to hear it. These difficulties constitute communication disorders that can affect a person's development and/or lifestyle in a negative way.

Audiology and **speech-language pathology** are professions that play primary habilitative and rehabilitative roles for children and adults with communication disorders. In this chapter, we briefly discuss both the professions of audiology and speech-language pathology in terms of scope of practice, educational/clinical preparation, and credentialing. Other than Chapter 10, our focus is on speech-language pathology for the remainder of the book. Throughout the rest of the text we often abbreviate speech-language pathologist as SLP to save space and avoid cumbersome writing.

WORK SETTINGS

Audiologists and speech-language pathologists often work closely in many settings with professionals such as physicians, neurologists, dentists, classroom teachers, psychologists, occupational therapists, physical therapists, nurses, and special educators. Communication disorders are among the most common impairments in medical as well as educational settings. This is one reason this text introduces communication disorders to audiologists and speech-language pathologists and to students in training for education and health professions. The more members of a rehabilitation team know about communication disorders, the greater the possibility of multidisciplinary cooperation in assessment and treatment. From the preceding list of professionals that cooperate with specialists in communication disorders, it may be obvious that speech-language pathologists and audiologists can be employed in a variety of settings. Although such settings can be broadly divided into clinical/medical and educational, we can discuss them more specifically. **Figure 1–1** illustrates that clinical/medical settings can include acute care hospitals, rehabilitation hospitals, community clinics, private practices, university clinics, and long-term care facilities. The second major category of educational settings is far simpler because it includes public school systems and private schools. This is rather deceptive because, in speech-language pathology, the majority of clinicians work in school settings.

We would like to spend a little time here briefly to characterize the clinical/medical settings. There are subtle differences among these facilities. First, **acute care hospitals** are the medical facilities that individuals with a critical need for care go to. For example, if a person experiences a stroke or heart attack, he would be taken to an acute care hospital. The length of stay at such a hospital is typically short, usually not more than a few weeks in duration. A major goal in such a hospital is to stabilize the patient and remove life-threatening conditions. At the end of that time, the patient either goes home or is transferred to a rehabilitation hospital for further treatment. Some acute care hospitals specialize in the pediatric population and are often known as children's hospitals. Some of these facilities offer both inpatient and outpatient services after a patient is discharged.

The second type of clinical/medical facility is a **rehabilitation hospital**. In a rehabilitation hospital, a patient receives medical treatment, but also a host of other therapies such as physical, occupational, speech-language, and respiratory is available. The length of stay at a rehabilitation hospital is typically less than two months. A third type of clinical/medical facility is the **community clinic**. In many urban communities, a clinic is set up by an organization (e.g., Sertoma International, Easter Seals). Such a clinic may include services such as physical therapy, occupational therapy, and speech-language therapy, but

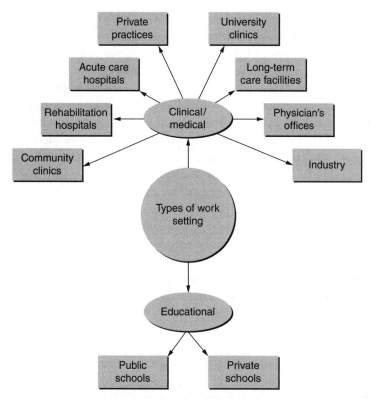

FIGURE 1–1 Types of work settings in audiology and speech-language pathology.

does not typically have an inpatient program where clients are housed residentially. Usually, the patients come for services to community clinics on an outpatient basis.

A fourth type of clinical/medical facility is called a **private practice**. This is an office set up by one or more professionals in audiology or speech pathology where outpatient services are provided. Imagine an office complex where the speech-language pathologist "hangs a shingle" and advertises services in speech and language assessment and treatment. It is like a doctor's or dentist's office that provides services. Sometimes professionals in private practice provide services to other facilities such as hospitals, day care programs, or Head Start programs. Usually, private practices comprise a limited number of professionals ranging from one to five; however, when a private practice develops to the point when it includes many specialists from different disciplines, it can turn into a community clinic.

The fifth kind of clinical/medical facility is a **university-based clinic**. If you are a major in communication disorders, you probably have one of these on your campus and it is an important part of your training program. University clinics provide clinical practicum for students in training to be audiologists and speech-language pathologists. These clinics usually see a full range of clients but do not typically have medical facilities or physicians on duty.

Thus, the patients seen in a university clinic are children and adults who seek assessment and treatment services as outpatients. Most of the services are provided by students in training under the supervision of certified professionals in communication disorders.

The sixth clinical/medical setting is the **long-term care facility**. These facilities are also known as nursing homes or assisted living centers. Patients in these facilities are residents who are typically not expected to return to independent living because of some persistent medical condition. The residents, however, still might require physical, occupational, respiratory, or speech-language treatment to increase their quality of life and allow them to be as independent as possible. The patients may also suffer from hearing impairment and require periodic reevaluation and maintenance of their hearing instruments.

The final two clinical/medical settings are usually reserved for specialists in audiology. Audiologists often are hired by physicians who specialize in otolaryngology (ear, nose, throat) because audiologic assessment and monitoring are essential to diagnosis and monitoring of treatment. It is far more common for an audiologist rather than a speech-language pathologist to be employed in a physician's office. Finally, many companies employ audiologists to monitor the hearing abilities of workers exposed to high levels of noise. The **industrial audiologist** assesses hearing acuity and prescribes hearing protection for workers as part of a program of hearing conservation.

It is clear from this discussion that audiologists and speech-language pathologists have diverse opportunities for employment in clinical/medical settings. Although educational settings may appear on the surface to be less diversified, there is more to these employment sites than meets the eye. First, educational settings vary from urban to rural. Working in a school system in a large city is quite different from being employed in a small town. One difference is in the number of colleagues available with whom to collaborate. Large city school systems may have more than a hundred speech-language pathologists to service the many schools in the urban area. Such systems have opportunities for professionals in many areas to collaborate in research, participate in continuing education, and devise innovative programs. Some school systems have taken the responsibility for serving the birth to 3 years population, and all school systems are responsible for children between the ages of 3 and 5. In rural school systems, it is possible that only one or two specialists in communication disorders are employed. Many states have school systems that are run by cities and other school systems that are run by counties. The age range of students served by the communication disorders specialists typically spans birth to age 21. Thus, it is not only children who receive services in school systems, but young adults as well. Another aspect of public school services is that the speech-language pathologist sees a full range of disorders. For example, disorders of voice, stuttering, articulation, language, and swallowing are all seen in public school settings. Furthermore, students with neurologic disorders such as cerebral palsy and head injury receive services in the public schools. In some school systems, the clinicians perform treatment and assessment in school buildings and children's homes, and they sometimes visit hospital settings to provide services under the aegis of the public schools. It is important to note that all services in public schools are provided free of charge, which is not the case in clinical/medical settings. Thus, the school system caseload offers a diversity of disorders, ages, and environments rivaling clinical/medical settings.

According to recent surveys (American Speech-Language-Hearing Association [ASHA], 2003), approximately 56 percent of speech-language pathologists work in school settings and 35 percent are employed in healthcare facilities such as hospitals and other residential facilities. The remaining 10 percent are either in private practice or university settings. Surveys report that 54 percent of audiologists (ASHA, 2003) are employed in nonresidential healthcare settings. Another 26 percent work in hospitals, and 11 percent in school systems.

THE PROFESSIONS OF AUDIOLOGY AND SPEECH-LANGUAGE PATHOLOGY

Audiologists focus on problems of hearing and largely perform diagnostic, habilitative, and rehabilitative services for both children and adults. The American Speech-Language-Hearing Association (2004) provides a summary of the scope of practice in both audiology and speech-language pathology. For both professions, more specific responsibilities are delineated in general areas. In this book, we only scratch the surface. There are six general areas of practice in the field of audiology:

1. *Prevention:* Audiologists conduct hearing conservation, **screening**, and education programs in an effort to prevent hearing impairment and promote hearing wellness. **Prevention** may also involve identifying adverse acoustic environments that can contribute to hearing loss.
2. *Identification (screening):* Audiologists attempt initially to identify people with hearing loss from birth throughout the life span. They also identify those with balance disorders and tinnitus (ringing in the ears).
3. *Assessment:* Whereas screening serves initially to identify those persons with hearing impairments, assessment involves a detailed examination of the entire auditory system from the ear canal to neurologic aspects of hearing. The audiologist uses many different technologically sophisticated devices to test the various parts of the hearing mechanism. Some of these involve use of pure tones and others use speech stimuli to determine exactly the type of signals the patient can hear and those that present difficulty. The results of a thorough assessment are used to develop a comprehensive treatment plan.
4. *Rehabilitation:* Audiologists fit appropriate hearing technology devices such as assistive listening systems and hearing aids as part of a management program. They also assess persons to determine whether a cochlear implant is appropriate, and if so, they participate in fitting and optimization of its use. Audiologists provide training in aural rehabilitation/habilitation, auditory training, speech reading, and strategies for effective communication. They also provide training for people with balance difficulties.
5. *Advocacy/consultation:* The audiologist provides advocacy for the rights of groups or individuals with hearing impairments and assists in obtaining funding for technology and/or treatment. Audiologists consult with other professionals, clients, families, agencies, the

government, and industry regarding hearing, auditory impairments, and management services.

6. *Education/research/administration:* Audiologists participate in professional education programs by teaching academic and clinical skills to students in training to be professionals in communication disorders. They also conduct basic and applied research on hearing, auditory impairments, assessment, and treatment to provide efficacy data on assessment and treatment protocols.

For a general explanation of screening, assessment, and treatment of persons with hearing impairments, refer to Chapter 10. As mentioned previously, the field of audiology is quite complex, and we cover it only enough to provide you with a flavor for what these professionals do in practice. Students in communication disorders who are interested in audiology as a specialty will have several courses specific to this field in their training program.

Speech-language pathologists diagnose and treat both problems of speech and problems of language. The disorders addressed by the speech-language pathologist fall into several broad areas, which include disorders of *voice, language, fluency, articulation,* and *swallowing.* Within each area are many specific types of communication impairments, and we describe these in separate chapters. For now, it is enough to know the general areas to allow us to briefly outline the scope of practice in speech-language pathology. Just as in audiology, there are six general components addressed in the ASHA (2004) scope of practice document:

1. *Prevention:* Speech-language pathologists promote communication wellness by promoting healthy lifestyles. Activities such as smoking cessation and wearing head protection in sports reduce the probability of laryngeal cancer and brain injury that could cause a communication impairment. Early detection and intervention programs with infants maximize communication abilities and reduce the level of handicap for individuals with disorders.

2. *Identification (screening):* The speech-language pathologist engages in screening procedures initially to identify persons with communication disorders. Screenings are especially important in the early **identification** of children with communication impairments but are also critical in identifying adults who suffer from speech, language, or hearing problems as a result of a variety of medical and neurologic conditions.

3. *Assessment:* After a person is identified as having a communication disorder, the speech-language pathologist conducts an in-depth evaluation to determine the extent of impairment and designs a program of treatment. The assessment may involve measurements by electronic devices, communication sampling, and administration of standardized tests.

4. *Treatment:* The speech-language pathologist provides intervention for adults and children diagnosed with speech and language disorders, which include the following possible management targets: articulation, motor speech disorders, apraxia, resonance disorders, voice disorders (e.g., disorders of pitch, loudness, quality), fluency disorders (e.g., stuttering, cluttering), language disorders (including syntax, semantics, morphology, phonology, pragmatics, literacy, and prelinguistic communication), cognitive disorders (e.g., attention, memory, problem solving), and feeding/swallowing disorders. The treatment can also include methods of augmentative communication using high- or

low-technology solutions such as laptop computers with speech synthesizers or simple communication boards.

5. *Advocacy/consultation:* The speech-language pathologist advocates for persons with speech, language, and swallowing impairments by serving as a member of collaborative teams, helping to secure funding for equipment/services, and serving as a consultant with other professionals.

6. *Education/research/administration:* Speech-language pathologists design and conduct public awareness programs on normal communication, communication disorders, swallowing impairments, and prevention of disorders. They conduct in-service training for other professionals and participate in the education and training of communication disorders specialists. Administrative duties involve managing clinical and academic programs.

It is easy to see that both audiologists and speech-language pathologists have much in common in terms of work settings and scope of practice. Both professions are intimately involved in prevention, identification, assessment, treatment, counseling, advocacy, administration, and research. The difference is that audiologists are focused on hearing, balance, and tinnitus, and speech-language pathologists largely concentrate on specific disorders of speech and language.

CREDENTIALING IN AUDIOLOGY AND SPEECH-LANGUAGE PATHOLOGY

Becoming an audiologist or speech-language pathologist is a complex process that is largely dictated by professional associations. The **American Speech-Language-Hearing Association (ASHA)** is a major professional organization made up of speech-language pathologists and audiologists. ASHA also includes the National Student Speech-Language-Hearing Association (NSSLHA) for students majoring in communication disorders. ASHA provides guidelines for the training of these professionals, which involves both academic and clinical skills. The academic and clinical requirements for becoming a communication disorders professional are quite complicated, and we discuss the process only generally in this chapter. To read the detailed requirements, go to http://www.asha.org/certification. Academically, in terms of degree requirements, a speech-language pathologist must obtain a master's degree (Master of Science, Master of Arts, Master of Communication Disorders) with a specialty in speech-language pathology, whereas an audiologist must obtain a doctoral degree (AuD; Doctor of Audiology). The degree program must be accredited by ASHA to ensure that it meets professional requirements. During the degree programs, speech-language pathologists and audiologists are required to obtain specific academic skills (specialized coursework) and demonstrate clinical skills in supervised practicum experiences. As you might predict, audiology programs are heavily weighted toward the study of normal hearing, hearing disorders, audiometric assessment, and aural rehabilitation along with courses in balance disorders. Speech-language pathologists study the normal aspects of speech, hearing, and language followed by coursework in how those areas can be disordered, assessed, and treated. Near the end of their training program, students in audiology and speech-language pathology must pass a national examination in their area of specialty. The student must also complete a year of working in the profession under the mentorship of a certified speech-language pathologist or audiologist. This is known as the **clinical fellowship year (CFY)**. In some audiology programs, this is included in the final year of the degree program. Speech-language pathologists typically complete their CFY during their first year of paid employment, with a certified professional agreeing to supervise them during that period. Thus, to be certified by ASHA, a student must (1) complete the required degree in the area of specialty at an accredited university program, (2) complete all academic and clinical requirements that are part of that accredited program, (3) pass a national examination in the area of specialty, and (4) complete a clinical fellowship year in the area of specialty. When all of this is completed, ASHA awards a **Certificate of Clinical Competence (CCC)** in either audiology or speech-language pathology. It should also be mentioned that the field of audiology has organizations other than ASHA that affect student training and professional development. One such group is the **American Academy of Audiology (AAA)**.

Certification is critical for speech-language pathologists and audiologists, but there is another credential typically required to practice. Each state has licensure requirements for audiologists and speech-language pathologists. In almost every state to provide clinical services, the professional must qualify for a state license. Fortunately, licensure requirements are typically identical to certification requirements, so professionals who have the CCC also qualify for a state license.

THE INFLUENCE OF PROFESSIONAL ORGANIZATIONS

As mentioned earlier, organizations such as ASHA set requirements for the training of professionals in communication disorders by accrediting university programs and prescribing academic and clinical experiences necessary to result in certification. ASHA also plays a role in establishing a code of professional ethics to which all speech-language pathologists must adhere. The code of ethics protects patients who receive services and ensures that clinicians act professionally and ethically in their practice. You can find the code of ethics at http://www.asha.org/docs/html/ET2010-00309.html. ASHA also serves a research function by publishing professional journals, offering grants for research, and holding continuing education workshops and conventions.

CASELOAD ISSUES FOR SPEECH-LANGUAGE PATHOLOGISTS IN EDUCATIONAL AND MEDICAL SETTINGS

EDUCATIONAL SETTINGS

One intent of this book is to provide classroom teachers, special education personnel, and SLPs interested in working in school settings with information on communication disorders so that they may better serve students with specific speech, language, or hearing problems. You may well wonder how many students in school settings have disorders of communication.

In the 50 states and the District of Columbia for the 2000–2001 school year, a total of 5,775,772 students (ages 6 to 21 years) received special education services (U.S. Department of Education, 2000). More than 50 percent of students being served by special educators in the public schools had learning disabilities as their primary handicap. Students whose primary impairment was speech or language accounted for 18.9 percent of the total served, and students with hearing impairments were 1.2 percent.

Clearly then, students with learning disabilities and communication disorders constitute the bulk of students with handicaps served in the schools, and other categories of disabilities (i.e., cognitive impairment, emotional disturbance, multihandicapped, orthopedically impaired, other health impaired and visually handicapped) are less prevalent. The astute reader will no doubt notice that all the incidence figures reported here are for children older than the age of 5 years. According to the law, schools must provide services for preschool children between the ages of 3 and 5 years. Many school systems have expanded this mandate to also include the birth to 3 years population. Because speech/language disorders are more prevalent in preschool-age children, this population expands the potential caseload of the school-based SLP considerably.

It is important to note that of the students who are classified as learning disabled, cognitively impaired, multihandicapped, and orthopedically impaired, a large proportion of these youngsters have an accompanying communication disorder in speech, hearing, or language. These students are classified according to their primary disability (e.g., cognitive impairment) and are not included in the 18.9 percent speech/language-impaired figure mentioned previously because this figure represents only those students whose primary classification is speech/language disorder. Thus, the SLP has a large number of cases who have speech, language, or hearing impairment as their primary disability, and also a very large population of other children whose primary classification represents another category, but who are likely to be receiving speech/language treatment as part of their special education program.

As a result of the large caseloads, the number of SLP positions in public school systems can be expected to increase nationwide. According to the U.S. Bureau of Labor Statistics, the employment rate for the profession of speech-language pathology is expected to grow significantly for the next decade. A 27 percent increase in job openings is predicted to compensate for the shortfall in available SLPs to serve ever growing caseloads of children and adults. All teachers, but especially elementary and special education personnel, can fully expect to have students with significant communication disorders in their classrooms at some time.

Results from the 2003 ASHA Omnibus Survey indicate that the average caseload size for speech-language pathologists working in schools full-time is 53, with a range from 15 cases to 110 cases. Average caseload size varies significantly by state. For example, on the ASHA Omnibus Survey of 2003, the lowest average caseload was North Dakota with 32, and the highest was Indiana with 75. As discussed later in this book, SLPs may use any of several available service delivery models. They see some students individually, others in groups; they accomplish some goals by integrating treatment into classroom activities. The 2003 ASHA Omnibus Survey indicates that speech-language pathologists have a mean of 49 individual sessions and 83 group sessions per month. Nearly 71 percent of their caseload consists of students older than the age of 6 years, 26 percent represents 3- to 5-year-olds, and almost 3.5 percent are in the birth to 2 years age group. Additionally, a wide range of severity of communication disorders is represented in the SLP's caseload: 23 percent of students exhibit severe impairments, 51 percent moderate impairments, and 26 percent mild impairments.

Subsequent chapters describe the various prevalence figures associated with each type of communication disorder. The frequency of occurrence, say, of language impairments is vastly different from that of voice disorders. The ASHA Schools Survey (ASHA, 2006) summarizes data with regard to representation of each disorder type in the typical SLP's caseload. **Table 1–1** shows this information. The percentages exceed 100 because of cooccurring disorders. For example, a student may exhibit both a language and articulation disorder. It is easy to see from Table 1–1 that the SLP must have expertise across many disparate areas. The implication for teachers is that this diverse group of students will also be present in their classes.

TABLE 1–1   Percentage of School-Based SLPs Who Provide Regular Services to Each Disorder Group and the Average Number of Clients Representing the Category on the Caseload

Diagnostic Category	% of SLPs Who Report Regularly Providing Services	Mean Number of Clients in Category on Caseload
Aphasia	6.0	4.5
Articulation/phonology	91.8	23.9
Attention Deficit Disorder	65.4	7.5
Autism/pervasive developmental disorder	77.4	5.0
Cognitive disorder	43.6	10.6
Swallowing disorder	13.8	4.0
Fluency disorder	67.5	2.5
Hearing disorder	45.8	3.2
Learning disability	72.4	16.5
Cognitive impairment	70.9	10.8
Motor speech disorder	4.7	4.1
Augmentative communication	50.8	4.8
Reading/writing	37.7	14.0
Language impairment	61.1	17.2
Verbal apraxia	59.4	3.1
Voice disorder	33.8	1.9

Source: Adapted from ASHA, 2006.

MEDICAL SETTINGS

For speech-language pathologists working in clinical or medical settings, ASHA provides statistics that give a snapshot of the typical caseloads (ASHA, 2007b). Regarding age groups, the 2007 healthcare survey revealed that 60 percent of clients in clinical/medical settings are adults, 12 percent are school age, 13 percent are preschool age, and 16 percent are infants/toddlers. **Table 1–2** shows the breakdown by disorder for clinicians working with adult and pediatric populations in clinical/medical settings.

LEGAL AND ADMINISTRATIVE ISSUES IN EDUCATIONAL AND MEDICAL SETTINGS

EDUCATIONAL SETTINGS: PUBLIC LAWS AFFECTING STUDENTS WITH COMMUNICATION DISORDERS

We briefly discuss each of these mandates because they provide a legal basis for provision of services to students with communication disorders in school settings. An understanding of the law helps to explain many of the procedures SLPs and teachers engage in during a school year.

Individuals with Disabilities Education Act (IDEA)   The Education for All Handicapped Children Act (PL 94-142) mandated in 1977 that all handicapped children between the ages of 3 and 21 years receive a free, public education that is appropriate to their needs. PL 94-142 has been amended five times over the years, and the guidelines were embodied in the **Individuals with Disabilities Education Act (IDEA)** of 1997.

TABLE 1–2   Percentage of Healthcare-Based SLP Regular Services to Each Disorder Group on the Caseload

Diagnostic Category	% Adult Areas of Intervention	% Child Areas of Intervention
Accent modification	1	—
Aphasia	17	—
Cognitive-communication	21	14
Motor speech	8	—
Swallowing/feeding	46	17
Voice/resonance	5	3
Articulation/phonology	—	24
Fluency	—	3
Language	—	35
Other	2	1

Source: Adapted from ASHA, 2007b.

Needless to say, disorders of communication can adversely affect educational achievement. Therefore, students with speech, language, or hearing disorders are covered under IDEA and are entitled to free and appropriate individualized services. All children with handicaps and their parents are guaranteed, under this law, **due process** with regard to identification, evaluation, and placement. This includes the identification, evaluation, and placement for disorders of communication as well as other handicapping conditions. These procedures are performed by a team of school professionals in cooperation with the student's parents. Although IDEA is a federal law, individual states are allowed latitude in developing rules and regulations to comply with it. Educational procedures, therefore, vary from state to state. Although this law has far-reaching consequences for the delivery of school services, we mention here only some of the key points of the law that affect the work of the speech-language pathologist.

The National Dissemination Center for Children and Youth with Disabilities (NICHCY) has a great Web site that includes a detailed training package on the law (http://www.nichcy.org). Part of the law specifies that a team of educational personnel and the parents must develop an **Individualized Education Program (IEP)**. In the case of a student with a communication disorder, the speech-language pathologist is a member of the team. The team also includes the parents, teachers, and, when appropriate, the student. The 1997 IDEA emphasizes that the regular classroom teacher participates in the IEP process. Although IEP forms differ among school districts, certain information must be contained in each. **Table 1–3** lists the IEP components adapted from the National Dissemination Center for Children and Youth with Disabilities.

TABLE 1–3 Components of the Individualized Education Plan

1. A statement of the present level of performance
2. A statement of annual goals
3. Short-term instructional objectives
4. Specific special education and related services to be provided
5. Extent of participation in the regular educational program
6. Projected date for initiation of services
7. Anticipated duration of services
8. Appropriate criteria to determine if objectives are achieved
9. Evaluation procedures to determine if objectives are achieved
10. Schedules for review
11. Assessment information
12. Placement justification statement
13. Some statement of how special education services are tied in to the regular education program

After being developed, the IEP is signed by the team members and is reviewed and typically updated annually. In 2004, the IDEA was reauthorized as the Individuals with Disabilities Education Improvement Act (PL 108-446). The most recent IDEA is piloting multiyear IEPs that include goals for three years and must be reviewed annually and at transition points. Of course, IEPs can be reviewed and revised more often at the request of a parent or teacher.

IDEA also stipulates that the student with a disability be provided educational services in the **least restrictive environment**. This means the student should be educated to the maximum extent possible in the regular class with normal peers, if the classroom has the least barriers to successful learning. A comprehensive evaluation must be conducted, and an IEP must be developed prior to the initiation of appropriate services.

PL 99-457   One of the first amendments to the Education for All Handicapped Act was **PL 99-457**. This served to broaden and strengthen the mandate for providing services to preschool children between the ages of 3 and 5 years.

This is an exciting and challenging aspect of the public school SLP's job for several reasons. First, considering the population of preschool children with disabilities as a whole, the vast majority have a communication delay even if their primary handicap is a hearing impairment, cognitive deficit, motor problem, or the like. Second, school systems do not have a captive audience in terms of identifying these children; they are not attending the public schools. Thus, locating, identifying, and screening preschool children with communication disorders necessarily entails much community and agency interaction. The school SLP can be a member of an early intervention team from the school system that is responsible for working with parents, day care centers, pediatricians, health departments, private practices, and other children's services. Through cooperative community efforts, preschool children with communication delay can be identified. IEPs for these children may reflect several agencies' roles and responsibilities in the provision of services. Service delivery for this population: (1) could be home-based, day-care-based, center-based, or a combination of these; (2) vary in intensity; and (3) may require more coordination with agencies and parents.

Infants and toddlers (ages birth to 3 years) must be screened and evaluated utilizing parents or caregivers. The early intervention team then must develop an **Individualized Family Service Plan (IFSP)** for the children who qualify. This is similar to the IEP developed for older children but, as stated in its title, the focus is on the child's family. The plan must be reviewed and revised as needed (at least every six months). The law encourages parent training, which obviously is necessary in the total treatment of these young children. Consequently, teachers and speech-language pathologists become more involved in the development and supervision of innovative parent training programs.

Section 504 of the Rehabilitation Act of 1973   Because public schools receive federal financial assistance, they are prohibited from denying a person with a disability the opportunity to participate or benefit from programs or services or otherwise limiting a qualified person with a disability in the enjoyment of any right, privilege, or advantage. Under **Section 504**, a person with a disability is defined as someone with a physical or mental impairment that substantially limits one or more major life activities. Some students who do not meet the categorical criteria for special education services under IDEA are entitled to reasonable accommodations under Section 504. For example, students who are identified as having Attention Deficit Disorder (ADD) or Attention Deficit-Hyperactivity Disorder (AD-HD) qualify for services under Section 504 and should have a "504 Plan" that delineates any accommodations the student needs.

The Americans with Disabilities Act   The **Americans with Disabilities Act (ADA)** was enacted July 26, 1990, and applies to public entities. This includes any state or local government and any of its departments, agencies, or other instrumentalities; thus, it applies to public schools. Specifically, all programs, services, and activities of schools are covered (i.e., field trips, parent meetings, standardized exams, lab classes). Participation in programs, services, and activities may not be denied simply because a person has a disability.

Communication has a special role in implementation of the ADA. Schools must ensure that communications with students who have hearing, vision, or speech impairments are as effective as for other students, and when necessary auxiliary aids must be provided. Auxiliary aids include services or devices such as qualified interpreters, assistive listening devices, telecaptioning, telecommunication devices (TDDs), videotext, taped textbooks, Braille materials, and large-print materials.

Are you still with us? We are aware that a discussion of laws and regulations is not the most entertaining fare for beginning students. It is important, however, that you know that the school-based SLP must operate under a fairly rigid set of guidelines set forth at the federal, state, and local levels. Performance of the job is not arbitrary, and many things the SLP does during the school year are prescribed by law.

CLINICAL/MEDICAL SETTINGS

Fortunately, there are not quite as many legal issues to cover for SLPs who work in clinical/medical settings. Some federal guidelines apply to hospitals and clinics just like they do to the public school system. For example, when dealing with infants and toddlers, SLPs in the clinical/medical setting also develop Individualized Family Service Plans (IFSPs) for use with the pediatric population. When dealing with adults, laws such as the Americans with Disabilities Act (ADA) also apply. Hospitals and clinics must show some degree of transparency in their procedures and paperwork and protect the confidentiality of patients. For example, in 1996, the Health Information Portability and Accountability Act (**HIPAA**) was passed as Public Law 104-191. This act establishes measures ensuring security and privacy of healthcare information that is maintained by both public and private healthcare providers. Confidentiality in school settings is just as critical as in medical environments. The Family Educational Rights and Privacy Act of 1974 (FERPA) is the law governing the confidentiality of information in school settings.

In clinical/medical settings, one administrative level of bureaucracy that is not present in school systems is the requirements of insurance companies and other third-party payers. SLPs working in medical settings must deal with the requirements of Medicare, Medicaid, and insurance companies. These third-party payers have very strict guidelines on what types of conditions they will pay for and how long treatment can continue to be subsidized. Thus, the SLP in a clinical/medical setting must be careful to document assessment and treatment activities very specifically so that reimbursement is possible.

Another aspect unique to medical settings is the pivotal role of the physician in ordering evaluations and treatment procedures for a given patient. This is clearly different from practice in educational settings in which parents and professionals determine eligibility for and the direction of services. However, it is important to note that doctors may be part of the educational team and in some cases must be included on such panels.

Medical settings also must operate under the guidelines of national and state organizations that accredit hospitals and other clinical facilities. All of these different levels of federal, state, and local control serve to dictate much of what the SLP in a clinical/medical setting must do on a daily basis.

THE ROLE OF THE SPEECH-LANGUAGE PATHOLOGIST IN THE SCHOOL SYSTEM

Public school SLPs hold unique and interesting positions within the school system hierarchy. Superintendents are responsible to the school board and, in turn, may have a number of assistant superintendents, depending on the size of the system. The special education director is responsible to the upper level of superintendents and oversees the provision of special education services in the entire school system. Under the special education coordinator in large school systems that employ 10 or more SLPs, usually one SLP is designated as the speech pathology coordinator and is responsible for managing speech pathology staff and services throughout the school system. In smaller systems, a senior SLP may be designated for leadership purposes, but usually all of the SLPs report directly to the special education coordinator, who then is responsible for the speech pathology program as well as other special education services. The SLP often works with more than one building principal because many SLPs serve multiple schools. In addition to daily interactions with teachers, SLPs frequently work with support personnel (psychologists, social workers, nurses, physical or occupational therapists, and so forth) and agency/community professionals.

The actual work settings and job responsibilities of speech-language pathologists within the school system can vary greatly. The following three vignettes illustrate this broad range.

VIGNETTE 1–1

Mr. James works at Glen High School and Marymont Junior High. His caseload consists of 8 students with hearing impairment who are working on curriculum language and social interaction skills; 6 students who stutter, ranging in severity from mild to severe; 14 students with specific learning disabilities (SLDs) who attend a communication skills class; 10 students who are in the program for the mentally handicapped and are working on functional communication skills necessary for vocational placement; and 2 students who are working for improved voice quality (one has nodules and the other is hypernasal).

VIGNETTE 1–2

Mrs. Sarnoff is an SLP for the Piedmont School District. She serves an elementary school in the mornings and a middle school in the afternoons. This allows her to see the severe cases every day. At the elementary school, she works in the early childhood class and the multihandicapped class using a collaborative consultation approach with the teachers. She integrates classroom curriculum content into all of the therapy sessions. This means that she must be in touch with the teachers, know what is being taught, and know which subject areas and skills are most in need of support. Ten of Mrs. Sarnoff's cases are preschoolers who come into the schools for speech and language services. She works closely with the parents, training them to facilitate their child's communication skills. Several of the children in the multihandicapped class use augmentative communication devices. Mrs. Sarnoff evaluated the children and was instrumental in obtaining the appropriate device for each child. Mrs. Sarnoff has had advanced training in this area and serves as a consultant to the region regarding augmentative communication.

VIGNETTE 1–3

The East Regional Early Intervention Team consists of a physical therapist, social worker, early childhood special educator, and speech-language pathologist. Katherine Smith, the SLP, works with the team in the infant and toddler program. The infants are brought to the Hope Center where the team works on the carpet with the parents by evaluating, demonstrating, and coaching to increase responsiveness of parent and infant. Infant referrals come from parents, neonatal high-risk nurseries, pediatricians, and agencies. Often, a member of the team is asked to come to the hospital neonatal intensive care unit to meet parents and begin a supportive relationship. Ms. Smith finds this to be an interesting aspect of her job. She also has organized a parent support group and attends these meetings as a facilitator. Ms. Smith works in the toddler class where an early childhood special educator works with the 2- and 3-year-olds on a daily basis. Ms. Smith has specific goals for each child and reviews these frequently with the teacher. They work together integrating communication and curriculum goals. All of the infants and toddlers have an Individualized Family Service Plan (IFSP) developed by the team and the parents after an assessment of family and child strengths and needs. Ms. Smith is also a member of the transition team that facilitates the movement of parents and children from one program to another (e.g., from infant to toddler program, from toddler to preschool program, from preschool to school-age services). She maintains records on all of the children and attends weekly early intervention team meetings, which often include persons from other agencies who are serving the parents and child (e.g., health department, children's services, human resources). If the parents of an infant with developmental delay cannot come to the Hope Center, or a toddler cannot be transported, Ms. Smith or another team member makes regular home intervention visits.

As you can see, there is great diversity within the public school setting; this is one of the exciting aspects of the profession of speech-language pathology. Yet all three SLPs share some common responsibilities. First, SLPs must manage each individual case from the initial screening or referral to a final determination that a maximum level of progress has been attained. Second, SLPs must manage their caseload as a whole by summarizing individual case data for compliance, planning, and reporting purposes. These summarized data, by school and total caseload, are given to the special education director who is responsible for program management. All SLPs are thus involved in three levels of management (individual student, caseload, and program levels) regardless of the size of their school system. Some of the specific responsibilities involved in planning, directing, and providing services to students with communication disorders are discussed next.

Case Finding   Case finding, most commonly called **child find**, refers to the preliminary identification of students with potential communication disorders. Case finding usually involves two procedures: screenings and/or referrals. Screenings are quick assessments of a student's communicative abilities; if a problem is suspected, a second screening may be scheduled or plans for a diagnostic assessment may be set into place. Some cases are identified by a referral from another professional. Sometimes parents refer their own children for screening. In most states, an active effort has been made to provide materials (e.g., flyers, posters) for the public that outline normal development in critical areas (e.g., language, social, self-help, hearing, cognitive) and symptoms that might indicate the need for a screening by a professional.

Procedures for locating preschoolers with potential communication disorders vary from "preschool roundups" in small towns to media blitzes in larger metropolitan areas. Mass screenings in the schools take an inordinate amount of time and really are not cost effective. It is much more prudent to put time and effort into quality teacher in-services, screenings upon teacher request throughout the year, and effective communication with teachers (good rapport, working relationships, and the like). In addition, the laws require that there be no lapse in services. Thus, speech and language services for children who are already identified must be initiated the first week of the school year, making mass screenings more difficult to conduct.

Referral is a widely used method of case finding. Anyone who has the student's welfare in mind and suspects a problem can make a referral. This includes parents, family doctor, school nurse, school counselor, principal, the individual student, and, of course, the teachers. The procedures and opportunities for requesting a screening or making a referral should be presented to teachers, parents, and other professionals periodically. The success of a referral system is dependent on the ability of teachers to identify potential disorders of communication. There is evidence that even without training, many communication problems can be effectively identified by teachers. On the other hand, teachers may not as readily be able to identify some disorders such as voice problems and subtle language problems (Sommers & Hatten, 1985).

Evaluation   The process of initial **evaluation** involves formal and informal testing of the student who has failed the screening or has been referred. Results of the assessment process usually yield a diagnosis (e.g., language disorder, fluency disorder, categorizing a student as performing within normal limits). If the student is diagnosed with a communication disorder, the evaluation includes an estimate of severity.

According to IDEA, each student with disabilities must receive a comprehensive multidisciplinary evaluation to determine whether the child is eligible for special education. Eligibility must be determined prior to placement in a special education program, and written parental permission is required for this testing. The speech-language pathologist must comply with the law and be sure that test instruments are valid, are not racially or culturally discriminatory, and are administered in the student's native language. Tests can be standardized (norm referenced, criterion referenced), nonstandardized (e.g., language sample), or, most appropriately, a combination of both.

The SLP may conduct the evaluation over several days and may focus on the suspected area of deficit in detail. The SLP should do a global communication assessment as well, including articulation skills, language competencies, and the normalcy of fluency, voice, and hearing. The SLP should also examine the speech mechanism to look at anatomic structure and function. Case history information from the parents, educational and behavioral observations from the teacher, and classroom observation of the student can be important. Additional information (such as level of cognitive functioning), obtained from school personnel, may be helpful in interpreting the assessment data.

It should be pointed out that assessment is ongoing. Once a student is found to be eligible and is subsequently placed in a treatment program, the speech-language pathologist and the classroom teachers must constantly monitor progress. These periodic reevaluations let the SLP know the success or failure of therapeutic techniques and the need to change or modify the program. The need for dismissal from services also is determined by this ongoing evaluation process.

Participation in Meetings for Case Staffing and Eligibility Determination The purpose of the initial evaluation is to obtain information regarding a student's communication skills that can be presented to the eligibility committee that will determine whether placement is appropriate in a speech, language, and/or hearing program in the school. After the testing, the SLP must be prepared to describe to the eligibility committee how a student's communication disorder interferes with educational performance and the student's ability to profit from classroom instruction. You may hear many tales of students who clearly have difficulties in school or with communication, whose parents are convinced that their child has a problem, and sometimes even the professionals who do the evaluation suspect an impairment, yet the child does not qualify for special education services. How can such a thing occur? One reason is that each school system operates under federal, state, and local guidelines. Eligibility determination ultimately is accomplished by combining these three levels of administrative regulations. It is not unusual for a child to qualify for services in one state, only to be ineligible when the family moves to another state. If a student is diagnosed with a particular problem, it is unfortunate if he or she cannot receive appropriate services just because of administrative regulations. Yet it happens often enough for parents to have formed support groups and for the legal profession to offer consultative services for parents who feel that the school system has not provided appropriate services to their children. Sometimes we just do not spend enough time and effort in evaluation of students. Ehren states:

> Eligibility often shapes caseloads in ways that seem inconsistent with the state of the art. In lieu of making a diagnosis, we ascertain whether the student meets eligibility criteria.
>
> Evaluation, then, becomes an eligibility determination process, rather than a process to describe a student's communication status. . . . First we need to make a diagnosis, next, recommend the need for service; then, discuss eligibility. Diagnosis should drive eligibility; eligibility should not dictate the diagnosis. Eligibility criteria should be viewed as the last hoop to jump through in identifying a student. (Ehren, 1993, p. 20)

Participation in staffing and placement decisions regarding the student is another responsibility of the speech-language pathologist. As a member of the placement team, the SLP reviews the data on individual students and participates in the development of the Individualized Educational Program (IEP) or Individualized Family Service Plan (IFSP) for each student. Parents must give written permission for placement prior to the initiation of services.

Delivery of Treatment Although called by different names—therapy, intervention, remediation, habilitation/rehabilitation services—*treatment* refers to the actual delivery of services. **Treatment** may be **direct**, when the speech-language pathologist works directly with the student, or **indirect**, when the speech-language pathologist works with others (such as the classroom teacher or parent) to develop, improve, or maintain communication abilities of the student.

Subsequent chapters of this book discuss the treatment principles for each of the disorders of communication SLPs frequently encounter in schools. In essence, however, treatment involves the instructional activities for the improvement of the communication deficit. The SLP must be accountable and able to show that the program of treatment is progress-directed by maintaining accurate student data. In some school systems, the SLP may be fortunate enough to have the assistance of paraprofessionals. **Paraprofessionals**, also known as communication aides, speech-language pathology assistants, or support personnel, can carry out some of the more routine treatment procedures established by the SLP. These aides are, however, limited by their educational qualifications and school system guidelines as to how much assistance they can render.

It is always the hope of the SLP that teachers support the speech-language treatment programs of their students. Teachers should participate whenever possible by working closely with the SLP (such as through sharing curricular topics, monitoring the use of techniques, assisting in carryover, and supporting in numerous other ways that are discussed throughout this book). Ideally, the classroom should be a real-life situation where the student can practice newly learned communication behaviors and strategies.

SERVICE DELIVERY MODELS

Whenever a child in a public school or clinical/medical setting receives treatment for a communication disorder it is almost always a team effort. A general guideline is that the more severe the case, the more team members will be involved. For example, a child who has cerebral palsy and a hearing impairment may require many different types of services from a broad range of professions (audiology, physical therapy, occupational therapy, SLP, classroom teacher, social worker, etc.). On the other hand, a child with a learning disability may be seen by the learning disability (LD) teacher, regular classroom teacher, and the SLP. Finally, a child whose only problem is misarticulation of the /s/ sound may be seen by only the SLP and classroom teacher. Teams can operate in a variety of ways in both educational and clinical/medical settings, and several common models are discussed here.

MULTIDISCIPLINARY, INTERDISCIPLINARY, AND TRANSDISCIPLINARY TEAM MODELS

Indirect as well as direct approaches to providing services typically involve parents, teachers, and other professionals acting as a team that participates in assessing, treating, and evaluating a treatment program. You can view the three models of team approaches on a continuum with **multidisciplinary** on one end, **transdisciplinary** on the other end, and **interdisciplinary** in the center (**Figure 1–2**). On the multidisciplinary end of the continuum, there tends to be less cooperation among team members in terms of planning and implementation of a remedial program. There is also less communication among team

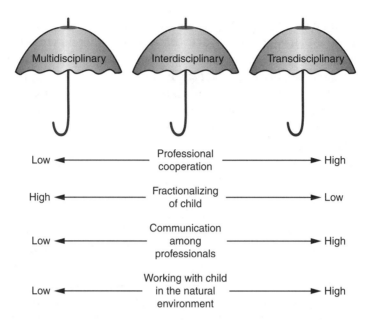

FIGURE 1–2 Models of team approaches.

members on this end of the continuum and more "fractionalizing" of the child, meaning the child is taken out of class for speech, then for work on a learning problem, then for counseling about academic adjustment, and so forth. As you approach the transdisciplinary end of the continuum, more group cooperation in planning and implementation and much greater communication exist. The team has incorporated many goals into the child's daily classroom routine, and perhaps team members have worked with the classroom teacher regarding how to use specific strategies in the child's daily activities. This accomplishes the educational objectives without constantly removing the child from the classroom.

One theme common to all three approaches is that they each use a variety of professionals. For instance, a regular classroom teacher, audiologist, SLP, psychometrist, and special educator may be involved with a case in all three approaches. In clinical/medical settings, even more professionals are involved. A second similarity is that all three approaches deal with both assessment and treatment of the child's problem. The differences among the approaches, however, are the focus of the present section. Initially, we discuss the multidisciplinary and interdisciplinary models.

The multi- and interdisciplinary approaches maintain the independence of each discipline in terms of doing separate evaluations and holding separate treatment sessions with the child. For planning purposes, both multi- and interdisciplinary approaches involve each professional making separate sets of annual goals and short-term objectives, although they comprise one Individualized Educational Program. When implementing the IEP, the multi- and interdisciplinary approaches either carry out the goals independently, or in the latter approach, incorporate some goals of other team members when possible. This tends to fractionalize the child and the program of treatment. It has often been said that it takes more than a staple punched through a pile of separate reports to make an integrated program. Yet, this is what often happens in a multidisciplinary approach. Even though the IEP may contain goals in many areas, often team members focus only on the goals that apply to their own disciplines. It is not uncommon for one professional to be unaware of the specific goals that another team member has targeted at a given point in time or of the child's progress in that area. Another criticism of these models is that it may not be clear exactly which member of the team is accountable for certain goals and evaluating programs.

In the transdisciplinary model, the professionals and family together develop the assessment and treatment options. It is important to remember, however, that regardless of the assessment/treatment model, the IEP must be developed jointly by professionals and family members. The transdisciplinary model merely emphasizes such interactions more than others. There is much consultation and discussion during the assessment period; team members may observe the child in a variety of settings in addition to collecting individual test data. The guiding philosophy is that team members are committed to working together *across discipline boundaries* to make the intervention effective. A prominent concern in transdisciplinary models is the notion of a primary service provider. In most cases, one professional sees the child more often than do other professionals. The classroom teacher, for instance, has many more opportunities to interact with a particular child and observe behavior than does the SLP. As such, the teacher and classroom environment have much to offer in terms of evaluation information for the SLP. Who knows more than the child's teacher about her typical communication skills, problem-solving strategies, consistency of language errors, intelligibility, fluency, and social skills?

The classroom environment and teacher are also primary considerations in the treatment of speech and language problems because the child uses communication skills in the classroom throughout the day. In most cases, the SLP sees children with communication disorders for individual sessions. This is especially true in the beginning phases of treatment. When the child leaves the classroom to go to speech therapy, the SLP must *contrive* activities that resemble real communication, especially in the later stages of treatment. It is difficult to justify spending time creating a natural environment for therapy when one already exists in the classroom. Often, children can effectively learn to use correct sentence structure, speech sounds, fluent speech, and good vocal habits in the confines of the speech room. However, as soon as the child returns to the classroom environment, he often forgets these skills. An enduring complaint of SLPs is that it is relatively easy to *establish* a new communication skill, but it is most difficult to *generalize* these skills to the child's natural environment. The classroom teacher, as a team member, can be of crucial assistance here.

If close communication between the SLP and the teacher occurs, the teacher can assist in facilitating generalization of newly established behaviors. For example, a child with a language problem who omits "is" from sentences such as "he is my friend" can easily be trained by the SLP to remember the "is" in therapy sessions. Yet, the child goes back to the classroom and continues to say sentences without including "is." If the teacher reminds the child to include "is" in classroom conversation, the child can rapidly learn that this piece of language is important and finally generalize it into daily communication. Cooperation of team members is not a one-way street. For example, imagine that a particular child scores low on vocabulary tests administered by the SLP, and the child should have some vocabulary enrichment. The SLP could consult with the classroom teacher and begin to train vocabulary words that are related to the child's academic work. For example, an SLP that we know was working with a student on building vocabulary and production of a correct /s/ sound. The SLP asked the teacher which areas of the child's academic performance were weak, and the teacher indicated that the boy was particularly struggling to understand how city government works. The SLP borrowed a textbook from the teacher and centered part of her therapy sessions around the topic of government, introducing related new vocabulary words and monitoring the child's /s/ sound during discussions they had about how the city was run.

This example underscores the symbiotic relationship between professionals. One final note about cooperation among professionals is necessary. Historically, professionals of various types have felt that certain training was their exclusive province. This type of "turfism" tends to be counterproductive. The most important goal is that the child develops skills, eradicates maladaptive behaviors, and learns specific information and strategies for problem solving. It makes no difference whatsoever if a child's grammar is corrected by the SLP, a teacher, or a parent. The critical point is that the problem is remediated. If a child learns certain concepts about classroom work from the SLP, she is further ahead, and the teacher should not feel that his or her territory has been encroached upon.

TYPES OF SERVICE DELIVERY OFFERED BY THE SPEECH-LANGUAGE PATHOLOGIST

The SLP working in the school environment can offer a continuum of services to help students with communication disorders. A number of terms are commonly used to refer to different types of services.

Direct/Indirect Services When the SLP works with children individually or in small groups, it is called direct service. These direct services can be done in the classroom, or they can be provided in a treatment room located elsewhere in the school building. When the SLP works with the student outside the classroom, either individually or in a group, this is sometimes called a pull-out model of service delivery. Most SLPs have offices/treatment rooms in which they can work with an individual child or small group for several treatment sessions per week. If the children are grouped, they are often chosen because they are all working on the same types of problems (e.g., groups of children with stuttering problems or language disorders). Whereas some SLPs are assigned exclusively to a single school building, others are itinerant and travel among several schools, providing services to each. Whether SLPs are itinerant or not, they must maintain close communication with all teachers regarding the students they see in treatment.

Direct services in which the SLP removes the students from the classroom environment have advantages and disadvantages. One positive aspect is that the SLP can work with the student in an environment free from distractions, and this is helpful in **establishment** of many communication behaviors (e.g., teaching a new speech sound to the child). Another advantage is that certain therapy approaches involving drillwork or specialized equipment can be more easily implemented outside of the classroom. On the other hand, if students are removed from the classroom several times a week, they can miss valuable academic lessons while in speech-language treatment sessions. Direct services provided in the classroom can be of help to both the student and the teacher. The SLP can help the teacher by assisting with classroom activities, giving them a communication slant that is beneficial to all members of the class. Direct services provided in the classroom assist in generalization of goals trained in a therapy room into the natural environment.

In most school systems, SLPs provide a mixture of direct and indirect services. They see some children exclusively with direct services, whereas others receive a combination of direct and indirect, and still others receive all of their treatment in the indirect mode. The configuration of services received depends on the caseload, teacher cooperation, the particular philosophy of the SLP, and guidelines set by the school system and state department of education.

Interestingly, the ASHA Schools Surveys conducted in 1995 and 2000 indicates the following:

> Except for the birth to 2 years age group, the most frequently used service delivery model was the traditional pull-out, followed by the classroom based model. For the birth to 2 years age group, the most used model was the collaborative consultation model.

Although it is true that many states currently emphasize use of indirect and collaborative models of service delivery, the ASHA data suggest that the majority of public school speech-language pathologists surveyed indicate that direct services are still prevalent.

Indirect Services: A Consultative/Collaborative Approach   Speech-language pathologists use a variety of assessment/treatment models to deal with both children and adults who have communication disorders (Frassinelli, Superior, & Meyers, 1983; Fujiki & Brinton, 1984; Marvin, 1987; Damico, 1987). As mentioned previously, in the traditional direct service model, the SLP removes the child from the classroom and sees him or her individually or in a group. Parents, teachers, and administrators have become so accustomed to this direct service model that they may find it unusual to deal with other modes of treatment, such as a consultative/collaborative mode. Basically, collaboration is a three-person (or more) chain of service. For instance, the consultant (SLP) provides professional service to the child indirectly through the teacher. Collaboration as a practice is not new. Speech-language pathologists have made suggestions to teachers and parents for decades regarding how they can assist in treatment progress. SLPs have now begun to realize that different children may require different levels of direct or indirect involvement with the SLP and that there is a continuum of services that SLPs can offer. Consultation models have been shown to be effective and workable in school systems and are especially important in **generalization** of communication skills to the natural environment of the classroom (Ferguson, 1991; Moore-Brown, 1991; Magnotta, 1991; Montgomery, 1992).

A teacher might ask, "For what kind of case would I be the primary interventionist?" One example might involve a child who is nonverbal in a preschool class. A primary goal for this child is to increase communication attempts through pointing and physically regulating the teacher (e.g., putting the teacher's hand on a toy to wind it up) in natural daily activities. This would be a difficult goal for the SLP to work on outside of the classroom. Yet, the teacher would not have to do anything extra for the child in terms of preparation beyond simply attending to the child's pointing during certain activities and allowing the child to physically regulate him or her to make needs known. The SLP then would evaluate the occurrence of communication attempts at different points in therapy and prescribe changes in teacher–child interaction.

In another example, the consultant (SLP) might do an in-service presentation on a topic in dialectal variation, such as the occurrence of African American English features in the language of minority children. A teacher attends the in-service and later has a student who indicates that he or she wants to learn to write some short stories in a Standard English form and eliminate elements of African American English from the story. The child also indicates a desire to learn to style shift, to speak Standard English on certain occasions and then shift back to African American English when desired. The teacher might agree to monitor the writing and speaking in certain situations and let the student know when dialectal features occur. In this case, the teacher really does all the assessment, intervention, and evaluation of the program with only some advice and information from the SLP consultant. Because this student is a dialect speaker, he or she does not have a clinically significant communication disorder, so no IEP is necessary in this case.

This collaborative model highlights enhanced communication and problem solving among professionals, and the plan for assessment and intervention actually springs from these discussions. It is probably a basic fact that people tend to participate more fully in an intervention program if they have had some role in determining its course. A teacher who has a good suggestion about how to approach a problem of a communication-disordered child in the context of the classroom will be more likely to carry out the plan than if he or she is asked to do a particular task by the SLP. When this child is served exclusively by the classroom teacher and the SLP acts as a consultant, the IEP must reflect the provision of indirect services only.

You can see that the continuum of services that the SLP could offer varies considerably in terms of teacher and SLP involvement. Almost any variation on the preceding models is possible and the particular configuration of treatment responsibilities for a particular child depends on some of the following variables:

1. Types of goals for a particular case and the child's point in the therapy program (whether the child is just beginning treatment or nearing dismissal)
2. Willingness of the SLP to be flexible in service provision
3. Willingness of the teacher to consider alternative models of service
4. Time available for consultation meetings for both parties

Although most children can benefit from direct service by the SLP, in many instances the SLP can best deal with cases by working collaboratively with the teacher or parents. Some other specific examples of cases that might be treated effectively with collaboration are illustrated next.

CASE I–I

One common example of a case suited to collaborative models is a child who habitually abuses his vocal cords by frequently yelling, screaming, and using the voice improperly. It is difficult to see how the SLP could monitor this behavior if the SLP sees the child only individually in an isolated therapy room. The teacher sees the child more than the SLP does and can monitor instances of vocal abuse and discourage them. The major input of the SLP would be to introduce to the child proper vocal hygiene practices, inform the teacher and parents of those practices, and monitor changes in the child's vocal quality over time.

CASE I–2

Any child who speaks in utterances less than three to four words in length is a natural candidate for indirect or collaborative treatment. These children require continuous stimulation of certain language forms and need to be reinforced naturally for use of correct language in real communicative situations (e.g., give the child objects she asks for; look at things she labels). The SLP could isolate this child and contrive activities similar to those already occurring in the classroom; however, this appears to be nothing more than reinventing the wheel. The teacher is with the child during her daily activities and can not only model appropriate language, but also reinforce the use of utterance types as suggested by the SLP. A very powerful technique known as *recasting* involves restating a child's incorrect utterance in a correct manner. For instance, if a child says, "Him my friend," a teacher or parent could say, "Yes, he is your friend." Many research projects have demonstrated that recasting can effectively promote the use of correct language forms in children with language disorders (Paul, 2007). This is a technique that does not take much extra time and that can be naturally incorporated into any interaction with a child.

CASE 1–3

A final example of appropriate use of indirect or collaborative therapy involves a child with any type of communication disorder who is in the generalization portion of speech/language therapy. The SLP can train the child's speech and language behavior only to a certain level, and then it is time for the child to use these new skills in natural situations. Some children can produce impeccable /s/ sounds in conversation with the SLP in the therapy room, only to misarticulate in the classroom or at home. Similarly, children who stutter are frequently fluent with the SLP but fail to use their fluency-enhancing techniques in real situations.

You might get the impression that collaboration is less complicated and takes less time than does providing direct services. Usually, this could not be farther from the truth. In fact, collaboration, when well done, can actually take more time than direct services do. Collaboration is not something that teachers and SLPs should dabble with. The process involves thoroughly assessing the child, establishing goals, determining who will be responsible for different aspects of the treatment program, and evaluating the effectiveness of the program (Frassinelli et al., 1983; Fujiki & Brinton, 1984; Marvin, 1987; Damico, 1987; Ferguson, 1991; Moore-Brown, 1991; Magnotta, 1991; Montgomery, 1992).

THE ROLE OF THE CLASSROOM TEACHER IN IDENTIFICATION, ASSESSMENT, AND TREATMENT

Consider the following vignettes of three teachers.

VIGNETTE 1–4

Mrs. Thomas has taught kindergarten for 12 years. She has been concerned for some time about little Rachel, who appears to have a great deal of difficulty following directions. Mrs. Thomas gave carefully sequenced instructions for making a pinwheel out of a stick, construction paper, and a metal pin. Rachel ended up with a "ball" of construction paper that was poised on the end of the stick like a perverted magic wand. Mrs. Thomas requested from the speech-language pathologist a hearing test for Rachel, and it was found that Rachel had a significant hearing loss caused by recurring ear infections. When she received an evaluation by an audiologist and wore her new hearing aid, she had little trouble with comprehending instructions.

VIGNETTE I–5

Mrs. Carson had dealt with Reginald for two years—once the first time through third grade, and again when he had to repeat that grade. She had put in literally hundreds of hours observing whom he liked and who liked him. She knew to whom he talked and the topics of conversation. She not only knew what he learned, but *how* he learned, what motivated him, what he could do, what he could not do, what made him cry, and who his favorite baseball player was. For instance, she knew that Reggie had difficulty in meeting a strange adult for the first time and that whenever he was asked to perform a task, it was always wise to present the instructions twice. After obtaining permission to evaluate, the new SLP asked if she could take Reggie for an hour to do some tests of his language ability. Unfortunately, she never asked Mrs. Carson any questions before removing Reggie for his tests. When the SLP brought Reggie back, she announced that he had failed all of the language tests and did not talk to her when she tried to obtain a conversational sample. Mrs. Carson was not surprised. Her input about how to deal with Reggie would have made the evaluation much more effective.

VIGNETTE I–6

Bob Brooks was a teacher who became uncomfortable whenever he thought of watching and listening to Emilio Chavez. Emilio had a severe stuttering problem and produced long, torturous blocks accompanied by facial grimaces and inspiratory gasps. Bob had discussed this with the SLP and knew it was not a good policy to avoid calling on a child who had a stuttering problem. So, now it was time to ask Emilio a question and see the look of a trapped animal quickly eclipse the child's face. Bob knew that Emilio was in speech therapy and the technique he was supposed to use was a slowed-down, stretched type of speech that prolonged vowel sounds to increase his fluency. As Emilio began to answer, he pressed his lips tightly together, and his head began to jerk in a series of rapid arrhythmic movements that lasted almost half a minute. Mr. Brooks finally said, "Remember to start out slowly and prolong the vowels like you do in speech class." Emilio stopped, tried to relax, and was able to answer the question appropriately with much less abnormality in his speech as he slowly glided from one vowel to the next.

These three vignettes illustrate the participation of teachers in three important aspects of dealing with communication disorders: identification of cases, evaluation of children's communication skills, and treatment of communication problems. In the examples involving case detection and treatment, the teacher succeeded in helping the communication-disordered child. In the case involving evaluation, the SLP failed to profit from the expertise of the teacher before evaluating a child. If she had only asked the teacher some questions, the evaluation would have been more efficient and would have provided more information. It is, of course, up to the individual classroom teacher, the school administration, and the

SLP to determine specific roles and duties in the real world. If teachers could incorporate even some of the information included in the present text into their daily interactions with children and SLPs, they could see gains in several areas. First, the children with communication disorders would be detected, evaluated, and treated more quickly and effectively. Second, SLPs would be able to perform their jobs more efficiently and be able to focus maximum effort on the cases that require the most attention. Third, teachers would be able to have an even greater impact on their students. Finally, as a member of the educational team, teachers would develop strong professional relationships with other disciplines.

Children in the public school system who are enrolled in special education comprise a highly heterogeneous group. These children represent almost every exceptionality, and public school professionals are expected to be able to diagnose and treat these problems and prescribe appropriate educational programs. In addition to representing a disparate variety of handicapping conditions, these children also manifest a full range in severity of their disorders. No single professional can hope to have expertise in assessment and remediation for every kind of physical, cognitive, language, speech, emotional, or educational problem. It is because of this diverse population and the monumental literature available about each type of disorder that public school professionals generally incorporate a team approach when dealing with special education cases. In subsequent chapters, we outline many specific ways that teachers and SLPs can cooperate in helping students with communication disorders.

THE ROLE OF THE SPEECH-LANGUAGE PATHOLOGIST IN MEDICAL SETTINGS

There is a general similarity in the functions of the SLP between clinical/medical and educational settings. As we stated earlier, the roles of case finding (screening), evaluation, treatment, and participation in staffing of cases define much of what a public school speech-language pathologist does during the course of a workday. SLPs working in clinical/medical settings perform similar functions. For example, a new patient admitted to an acute care hospital after suffering a stroke will probably be screened by the SLP for speech, language, and swallowing disorders. If difficulties in any of these areas are detected, a more thorough evaluation will be conducted and treatment will be recommended if indicated. One big difference in clinical/medical settings as compared to schools, however, is that the patient's physician must order evaluation and treatment before these can be conducted.

SLPs in clinical/medical settings perform screenings, evaluations, and treatment in much the same way as their counterparts in the school system do. Evaluations comprise standardized tests, nonstandardized tasks, and use of facility-specific checklists. Treatment in clinical/medical settings may differ based on the type of facility, but considering the clinical/medical settings as a whole, many types of therapy can be found. For instance, some facilities offer group therapy for language disorders in adults who suffer from brain injury, stroke, or dementia. SLPs also provide direct one-on-one therapy in most clinical/medical settings. All three of the treatment models discussed earlier are used in clinical/medical settings. Collaborative consultation may be used in clinical/medical settings, but instead of involving teachers in the treatment, physical therapists, occupational therapists, nurses, and family members contribute to speech and language goals.

THE ROLE OF HEALTHCARE PROFESSIONALS IN IDENTIFICATION, ASSESSMENT, AND TREATMENT

Depending on the type of clinical/medical facility, there is almost always an opportunity for healthcare professionals to play a role in speech, language, or swallowing assessment and treatment. First of all, healthcare professionals should always be thinking of speech, hearing, language, and swallowing when they see a patient so that they can share any concerns with others on the medical staff. If a nurse is having trouble communicating with a new patient, the nurse can request a screening. Thus, the first person to encounter a patient with a communication disorder is often a healthcare professional other than the SLP.

The thorough assessment of a patient requires input from a variety of sources. The speech-language pathologist is interested in discussing the patient's communication with other healthcare professionals involved in the case. If the physical therapist (PT) has evaluated the patient prior to the SLP, the SLP can talk with the PT to see how the patient interacted. Which words did the patient use? Did the patient form sentences? Did the sentences make sense? Was the speech slurred? Healthcare professionals can answer many questions and provide valuable information to the SLP. If a swallowing evaluation is scheduled, the SLP may want to talk with the nursing staff about the patient's ability to eat or drink certain foods and beverages. These are only a few examples of how the healthcare staff can provide important information to the SLP and contribute to the evaluation of a patient's communication.

Depending on the type of clinical/medical facility, the patient's length of stay, and whether the patient is an inpatient or outpatient, healthcare professionals also can play an important role in the treatment process. If a patient is in a rehabilitation hospital for a reasonable length of time, the professionals at the facility have the opportunity to work as a team on treatment goals. In most facilities, patients are "staffed" in a meeting of all relevant professionals who discuss their goals and progress that has occurred. These staffings occur frequently and on a regular basis. Think of how valuable it can be to hear the PT, occupational therapist (OT), respiratory therapist, nurse, and speech-language pathologist discuss what levels of competence the patient has reached and what others can do to facilitate progress. During such a meeting, the SLP might tell the others which types of cues are the most efficient to help the patient retrieve vocabulary during interactions. The OT might communicate to other professionals which activities of daily living (e.g., eating, drinking, dressing) the patient should be expected to perform on his own and how to help if he has difficulty. All professionals who interact with the patient can play a role, no matter how small, in achieving each other's goals for that patient.

This chapter provides an overview of several topics. First, we introduced the professions of speech-language pathology and audiology. We discussed work settings, caseload issues, credentialing, and professional organizations. Next, we dealt generally with legal and administrative issues that dictate the day-to-day operations of speech-language pathology and audiology programs. Finally, we discussed the role of the SLP in educational and clinical/medical settings and tried to provide an overview of how teachers and healthcare professionals could contribute to identification, assessment, and treatment of communication disorders. The rest of this text focuses on specific kinds of communication disorders and how they are identified, assessed, and treated in educational and clinical/medical settings.

Terms to Know

Communication	Individuals with Disabilities Education Act
Language	(IDEA)
Speech	Due process
Audition	Individualized Education Program (IEP)
Audiology	Least restrictive environment
Speech-language pathology	PL 99-457
Acute care hospitals	Individualized Family Service Plan (IFSP)
Rehabilitation hospital	Section 504 of the Rehabilitation Act
Community clinic	Americans with Disabilities Act (ADA)
Private practice	HIPAA
University-based clinic	Child find
Long-term care facility	Referral
Industrial audiologist	Evaluation
Screening	Treatment
Prevention	Direct treatment
Identification	Indirect treatment
American Speech-Language-Hearing	Paraprofessionals
Association (ASHA)	Multidisciplinary
Clinical fellowship year (CFY)	Transdisciplinary
Certificate of Clinical Competence	Interdisciplinary
(CCC)	Establishment
American Academy of Audiology (AAA)	Generalization

Study Questions

1. Discuss the importance of federal special education laws from PL 94-142 to IDEA 2004. What are some of the main points of each public law?
2. What is an Individualized Education Program? What are some of its component parts? How is the IEP developed?

3. Why is it important that teachers make referrals to speech-language pathologists? What are the requisite skills needed to be able to make these referrals?
4. Differentiate between direct and indirect treatment services.

Bibliography

American Speech-Language-Hearing Association. (1984). Guidelines for caseload size for speech-language services in the schools. *Asha, 26,* 4, 53–58.

American Speech-Language-Hearing Association. (1992). *1992 Omnibus survey caseload report: SLP.* Rockville, MD: Author.

American Speech-Language-Hearing Association. (2003). *2003 Omnibus survey caseload report: SLP.* Rockville, MD: Author.

American Speech-Language-Hearing Association. (2004). *Scope of practice in audiology.* Rockville, MD: Author.

American Speech-Language-Hearing Association. (2006). *2006 schools survey: Caseload characteristics 1995–2008.* Rockville, MD: Author.

American Speech-Language-Hearing Association. (2007a). *Scope of practice in speech-language pathology.* Rockville, MD: Author.

American Speech-Language-Hearing Association. (2007b). *SLP health care survey: Caseload characteristics.* Rockville, MD: Author.

Damico, J. (1987). Addressing language concerns in the schools: the SLP as consultant. *Journal of Childhood Communication Disorders, 11,* 17–40.

Ehren, B. (1993). Eligibility, evaluation and the realities of role definition in the schools. *American Journal of Speech-Language Pathology, 2,* 1, 20–23.

Ferguson, M. (1991). Collaborative/consultative service delivery: An introduction. *Language, Speech & Hearing Services in Schools, 22,* 147.

Frassinelli, L., Superior, K., & Meyers, J. (1983). A consultation model for speech and language intervention. *Journal of the American Speech-Language-Hearing Association, 25,* 11, 25–30.

Fujiki, M., & Brinton, B. (1984). Supplementing language therapy: Working with the classroom teachers. *Language, Speech & Hearing Services in Schools, 15,* 98–109.

Magnotta, O. (1991). Looking beyond tradition. *Language, Speech & Hearing Services in Schools, 22,* 150–151.

Marvin, C. (1987). Consultation services: Changing roles for SLPs. *Journal of Childhood Communication Disorders, 11,* 1–16.

Montgomery, J. (1992). Implementing collaborative consultation: Perspectives from the field. *Language, Speech & Hearing Services in Schools, 23,* 363–364.

Moore-Brown, B. (1991). Moving in the direction of change: Thoughts for administrators and speech-language pathologists. *Language, Speech & Hearing Services in Schools, 22,* 148–149.

Paul, R. (2007). Language disorders from infancy through adolescence. St. Louis, MO: Mosby Elsevier.

Sommers, R. K., & Hatten, M. E. (1985). Establishing the therapy program: Case finding, case selection, and case load. In R. J. Van Hattum (Ed.), *Organization of speech-language services in schools.* San Diego, CA: College-Hill.

U.S. Department of Education. (2000). *To assure the free appropriate public education of all children with disabilities: Fourteenth annual report to Congress on the implementation of the Individuals with Disabilities Education Act.* U.S. Department of Education: Washington, DC.

NORMAL ASPECTS OF COMMUNICATION

To better understand the communication disorders reviewed in the following chapters, it is helpful first to understand some basic aspects of normal communication. Human communication is a very complex process, many aspects of which are not yet fully understood. It is not even possible to talk about "normal" communication without specifying for whom it is normal. The ability to communicate is a developmental skill. People do not expect an infant to be able to communicate as well as a first-grader, and they do not expect a first-grader to communicate as well as an adult. Children exhibit different levels of communication skills at various stages of their development. Parents, teachers, and speech-language pathologists (SLPs) who deal with young children on a regular basis should be aware of these different levels of communication skills because expecting too much can lead to frustration on the part of the child and expecting too little can result in a failure to identify early signs of a communication disorder.

Several terms used throughout this book are important for you to understand. These terms are **communication**, **language**, and **speech**. Many people use these terms interchangeably, which can lead to confusion. SLPs must understand the specific skill described by each term and use the terms correctly as must others who work with people with communication disorders.

COMMUNICATION

Communication is the broadest of the three terms and refers to an exchange of ideas or feelings. Speech and language are means of communicating, but human beings communicate in many other ways too. Artists communicate through art. A painting or a sculpture can communicate feelings or ideas in a very effective manner. Others with less artistic skill can communicate through gestures, body positions, or facial expressions. A tight jaw and a clenched fist communicate one meaning, while a smile and a wink communicate quite another. The most common way for human beings to communicate, however, is the way we are communicating now, through language.

LANGUAGE

Language can be defined in many ways. Perhaps the best definition of language for the purposes of this chapter comes from Bloom. She defines language as: "A code whereby ideas . . . are represented through a conventional system of arbitrary signals for communication" (Bloom, 1988, p. 2). According to this definition, to communicate through language, a person must first have an idea, and then arrange some symbol system in such a way that another person can process those symbols and draw from them the intended meaning.

Several conditions must be met to communicate using language. First, the person sending the message must have an idea to communicate. For example, if you are asked to discuss agricultural practices in Estonia prior to World War I, you probably would have some difficulty because you may not have much of an idea on that topic to communicate. As children grow, their knowledge and understanding of the world also grow. As a result, they have more ideas to express and more topics to communicate. A second condition is that the communicator must be familiar with the symbol system used to express ideas. If you have studied a foreign language, you know that it is easier to say what you want to say in your native language than in the new language, even though your idea is the same. It takes time and practice to master a new symbol system. As you will see in Chapter 3, children master their language symbol systems in developmental stages.

It is important to remember that language is not only expressed, but for communication to occur, language must also be received. When people send a message, they are using **expressive language**; when they receive a message, they are using **receptive language**. We are communicating with you (we hope) through language right now. We are using expressive language, putting our ideas into symbols. You are using receptive language, processing those symbols so that you can understand our ideas. If you understand our ideas, we have communicated. The process involved in expressive language is **encoding**, putting ideas into code, and the process involved in receptive language is **decoding**, taking ideas out of code.

To communicate through language, both the encoder and the decoder must know the same code. If you speak only English and you try to explain something to someone who speaks only Mandarin Chinese, any communication would probably result from gestures and facial expressions rather than from language because you do not share a common linguistic code with your listener. It does not matter how slowly or how loudly you say the words. The other person will not be able to understand you because she does not have knowledge of your code. Even if the person to whom you are trying to communicate speaks English, if that person does not have knowledge of the words you are using, you will not communicate your idea to the listener. For example, if someone told you that he wanted you to "defenestrate my guzmania," you might not know that he wanted you to take a plant (a guzmani) and throw it out a window (defenestration). If you did not have the confidence to admit that you did not understand the direction, you might do nothing or do something completely unrelated to the instruction. Now imagine a child in an educational setting who does not have sufficient vocabulary to understand the teacher's instruction. That child is in the same situation of not knowing what to do, and her inappropriate response might be misinterpreted by the teacher as disobedience or failure to pay attention.

Because language is such a broad topic, it is sometimes helpful to specify certain aspects or subcomponents of language. Five subcomponents are typically identified: semantics, syntax, phonology, morphology, and pragmatics.

Semantics is the component of language having to do with meaning. The words and sentences people use must have meaning if they are to communicate. If a speaker uses an incorrect word to express an idea or if a listener does not understand the meaning of a word, information may not be conveyed accurately. Certainly one of the more observable aspects of a person's semantic ability is vocabulary. Individuals' vocabularies expand throughout their lives. Hopefully, you are adding to your vocabulary as you read this chapter. During childhood, however, vocabulary grows rapidly. Between the ages of 2 and 4 years, it seems as if children learn a new word every day.

As with all components of language, the semantic component has both an expressive and receptive aspect. Like adults, children usually understand more words than they use. It is not correct to assume that a child does not understand a word simply because he never uses it. On the other hand, because a child uses a word in one context does not mean that he understands all of the possible meanings associated with that word or even is aware that the word has other meanings. The phrases a "loud" jacket, a "sharp" student, or a "school" of fish might not convey the same meaning to a child that they do to an adult. In the same way, idiomatic expressions such as "You're pulling my leg" or "She went to pieces" may suggest some unusual images to a child who knows all the words but on a less abstract level. Additionally, some of a child's first words may be applied more broadly than they are in the adult form of the language. For example a child might call all women "Mommy" or all animals "kitty." This is called overgeneralization. As children's language skills increase, they apply labels more specifically.

Syntax is the component of language that has to do with the way words are put together to form sentences. This includes rules regarding the acceptable order of words in sentences. Syntax is related to those skills referred to as grammar. As children develop, their skills in the area of syntax improve. Children begin with single words and move to two- and three-word utterances. Gradually, they are able to use questions, tenses, different forms of the verb "to be," compound and complex sentences, and other advanced syntactic structures. Consider the complexity of the following sentence: "By this time next year, you will have been in first grade for three months." A student who is not yet able to deal with such complex sentence structure will not be able to decode the message adequately. Just as SLPs see overgeneralization in semantic development, they sometimes see overgeneralization of basic syntactic rules to irregular forms. For example, a child might apply the rule of adding *s* to form a plural to a word such as *foot*, resulting in a sentence such as "I have two foots." Or a child may apply the rule of adding *ed* to indicate past tense and say, "I drawed a picture."

Phonology is the component of language that deals with putting sounds together to make words. The sounds of a language are called **phonemes**, and there are certain ways in which phonemes can and cannot be combined to make words. For example, in English, certain consonants can be combined in a cluster at the beginning of words, such as fr in *from*, bl in *blue*, and scr in *scream*, but English speakers never begin a word with a pb or a dg combination. In the early stages of phonologic development, it is quite common for children to reduce consonant clusters to a single consonant, so a word such as *green* may be produced as "geen," and *stop* may be produced as "top." In very young children, this is part of the normal development of phonology.

Morphology deals with the use of morphemes. A morpheme is the smallest unit of language that conveys meaning. A word such as *boy* is a morpheme. When the phoneme s is added to the word *boy*, the s means more than one. In this case, because the s conveys meaning, it is also a morpheme. In addition to signifying a plural form, an s can also indicate a possessive form when it follows an apostrophe, but in either case, the s has to be attached to another morpheme to have meaning. Morphemes that have to be attached to other morphemes are called **bound morphemes** and include plural and tense markers, as well as prefixes and suffixes such as un in *undress* and ly in *quickly*. Morphemes such as *boy* that are meaningful when standing alone are called **unbound** or **free morphemes**. A child's language development is often reflected in the number of morphemes he or she uses in each utterance.

Pragmatics has to do with the effective use of language in various contexts. Skills such as appropriately initiating a conversation, taking turns during conversation, and assessing how much information your listener needs to be able to understand your message are all part of pragmatics. It is very common for children to think that everyone shares their knowledge of people, places, and things. When asked, "Where did you go on vacation?" a child might say something like, "Billy's house." It is then left to the listener to ask, "Who is Billy?" and, "Where does he live?" As pragmatic skills increase, the child can answer such a question by saying, "I went to visit my cousin Billy in Ohio."

There are two features of language that are important to point out. Language is **rule based**, and it is **generative**. By rule based, we mean that there are certain rules that all speakers of a language know and obey. These are not the rules you learn in junior high English class regarding split infinitives and dangling participles, but rules of which you may not even be aware. You simply know them as a speaker of your language. Some examples can help illustrate this point. You know that the prefix in means not. So, if something is not accurate, it is inaccurate, and if it is not tolerable, it is intolerable. But what if something is not possible? You do not say **in**possible; you say **im**possible. Why does the n become an m in this word? While you make the change somewhat automatically, you may not understand why you make the change. (It is simply more efficient to move from an m to a p than from an <u>n</u> to a <u>p</u> because the lips are together for <u>m</u> and <u>p</u> but apart for <u>n</u>.) Here is another example of a phonological rule: Each of the following are words in English, with one exception. Which one is not a word in English?

1. Monogenesis
2. Palpus
3. Rowel
4. Fugacious
5. Sssssseeeellpn

It shouldn't take very long for you to select number 5. Sssssseeeellpn is clearly not a word in English. It is likely that some readers might have difficulty defining words 1 through 4. But even if you do not know the meaning of the words (there is no semantic component to guide you), you can still identify the nonword. What is the phonologic rule that the first four terms obey but that the fifth violates? After some thought, you might be able to say something about the syllable structure or too many consonants together without a vowel, but you probably cannot state a rule that you memorized at some time in your educational history. As a speaker of English, you knew immediately that choice 5 was not a word. If you change the order of the letters so that "sssssseeeellpn" becomes *sleeplessness*, you now recognize it as a word all too familiar to most college students.

Here is an example of a syntactic rule. Which of the following is an acceptable sentence?

1. The old miles were lived clearly on a clean plate.
2. Plate on old the clearly lived miles a clean were.

As in the previous example, it should not be hard for you to choose. Number 1 is a sentence, whereas number 2 is simply a jumbled string of words. What makes number 1 a sentence and number 2 a nonsentence? Once again, although it might be very difficult to rattle off a rule, you know that the sequence of words in number 2 does not qualify as a sentence. The words in number 1, on the other hand, do form a sentence, even though the sentence is without meaning. As children develop their language skills, they must learn the rules of the language. During early stages of development, they do not know all of the adult rules, or they may operate under a different set of rules that allows them to communicate, but in a simpler fashion than adults. Consider the child who refers to his feet as "foots." Here is a child who has learned the rule: "If more than one, add <u>s</u>." Assuming normal language development, the child will learn the exceptions to that rule later.

The other characteristic of language is that it is generative. Once you learn the rules of the language, you can make and understand sentences that you have never heard before. You probably never before heard the preceding sentence, but you can understand it. The last time you took an essay test, you probably created sentences that you never used before (and in some cases may never use again). Children display this generative aspect of language very early in their development when they make sentences such as "all gone milk." Parents may repeat this utterance, but in most cases the sentence was first created by the child.

An example of how children use their knowledge of linguistic rules to generate novel sentences was proved by the son of one of the authors. After a request that he "behave," the boy responded, "But, Dad, I am being have." It is this generative aspect of language, the ability to create new sentences that makes language such a powerful tool for communication.

Language is most frequently expressed through two avenues: writing and speaking. The more common avenue for most people is speech.

SPEECH

Speech is the process of producing sound patterns to communicate. For most people, speech is a relatively effortless process. However, speech is a complicated action requiring the coordination of several processes. Five basic processes associated with speech are: **respiration**, **phonation**, **resonance**, **articulation**, and **cerebration**. Although these processes work together to produce speech, it is helpful to describe each separately.

RESPIRATION

Respiration is the inhalation and exhalation of air from the lungs. Quiet breathing, as you are probably doing now, is an automatic function. When your body senses the need for oxygen, your chest cavity expands by the contraction of chest muscles and the **diaphragm** (the muscle that separates the chest cavity from the abdominal cavity). Expanding the chest cavity causes the lungs to expand. The increased size of the lungs results in lower pressure inside the lungs than outside, and air rushes in to balance the pressure. When you exhale, you relax the diaphragm and chest muscles, allowing the lungs to return to their resting position. As the size of the lungs decreases, the pressure inside becomes greater than outside, and air is forced out until the pressure inside the lungs once again equals the pressure outside.

Beyond exchanging carbon dioxide and oxygen, respiration also serves as the driving force for speech. Breathing for speech is a much more complicated process than quiet breathing is. When using connected speech, speakers allow only brief pauses to "take a breath." Inhalation for connected speech then must be faster than inhalation for quiet breathing. Exhalation for speech is even more complex. Connected speech requires frequent changes in loudness and stress patterns. All of these changes require adjustments in the amount of air pressure provided by the respiratory system. Too much pressure results in speech that is too loud or in stress being placed on the wrong syllable. Too little pressure results in speech that is hard to hear or difficult to understand. Sometimes, speakers are almost "out of air," but they don't want to pause to take a breath. So, they force out air beyond the point where they would ordinarily stop to inhale. All of these adjustments must be done quickly enough to support rapid connected speech, and all must be coordinated with the activity of the other speech structures. Several abdominal, chest, and back muscles are used during exhalation for speech to provide just the right amount of air at just the right time to support a smooth flow of speech.

As air leaves the lungs, it travels through the trachea. Directly atop the trachea is a structure composed of cartilage and muscle, which some people call the voice box, but which we shall call the **larynx** (lar-ingks). The larynx has several functions. One function is to prevent food or liquids from entering the trachea and the lungs. The explosive coughing that you experience after swallowing something "the wrong way" is a result of the larynx fulfilling its role as protector of the lower airway. Another function of the larynx is the production of **voice**. The process of producing voice is called phonation and is the next basic process of speech to be discussed.

PHONATION

Phonation is the production of voice (be careful not to confuse *phonation* with *phonology*). Voice is produced in the larynx. **Figure 2–1** shows the position of the larynx in relation to the lungs and trachea. The larynx forms what many people refer to as the "Adam's apple."

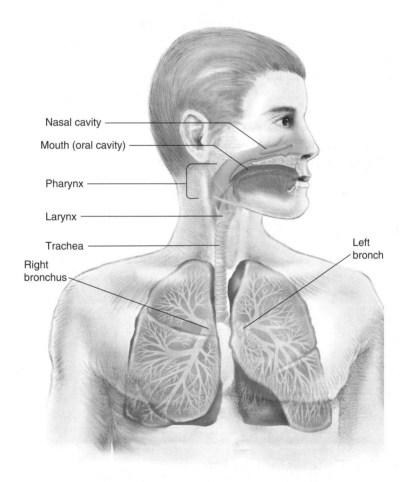

FIGURE 2–1   Relative position of the lungs, larynx, and pharynx.
Source: Chiras, D. (2008). *Human Biology* (6th ed., p. 153). Jones & Bartlett Learning. Reprinted by permission.

If you place your finger on the side of your Adam's apple and produce a prolonged "eeeeeee," you should feel some vibration. What you feel is the rapid vibration of the vocal cords, or more accurately the **vocal folds**. The vocal folds are two bands of muscle that run horizontally from the front to the rear of the larynx (see **Figure 2–2**). Air from the lungs sets these muscles into vibration. This vibration of the vocal folds produces voice.

The position and action of the vocal folds are sometimes difficult to visualize. It may be helpful to use the following hand analogy. With your index and middle fingers, make the letter *V*. Now hold your fingers in a horizontal plane so that you are looking at the fingernail side. You now have an analogy of the vocal folds. They are attached in a V shape in the front but are free to move together and apart at the rear. During quiet breathing, the vocal folds are apart, or **abducted**, allowing air to pass into and out of the trachea and lungs. To produce voice, the vocal folds must be brought together, or **adducted**, following inhalation. In this position, the vocal folds lie in the path of the exhaled air. The airflow from the lungs sets the adducted vocal folds into vibration, causing a buzzing sound that serves as the basis for what will eventually be heard as voice. The rate of vibration, or cycles per second, determines the **frequency** of the voice.

Listeners perceive frequency as **pitch**. A high-pitched voice is associated with faster vibratory rate (more cycles per second), and a low-pitched voice is associated with a slower rate of vibration (fewer cycles per second). Although a rubber band is not a perfect analogy for a vocal fold, it may help to clarify the pitch-changing mechanism of the larynx. As a child, or in an idle moment as an adult, you've probably plucked a rubber band, producing a sound. As you stretch the rubber band, it becomes longer, thinner, and tighter (or more tense), and the

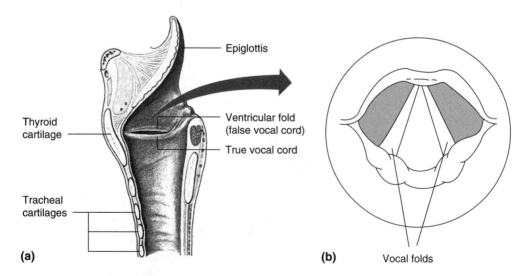

(a) Epiglottis
Thyroid cartilage
Ventricular fold (false vocal cord)
True vocal cord
Tracheal cartilages

(b) Vocal folds

FIGURE 2–2 The larynx and vocal folds.
Source: (a) Chiras, D. (2008). *Human Biology* (6th ed., p. 154). Jones & Bartlett Learning. Reprinted by permission. (b) Illustration by Mark J. Moran.

sound produced by plucking it increases in pitch. That is roughly what happens to the vocal folds when a speaker increases vocal pitch. When you raises your pitch, you stretch the length of the vocal folds, which makes them thinner and increases the tension. A low pitch is associated with shorter, thicker, more lax vocal folds. Although there is no significant pitch difference in the voices of young boys and girls, adult males have a lower pitch than do adult females. The pitch difference between the sexes in adults is a result of the growth of the larynx during puberty. Chapter 3 contains more information about the changes in pitch across the life span.

In addition to pitch, another aspect of voice that speakers frequently alter is loudness. Just as pitch is the perceptual aspect of frequency, **loudness** is the perceptual aspect of **intensity**. Intensity is controlled primarily by the amount of air pressure with which the vocal folds are blown apart. Imagine that you are going to yell to a friend across a parking lot. Your friend is far away and the parking lot is noisy, so you have to yell loudly. What is the first thing you do as you prepare to yell? For most people, the answer is to take a deep breath. The large volume of air in the lungs resulting from the deep inhalation, along with forceful contraction of abdominal, chest, and possibly back muscles, provides the powerful exhalatory air stream needed for a loud voice.

Pitch and loudness by themselves do not completely describe a person's voice. Two people producing a sound at the same pitch with the same loudness still sound different from each other. The factor that gives each person's voice a certain uniqueness is the factor of **voice quality**. Voice quality is not as easy to define as pitch and loudness. Whereas pitch and loudness are each perceptual aspects of single physical characteristics (frequency and intensity), quality is the perceptual aspect of several physical characteristics. To complicate matters further, SLPs are not certain of all the physical characteristics that contribute to quality. Whereas pitch can be described as high or low and loudness can be described as loud or soft, a number of terms are used to describe quality. Terms such as *hoarse, harsh, breathy, rough, raspy, rich, mellow, flat*, and *throaty* all are attempts to describe voice quality. Although professionals do not understand all of the factors that affect voice quality, most authorities agree that voice quality is related to the process of phonation and the next process to be discussed, resonance.

RESONANCE

The sound that you hear as a person's voice is not the same sound that that person produces at the larynx. The sound has to pass through the **vocal tract**, which is the area from the larynx to the end of the lips or, sometimes, the end of the nostrils (see **Figure 2–3**). The size and shape of the vocal tract has an effect on the sound that listeners finally hear. The effect of the size and shape of the vocal tract on the sound that passes through it is resonance. A common childhood activity provides an example of resonance. Children often amuse themselves and others by talking into the cardboard tube from which paper towels or plastic wrap is dispensed. Holding the tube in front of the mouth results in a

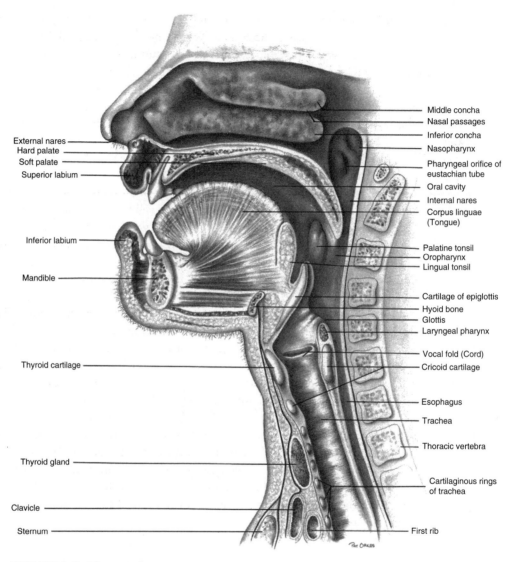

FIGURE 2–3 The vocal tract.
Source: Donnersberger, A., & Lesak, A. (2000). *A Laboratory Textbook of Anatomy and Physiology.* (7th ed., p. 332). Jones & Bartlett Learning. Reprinted by permission.

different sound than is produced without the tube. Holding the tube in front of the mouth effectively lengthens the vocal tract, and the sound that finally is released into the air is quite different from the sound that would have been released at the lips. Perhaps the most important aspect of resonance to understand is oral versus nasal resonance. For most speech sounds in English, the nasal cavity is closed off from the oral cavity by the upward and backward movement of the soft palate, or **velum**. Only the m, n, and ng sounds are produced with the velum down (open). If other sounds, especially vowels, are produced with the velum down, the voice has a nasal quality and the person sounds as if she is "talking through the nose." If an obstruction in the nasal cavity prevents the sound from passing through the nose on m, n, and ng, the person has a denasal quality and sounds as if she has a head cold. Problems of nasal resonance are discussed further in later chapters.

In the vocal tract, speech sounds, or phonemes, are produced by means of the next process to be discussed, articulation.

ARTICULATION

As mentioned in the previous discussion of language, phonology deals with the rules for putting speech sounds together to make words. Articulation is the physical production of the speech sounds. Speech sounds are produced by altering the flow of air from the lungs. The way in which the speaker alters the airflow and the place in which it is altered determines which sound is produced. The body structures speakers use to alter the flow of air through the vocal tract are called **articulators**. Some articulators are movable and some are immovable. The articulators are listed in **Table 2–1**.

Before we discuss individual speech sounds, we have a problem to solve. We are talking about speech sounds, but because we are communicating through written language, we must use a written symbol to represent each speech sound. Unfortunately, English is not a phonetic language. By that, we mean that the letters of the alphabet do not always represent the same sound. For example, the c in *Cindy* is produced as an s, but the c in *candy* is produced as a k, and the two c's together in *Gucci* are produced as a ch. In other cases, the same sound may be represented by several different letters. The f sound can be represented by the letter f, but it is also represented by the ph in *Philadelphia* and the gh in *enough*. In these examples, we have been able to identify the sound we mean by referring to another letter, but that is not always the case. What sound does the s represent in *vision*? How can we differentiate the th in *the* from the th in *think*?

It is difficult to describe the sound without producing it. That is one of the limitations of written language: We cannot make the sounds we wish to describe. In the field

TABLE 2–1 The Articulators

Movable Articulators	Immovable Articulators
Lips	Teeth
Mandible	Alveolar ridge
Tongue	Hard palate
Soft palate (velum)	
Larynx	
Pharynx	

of communication disorders, professionals solve this problem by using the International Phonetic Alphabet. In this alphabet, there is a symbol for each speech sound, and each symbol represents one and only one speech sound. It is beyond the scope of this text to discuss the International Phonetic Alphabet, so when the written letter does not represent clearly the sound we intend, we use a key word as an illustration (e.g., j as in *joy*). That way, we can use your speech to communicate our message.

There are two major categories of speech sounds, or phonemes: vowels and consonants. Consonants are produced with a greater degree of obstruction in the vocal tract than are vowels. To produce a consonant sound, speakers must use two articulators to obstruct the flow of air in just the right way to produce the sound that listeners recognize as a consonant. Consonant sounds are distinguished from each other on the basis of three production features (see **Table 2–2**). The **manner of articulation** describes *how* the airflow is altered. The air can be completely blocked and then suddenly released, as is the case for p, b, t, d, k, and g. Because these sounds often have an explosive quality to their production, they are sometimes called **plosive** consonants, but they are not always exploded. For example, in the word *hat*, the final t is rarely exploded, especially in connected speech such as "I wear a hat in the winter." The aspect that all of these consonants do have in common is the complete stoppage of air at the beginning of production. Therefore, we refer to these sounds as **stop consonants**.

Another way to alter airflow to produce a speech sound is to force it through a narrow opening. Forcing air through a narrow opening results in a friction noise, and consonant sounds made this way are called **fricatives**. Examples of fricatives are f, v, th (voiced as in *the* and unvoiced as in *thin*), s, z, sh and h, and the sound made by s in the word *vision*. Some sounds combine features of stops and fricatives and are called **affricates**. In English,

TABLE 2–2 Manner, Place, and Voice Characteristics of Consonants

Place	Manner				
	Stop	**Fricative**	**Affricate**	**Nasal**	**Semivowel**
Bilabial	p, b*			m*	w*
Labiodental		f, v*			
Linguadental		th (*thin*), th (*the*)*			
Lingua-alveolar	t, d*	s, z*		n*	l*
Linguapalatal		sh s (*vision*)*	ch, j (*joy*)*		r*, y*
Linguavelar	k, g*			ing*	
Glottal		h			

*Indicates voice.

there are two affricates: the ch sound as in *church*, and the dg sound at the end of the word *fudge*.

As mentioned earlier, most speech sounds in English are made with the nasal cavity closed off from the oral cavity by the velum. There are three sounds in English made with the velum open, allowing sound into the nasal cavity. These consonants, m, n, and ng, are called **nasals**. A group of consonants are made with the vocal tract too constricted to be vowels but not as constricted as the other consonants. These sounds are called **semi-vowels** because they are vowel-like but are still considered consonants. Semi-vowels are l, r, w, and y.

The second production feature used to distinguish among consonants is the **place of articulation**. The place of articulation indicates *where* in the vocal tract the alteration of the airstream occurs. Place of articulation is determined by the articulators used to produce the sound. For example, p, b, and m are made with both lips together and are therefore called **bilabial** (two-lip) sounds. Putting manner and place characteristics together, p and b are bilabial stops, while m is a bilabial nasal. The sounds f and v are made with the lower lip between the teeth, so these sounds are **labiodental**. The th sounds are made with the tongue between the teeth and are called **linguadental**. The ridge immediately behind the upper front teeth is the **alveolar ridge**. Several sounds are made with the tongue touching the alveolar ridge. These sounds, t, d, s, z, and l, are called **lingua-alveolar**. Moving back, the next place of articulation involves the tongue contacting the hard palate. Sounds made in this place, sh, ch, the s sound in *vision*, and the j sound in *joy*, are called **linguapalatal** sounds. The k and g are made with the tongue against the soft palate. We have already used *palatal* to mean hard palate, so for these sounds we use the term *velar* (referring to the velum). The k and g are **linguavelar** sounds. (Note the spelling difference between alveolar and velar). Finally, at least one sound, h, is made at the glottis (the space between the vocal folds), so it is known as a **glottal** sound.

The third production feature used to distinguish among consonants is **voicing**. Voicing indicates whether the vocal folds are together and vibrating or apart and not vibrating during the production of the sound. Some consonant sounds are voiced (vocal folds vibrating), while others are voiceless (vocal folds not vibrating). Voiceless consonants are p, t, k, s, th (as in *think*), sh, ch, and h. Voiced consonants are b, d, g, m, n, ng, v, z, th (as in *the*), j (as in *joy*), l, r, w, and y. Sounds that have the same manner and place of articulation but differ in voicing are called **cognates**. For example, s and z are both lingua-alveolar fricatives, but s is voiceless and z is voiced. Therefore, z is the voiced cognate of s. The phonemes are organized by manner, place, and voice characteristics in Table 2–2.

Vowels are not as easy to classify as are consonants. Vowels tend to be more continuous with each other, while consonants are more discrete. We cannot use the manner or voice features to distinguish among vowels because all vowels are made in the same manner (the manner of vowel production is called **vocalic**) and all vowels are voiced. That leaves only place. Although we have said that vowels are produced with a relatively unobstructed vocal tract, the articulators do assume certain positions to produce each vowel. Vowels are classified according to tongue position. To have a sense of the tongue positions for vowels, say the vowel ee as in *feet*, and then quickly change to oo as in *too*. Do this several times and note the direction in which your tongue moves. When you say ee your tongue should be toward the front of the mouth, and when you say oo it should move to the back. The ee is a **front vowel**, the oo is a **back vowel**. Now do the same thing with ee and a as in *at*. You should sense movement of the tongue from high in the mouth for ee to low in the mouth for a. Therefore, ee is a **high vowel** and a is a **low vowel**. It is on the basis of high–low and front–back that SLPs distinguish among vowels. Vowel classifications are presented in **Table 2–3**.

A **diphthong** is a sound produced by the joining of two adjacent vowel sounds in the same syllable. The sounds represented by the ow in *cow*, the oy in *boy*, and the i in *mine* are the three primary diphthongs in English.

The muscle movements required to make the speech sounds and the rules used to put the sounds together to make words are governed by the nervous system. The critical role of the nervous system is discussed as the process of cerebration.

CEREBRATION

Cerebration refers to the role of the nervous system in producing speech. The nervous system plays two distinct roles in speech. First, the cognitive-linguistic role involves supplying the ideas to be communicated and managing the rules that are to be used to communicate those ideas. The other role involves the motor aspect of speech. The impulses that move and control the muscles of respiration, phonation, and articulation originate in and are carried by the nervous system. The nervous system can be divided into two portions: the **central nervous system (CNS)** and the **peripheral nervous system (PNS)**. The CNS consists of those parts of the nervous system encased in a bony covering: the brain and spinal cord (see **Figure 2–4**). What is typically called the brain is actually several structures. The uppermost section is the cerebrum. The outer covering of the cerebrum, the **cerebral cortex**, is where most of the processing activity takes place. The cerebrum is divided into two halves, or hemispheres. It appears that these hemispheres have different functions. In most people, the left hemisphere is associated with intellectual functions including

TABLE 2–3   Vowel Classifications

	Front	Central	Back
	meet		too
	hit	but	foot
High to Low	made	her	no
	red		law
	hat		father

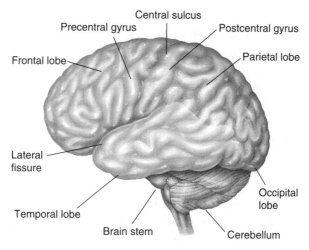

Central sulcus

Precentral gyrus

Postcentral gyrus

Frontal lobe

Parietal lobe

Lateral
fissure

Occipital
lobe

Temporal lobe

Brain stem

Cerebellum

FIGURE 2–4 The brain.
Source: Chiras, D. (2008). *Human Biology* (6th ed., p. 199). Jones & Bartlett Learning. Reprinted by permission.

language and speech. The right hemisphere is associated more with spatial relations, musical patterns, and nonlanguage functions. Each hemisphere is further divided into four lobes: the frontal, parietal, occipital, and temporal lobes (see Figure 2–4). The frontal lobe is associated with speech, and the temporal lobe is associated with hearing. The cerebral cortex sends signals to and receives signals from the rest of the body via nerve fibers.

The PNS consists of the parts of the nervous system that exit the bony covering and carry signals to and from the muscles and organs. Fibers called **cranial nerves** carry signals to and from the muscles and organs of speech and hearing. The cranial nerves originate in the brainstem and innervate (i.e., carry signals to and from) most of the muscles above the shoulders. There are 12 pairs of cranial nerves (one member of each pair on each side of the body). The cranial nerves are quite complex and innervate nonspeech structures as well. These nerves serve as the connection between the nervous system and the speech structures.

The five processes of respiration, phonation, resonance, articulation, and cerebration allow human beings to put language into coded sound patterns. But communication cannot take place unless there is a way for others to decode those sound patterns. The way in which listeners usually decode the speech signal is through their sense of hearing.

HEARING

Recall from the earlier discussion that speech is a sound pattern. The sense used to receive sound is hearing. For listeners to hear a sound, three elements must be present. Small (1973) describes these elements in the following manner: First, there must be a sound source.

This could be a car horn, a falling tree, or the speech-production mechanism. Second, there must be a conducting medium to carry the sound away from the source. For speech, the medium is usually air, but if you've ever put your ear to a railroad track or lived in an apartment with thin walls, you know that sound can travel through materials other than air. Finally, there must be a mechanism to receive the sound. The mechanism that allows listeners to receive sound is the **auditory** system. The part of the auditory system with which you are most familiar is the ear. The ear changes the sound waves created by the speaker and carried through the air into nerve impulses. These nerve impulses are then sent to the brain to be interpreted or decoded.

We must mention two aspects of sound at this point: frequency and intensity. Recall from the earlier discussion of voice that frequency is the aspect of sound that listeners perceive as pitch. Frequency is measured in units called **hertz (Hz)**. Intensity is the aspect of sound listeners perceive as loudness. Intensity is measured in **decibels (dB)**.

The ear consists of three parts: the **outer ear**, the **middle ear**, and the **inner ear**. The parts of the ear are shown in **Figure 2–5**.

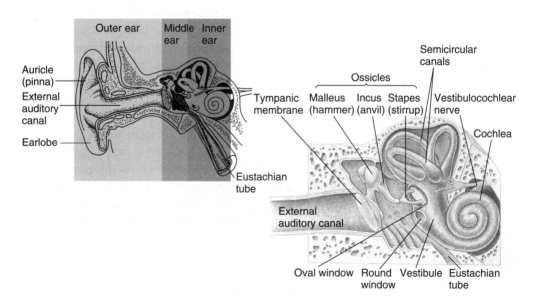

FIGURE 2–5 The outer, middle and inner ear.
Source: Chiras, D. (2008). *Human Biology* (6th ed., p. 226). Jones & Bartlett Learning. Reprinted by permission.

THE OUTER EAR

The outer ear is made up of the part of the ear you see on the side of the head. This structure, made mostly of cartilage covered by flesh, is the **pinna**, also called the **auricle**. Inside each pinna, leading into the head, is a canal known as the **external auditory meatus**. Within the external auditory meatus are two structures that aid in protecting the ear from dust and other tiny particles. These structures are tiny hairs, which are visible upon close inspection of the ear, and tiny glands which secrete **cerumen**, a substance better known as ear wax. Cerumen serves an important function in protecting the ear from foreign particles. The outer ear does not play as important a role in hearing as the other parts of the ear. The pinna apparently serves to gather the sound waves from the air and funnel them down the canal to the middle ear.

THE MIDDLE EAR

At the end of the external auditory meatus is a thin membrane known as the ear drum, or, more properly, the **tympanic membrane**. The tympanic membrane separates the outer ear from the middle ear but is considered here as part of the middle ear. Behind the tympanic membrane is a cavity known as the middle ear space. There are several structures within the middle ear space, the two most important of which are the **Eustachian tube** and the **ossicles**. The middle ear space would be airtight except for the fact that it is ventilated by the Eustachian tube. The Eustachian tube leads from the middle ear to the **pharynx** (upper throat area) and allows air into and out of the middle ear space. This ventilation serves to balance pressure on each side of the tympanic membrane. You have probably experienced your ears "popping" in an airplane or as you drive up or down a mountain road. As altitude increases, the air pressure decreases. The result is more air pressure in the middle ear than on the outside. This can be painful and cause reduced hearing sensitivity. As you yawn, talk, or chew gum, the Eustachian tube opens, allowing air to escape from the middle ear until the pressure is balanced. With a decrease in altitude, the pressure outside becomes greater, and the Eustachian tube opens to allow more air into the middle ear. As discussed in Chapter 10 on hearing problems, Eustachian tube malfunction and resulting middle ear disorders are quite common among children.

The other major structure of the middle ear is a chain of tiny bones. As you no doubt learned in elementary school, there are three bones in the middle ear. These bones are sometimes called the hammer, anvil, and stirrup because of their appearance, but the true names of these bones are the **malleus, incus**, and **stapes**. Together, these bones are known as the ossicles, or the **ossicular chain**. The ossicles are attached to the tympanic membrane on one end and to a portion of the inner ear known as the **oval window** on the other end. As sound waves travel down the external auditory meatus, they hit the tympanic membrane, causing it to vibrate. The vibration of the tympanic membrane, in turn, sets the ossicular chain into motion, causing it to push in and out on the oval window, transmitting the pressure wave to the inner ear.

THE INNER EAR

The inner ear consists of two portions: the **vestibular** portion, which is related to balance, and the **cochlea**, which is associated with hearing. In the cochlea the pressure wave is changed to a nerve impulse by the action of a specialized structure called the **organ of Corti** (see **Figure 2–6**). The organ of Corti extends almost the entire length of the snail-shaped cochlea. The cochlea is filled with fluid in which the organ of Corti rides.

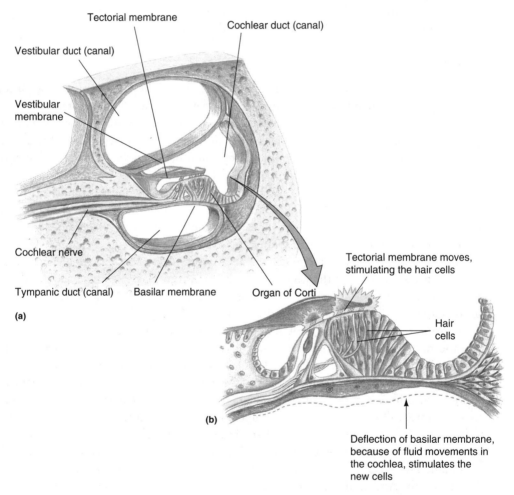

FIGURE 2–6 A cross section through the cochlea showing the position of the organ of Corti (a), and a closer view of the organ of Corti (b).
Source: Chiras, D. (2008). *Human Biology* (6th ed., p. 227). Jones & Bartlett Learning. Reprinted by permission.

When the ossicles of the middle ear move in response to sound, they create waves in the cochlear fluid. The waves cause **hair cells** in the organ of Corti to move in a shearing action. The shearing of the hair cells produces the nerve impulses that are carried along the auditory nerve and eventually to the brain. The organ of Corti is structured in such a way that different parts of the organ respond to different frequencies. The outer portion responds to high frequencies, and the inner portion responds to low frequencies. This is a very fortunate arrangement for receiving speech sounds. The frequency range of human hearing is approximately 20 to 20,000 Hz. Most speech sounds have the bulk of their energy between 500 and 2000 Hz. Because speech frequencies are closer to the low end of the range than to the high end, the portion of the organ of Corti that responds to these frequencies is near the inner, most well-protected portion. This arrangement provides maximum protection for the portion of the cochlea most important to speech.

After the organ of Corti converts the sound wave to a nerve impulse, that impulse is carried over nerve fibers up to the temporal lobe of the cerebral cortex. The right ear sends signals to the left temporal lobe, and the left ear sends signals to the right temporal lobe. Once the nerve impulse reaches the cortex, it can be processed so that meaning can be attached. What was once a pressure wave in the air, and then a series of nerve impulses, is perceived as poetry, humor, anger, obscenity, or any other message that can be conveyed through speech. What was once an idea in one person's mind becomes an idea in another's mind. Communication has occurred.

Even from this rather brief discussion you can see that the ability to communicate effectively through language and speech is a complex skill, requiring the coordination of several physical and intellectual functions. As with any complex process, there are many opportunities for things to go wrong. All listeners and speakers occasionally stumble over a sound or have difficulty finding the right word. Their voice sometimes deserts them, and they sometimes hear noises that exist only in their head. *Normal* does not mean perfect. There are, however, problems with communication that are outside the range of normal, problems that must be considered communication disorders. The rest of this book deals with those communication disorders.

Terms to Know

Communication	Phonology
Language	Phonemes
Speech	Morphology
Expressive language	Bound morphemes
Receptive language	Unbound or free morphemes
Encoding	Pragmatics
Decoding	Rule based
Semantics	Generative
Syntax	Respiration

Phonation
Resonance
Articulation
Cerebration
Diaphragm
Larynx
Voice
Vocal folds
Abducted
Adducted
Frequency
Pitch
Loudness
Intensity
Voice quality
Vocal tract
Velum
Articulators
Manner of articulation
Plosive
Stop consonants
Fricatives
Affricates
Nasals
Semivowels
Place of articulation
Bilabial
Labiodental
Linguadental
Alveolar ridge
Lingua-alveolar
Linguapalatal
Linguavelar
Glottal
Voicing

Cognates
Vocalic
Front vowel
Back vowel
High vowel
Low vowel
Diphthong
Central nervous system (CNS)
Peripheral nervous
   system (PNS)
Cerebral cortex
Cranial nerves
Auditory
Hertz (Hz)
Decibels (dB)
Outer ear
Middle ear
Inner ear
Pinna
Auricle
External auditory meatus
Cerumen
Tympanic membrane
Eustachian tube
Ossicles
Pharynx
Malleus
Incus
Stapes
Ossicular chain
Oval window
Vestibular
Cochlea
Organ of Corti
Hair cells

Study Questions

1. Identify and describe the five basic processes of speech.
2. Compare and contrast quiet breathing and breathing for speech.
3. Describe the mechanism by which a speaker increases vocal pitch, loudness.

4. How do vowels differ from consonants? How are consonants classified? How are vowels classified?
5. Provide several examples of words in which the same letter represents different sounds. Provide examples of words in which different letters represent the same sound.
6. Describe the cognitive and the motor function of the brain in spoken communication.
7. Identify the major structures of the ear and describe their role in normal hearing.

Bibliography

Bloom, L. (1988). What is language? In M. Lahey (Ed.), *Language disorders and language development*. New York, NY: Macmillan.

Small, A. (1973). Acoustics. In F. Minifie, T. Hixon, & F. Williams (Eds.), *Normal aspects of speech hearing and language*. Englewood Cliffs, NJ: Prentice Hall.

3

COMMUNICATION DEVELOPMENT THROUGH THE LIFE SPAN

When most people think of the development of communicative ability, their focus is typically on childhood. Certainly, it is true that the most significant and dramatic developments take place between birth and 6 years of age. A child goes from not being able to communicate intentionally at all to using complex sentences in the space of six years. Authorities in language acquisition maintain that normal language development continues through the teenage years, albeit the changes are more subtle and complicated during that period. By the time a person graduates from high school, he or she not only can speak the language of the culture, but also can write, read, and spell. Thus, it might appear to many casual observers that normal changes in communication are complete by the late teenage years. Yet, researchers have shown that there are changes in communication that continue to occur with aging.

As we discuss in this chapter, the most critical and dramatic changes in the development of language and phonology do, in fact, occur in childhood. But it is also important to document normal changes in communication that are seen in older adult populations. There are changes in voice, fluency, hearing, language, and memory that are part of normal aging and should be expected. It is important for professionals to take these changes into account when assessing or working with older adults. For example, normal adults experience a degradation in their ability to hear high-frequency (pitch) sounds as they become older. The whole idea of "normal hearing" must take into account these inevitable changes that occur with age. Similarly, normal adults may have more difficulty retrieving words as they become older. These are not necessarily "disorders" but may be part of the normal evolution of communication as a person ages. In this chapter, we begin by discussing the dramatic changes that occur in language and phonological development in early childhood. The second part of the chapter documents changes in voice, fluency, language, and hearing that are part of normal development and aging.

LANGUAGE DEVELOPMENT IN CHILDHOOD

People often take for granted the process of a child learning how to talk. A newborn child cannot speak, yet in the space of only one year says her first words. Four short years later, she has learned most of the basic language structures of the culture. Although the language acquisition process continues well beyond this age (Nippold, 1988), in a relatively short time the child has moved from being nonverbal to producing complex and compound sentences involving embedding and conjoining. This takes place with little direct help and often a great deal of distraction. When children reach school age, they can produce almost all of the basic sentence structures and speech sounds that are used by adults. Some, as discussed in this text, do not acquire language and speech sounds normally, and this affects their ability to perform socially, communicatively, and academically.

The present chapter is designed to provide you a basic understanding of the order in which language and speech sounds are acquired by normally developing children. We present this information for two main reasons. First, in assessment of a child's language and sound system speech-language professionals must determine where the child is in the developmental process. So, when we talk about various language and articulation assessment measurements in later chapters, a basic knowledge of development will be helpful. Second, the speech-language pathologist (SLP) uses the normal developmental order as a major consideration in selecting therapy targets to work on with children who have language or articulation disorders. The first part of the chapter deals with language development and acquisition of the sound system in childhood. The final portion of the chapter discusses normal changes in hearing, vocal production, language, and fluency in adults as they go through the aging process.

EARLY COMMUNICATIVE DEVELOPMENT: GESTURES AND LANGUAGE

This section provides a basic appreciation of the process and order of early communication development. We include this portion because without an understanding of the aspects involved in communicative development you cannot understand the types of children with limited language, how they are assessed, and how they are helped in intervention. We must say at the outset that the acquisition of communication is an extremely complex unfolding of highly interrelated abilities that is not fully understood. Speech-language professionals do know, however, that certain components must be in place for the developmental process to occur and know the basic order in which some of these aspects mature. Thus, the process of early communicative development may be grossly divided into two parts: (1) the basic building blocks of communicative development, and (2) the development of verbal communication. We briefly discuss each of these two important areas.

Basic Building Blocks of Communicative Development A contractor knows that the integrity of the house being built depends on a firm foundation. If the structure is built on footings that are not level or that are cracked in places, problems will become apparent as the building progresses.

Similarly, in the development of communication, a number of basic building blocks exist on which the language acquisition process rests. We use the acronym BACIS (pronounced like *basis*) to reflect the basic building blocks or the basis of communicative development. **Figure 3–1** shows the bases of communicative development and mentions some specific acquisitions in each area. Read the figure from the bottom to the top. The five areas, biological, access to a language model, cognitive ability, intent to communicate, and social ability, need to be in place prior to communication development. Upon these bases, actual communication develops from early gestures to the later use of complex sentences. It is important to mention here that the building blocks for communication are developing

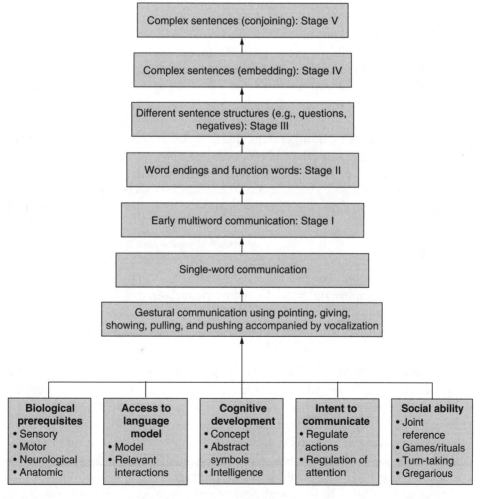

FIGURE 3–1 The BACIS of language development and steps in the language acquisition process.

simultaneously and influence each other in development. For instance, motor development allows a child to explore the environment, and this exploration facilitates cognitive and social development. We briefly discuss each building block area.

Biological Bases   Many prerequisites of language could be considered biological in nature.

1. *Sensory abilities:* To develop communication it is imperative that a child possesses adequate abilities to sense information from the environment. This is important because people listen to others producing language, and they see what they are communicating within the environment. Thus, normal vision and hearing are critical for the development of language. It is not surprising that research over the years has consistently shown that children with hearing or even visual impairments are at risk to develop communicative abilities at a slower rate and are high priority for early intervention.
2. *Motor abilities:* When humans use the speech mechanism to produce language, very complex adjustments must take place. As discussed in Chapter 2, the articulators move very rapidly to produce the variety of speech sounds in English. Children who do not have voluntary control of their speech mechanism do not develop oral language. Children with cerebral palsy, for instance, often have fine motor coordination difficulties, and some may never be able to produce oral language intelligibly. They may, however, be able to use a communication board or some electronic device to transmit their ideas to others. If a child is going to learn the oral production of language, motor ability must be intact.
3. *Neurological status:* Language appears to be a skill that is developed only in species having the largest and most complex brains. When the human brain is damaged, typically the most complex skills are lost first. For instance, if an adult has a stroke, the first abilities that are impaired are fine motor coordination, language, and speech. If a child suffers brain damage prior to or during the birth process and begins life with a neurologic impairment, you can almost always predict problems in developing communication.
4. *Anatomic structure:* For normal oral production of language, the speech mechanism needs to be complete and intact. Children who are born with abnormalities of the mouth, face, or vocal tract experience difficulty in orally producing language, as mentioned in Chapter 11 in the discussion of cleft palate.

Access to a Language Model   For children to learn the language of their culture, they must have access to caregivers who model simplified language in relevant, appropriate situations. It only makes sense that a child must have a pattern to follow in communication development. In extreme cases of children who were raised by psychotic parents or even by wolves in the wild, the result is the absence of linguistic verbal communication (Brown, 1958; Curtiss, Fromkin, Krashen, Rigler, & Rigler, 1974). If there is no one to act as a model in using language, a child learns no language. A great deal of research shows that parents tend to simplify the length and complexity of their language when talking to children (Owens, 2008). The normal language–learning child listens attentively to parents or other caregivers during play and soaks up the new words and sentences like a little sponge. Without these interactions, the child would not develop language.

Cognitive Ability   Cognition is a very complex area, and the specific relations between language acquisition and cognitive development are only just being discovered. Although speech-language professionals are not certain about the exact nature of the cognition–language relationship, they do know that certain cognitive attainments seem to be associated with language acquisition. Cognition is related to language development in several important ways.

1. *People talk about concepts.* Cognitive development has to do with the increasing ability of a child to mentally represent objects, actions, and events in the world. Most often, researchers talk about the development of concepts. For instance, English speakers have a concept of "animal" that includes all types of species, and you can divide the concept into domestic and wild animals. You can also divide domesticated animals into different types of pets (e.g., dogs, cats, hamsters, fish, birds). The point here is that people have a mental construct having to do with nonhuman, animate beings. With language, they can talk about all aspects of their concept of animals using specific words and word combinations that are appropriate to that concept (e.g., jaguar, poodle, Himalayan, purr, bark). Essentially, humans develop language to be able to talk about the concepts they have of the world. Without the development of concepts, people really would have nothing to talk about. So, concepts must develop prior to language (or at least simultaneously). As individuals develop language, their linguistic ability then helps to refine their concepts.

2. *Language is an abstract symbol system.* The more cognitive development a child experiences, the greater is that child's ability to appreciate abstractions. If something is abstract, it may not be totally clear to a person. For instance, a piece of abstract art depicting a man riding a bicycle may not really resemble a photograph of a man riding a bicycle. If a word is abstract, it may not be easily visualized mentally (e.g., *honor, hypothesis*), but if a word is concrete, it can be more readily pictured in the mind (e.g., *dog, sun*). Language is a system of very abstract symbols. The word *dog* does not look like a canine or sound like one. Additionally, the word disappears almost as soon as it is uttered because speech is a transitory signal. Similarly, the written word *dog* is abstract and unrelated to the physical attributes of an actual dog. Because language symbols do not represent the real world in a concrete way, it is necessary for people to develop higher or more complex brain functions. If a person is incapable of abstract reasoning, she will be impaired in her ability to develop language.

3. *Language requires minimal levels of cognitive development.* The developmental psychologist Jean Piaget studied cognitive development in children and found that during the first two years of life children pass through six stages of what he called the "sensorimotor period" (Piaget, 1952, 1954, 1970). The sensorimotor period is a time

when children physically manipulate the environment and gradually learn to manipulate reality mentally. Tests can locate children in the six stages of the sensorimotor period, and much research has been done to determine which stage is most associated with the onset of language. Many studies report that a child must be at least in stage 4 to use gestural communication for intentionally making needs known and must attain at least the beginning of stage 5 to use verbal language (McCormick, 1984; Owens, 2008). Thus, in the literature there are no reports of children before stage 4 of the sensorimotor period using verbal language, and this fact suggests that at least a minimal level of cognitive development must be necessary for language to be acquired. You can also see evidence in children's behavior of post–stage 4 attainments in their play. Children who have the cognitive ability to develop language can use toys and objects appropriately, mentally represent a missing object (object permanence), use something as a means to achieve a particular end (use a stick to reach a distant object; means-end concept), and have the ability to imitate the gestures and vocalizations of a model. One of the surest indications that a child is cognitively ready to develop language is the presence of symbolic (pretend) play. If a child can pretend that a block of wood is a car, he is demonstrating the ability to use symbols that have some degree of abstraction because the block does not really look like an automobile. Children with severe cognitive impairment show their levels of cognitive development in their play and interaction with other objects. It is not unusual to find children below stage 4 of the sensorimotor period whose play is primarily characterized by mouthing, banging, shaking, and throwing objects. They rarely use an object or toy appropriately and may not solve problems in play involving the means-end concept or perform symbolic play. Thus, it appears that there must be a minimal level of cognitive development for a person to understand the world, develop concepts, and acquire abstract language symbols.

Intent to Communicate　A child will never develop language unless she possesses a reason or intent to use communicative symbols. In short, people talk because they have a particular goal in mind to either (1) influence the actions of a listener, or (2) influence the attention/attitude of a listener (McClean & Snyder-McClean, 1978). When you think about it, these two broad reasons to talk really can account for much of what you say during a day. Believe it or not, before a child reaches a specific point in cognitive development (stage 4), it is said that no "intentionality" exists (McCormick, 1984). That is, a child prior to stage 4 does not really "intend" to do anything or plan it ahead of time; the behavior just occurs. As children develop cognitively, they can mentally represent objects and events to a greater extent and manipulate reality mentally instead of physically. They can actually *plan* to do something because they work it out mentally prior to doing it. Thus, at stage 4 a child can *intend* to influence the activities and attention of adults and use gestures as a *means* to accomplishing this *end* (as in the means-end concept referred to earlier). Children with severe cognitive impairment may reach only stages 1–3 of sensorimotor development, and because they do not have the cognitive development to anticipate or plan an event, they do not have intent to communicate. These children may never actively try to communicate with adults, even though adults often attribute communicative intent to them. For instance, a child with a severe impairment may produce a vocalization while clapping hands, and the adult may say, "He wants me to turn on the music now." In reality, this child may just be clapping and vocalizing, and the adult treats it as a communicative intent. Also the child may have a simple association between music and clapping; however, the clapping may not be done as intent to communicate anything.

Social Abilities   Many social abilities are prerequisite to the acquisition of language.

1. *Joint referencing:* During play, parents and children look at the same objects and events. This is called *joint referencing* because the parents and children are jointly sharing visual regard for the same object or event. It is during joint referencing that caregivers talk to children about what they are seeing and doing and provide language stimulation or language modeling. The child profits from this language stimulation in relevant interactions by learning vocabulary and the rules of language (Owens, 2008).
2. *Games and rituals:* Parents also teach language to children in the context of certain games and rituals such as those you might see at family gatherings, malls, Laundromats, and other places. For instance, the parent may say to a child, "Say hello to Aunt Martha," "say thank you," "say trick or treat." Parents also engage with their children in routine language stimulation events such as joint book reading or naming games. These activities serve to provide the child with consistent and repeated exposures to the appropriate use of language and may aid in language acquisition.
3. *Turn-taking:* Language is a reciprocal activity. People take turns in conversations. Children learn turn-taking skills in early play routines with parents, and they demonstrate these same reciprocal skills in their first conversations with their caregivers.
4. *Desire to attend to and be with people:* Human communication involves wanting to interact with other people. People have a basic desire to be gregarious and want to influence the attitudes, attention, and activities of other people. If a child does not have a basic desire to interact with people, there is no need for language to develop. For instance, children who have been diagnosed with autism are often characterized as being "in a world of their own" and may not readily develop social relationships with others (Rutter, 1978). If a child has no use for even nonverbal interaction, it is doubtful that language will be a major priority because it is used to touch other people. Thus, children who like to be isolated, do not make eye contact with adults, or do not enjoy reciprocal play activities probably will not develop language at the appropriate age.

It is easy to see that the BACIS of language can be in place when children are communicating through the use of gestures and vocalizations. The BACIS is a platform on which verbal language is built, and normally developing children all demonstrate BACIS elements as they approach the end of their first year of life.

EARLY DEVELOPMENT OF THE LANGUAGE FRAMEWORK

We have already said that specific building blocks (BACIS) need to be in place to provide a firm foundation for the development of the complicated language rule system. If one of the building blocks is missing or defective, the resulting linguistic framework will be distorted or at least be more difficult to erect on the inadequate foundation. Let us say, however, that the child *has* the BACIS for language development. How do language and communication begin to emerge? This section describes communication in the nonverbal, single-word, and early multiword periods in very general terms.

The Nonverbal Period   Communication in the nonverbal period typically occurs somewhere between 7 and 14 months in normal children and consists mostly of gestures and vocalizations. There is considerable variability in the age a child begins nonverbal communication and also in the duration of the nonverbal period. In the nonverbal period, the child uses gestures of pointing and physical regulation of adults to make needs known. Toward the end of this period, the child accompanies the gestures and physical regulations with vocal productions that are not words. For instance, a child might say "ba" while he is pointing at something or "uh . . . uh" while pulling the parent toward a desired object. The major point here is that the child is expressing intent to communicate, and this intent is now coupled with vocal productions. Generally, children communicate this way to (1) regulate adult action (e.g., obtain an inaccessible object using the adult as a means) or (2) regulate adult attention (e.g., obtain adult attention using objects or sounds as a means, as in banging a toy repeatedly until an adult looks or comments). Other gestures or social communications during this period involve pointing, showing, giving, and repeating an action to enlist adult attention.

The Single-Word Period   Gradually, the child replaces the vocalizations produced in the nonverbal period with actual *approximations* of adult words. This can occur anytime from 9 to 18 months of age in normally developing children, and there is also considerable variability in the age children reach this stage. We say the words are approximations because they may not fully resemble the productions of adults and are missing some components. Later in this chapter, we discuss phonologic development and the notion that early word productions may be simplified or reduced in characteristic ways. Early single words are usually consonant–vowel (CV) combinations such as "ba" for *ball* or "da" for *dog*. These are regarded as approximations instead of just vocalizations because they are used in the appropriate context (e.g., when a ball or dog is around), and they resemble the adult production in terms of the initial sound. Other early words may be CVCV combinations such as "dada" for *daddy* or "wawa" for *water*.

Children accumulate their early vocabulary slowly at first, and then experience a vocabulary spurt or a big increase in the number of words they can say. The average age of the vocabulary spurt is around 18 months (Owens, 2008). There also is a steady increase in the number of words these children *understand* during the single-word period. Comprehension of words is always ahead of the production of words, and research suggests that children in this period understand about four times more words than they produce (Benedict, 1979). The size of the expressive vocabulary in the single-word period increases until the vocabulary spurt; at this time, the child has a vocabulary of about 50 different words. Studies have shown that these early 50-word vocabularies are primarily composed of general and specific nouns (*ball, car*, names of people, and such) but also include action words (*go, run*), personal-social words (*yes, no, bye-bye*), modifiers (*big, dirty*), and even some minimal use of function words (*in, a*). At the point when children possess the 50-word vocabulary, they make their first attempts at combining words.

Early Multiword Productions   Many researchers in language acquisition have studied early word combinations produced by children, and they generally agree that specific types of combinations seem to emerge consistently, regardless of the child's culture, sometime between 15 and 30 months of age. That is, all over the world, children begin to use the same types of word combinations to talk about objects, events, and relationships in their lives, regardless of the language they are learning. This is often cited as further evidence that children learn to talk about concepts and experiences that they have developed in the sensorimotor period of cognitive development. Some of the basic word combination types and examples of each are listed in **Table 3–1**.

You can easily see that the relationships children talk about in their early word combinations are things that they have seen and participated in during the first two years of life. Also, note that most of the function words (articles, prepositions) and word endings (*-ing, -ed, -s*) are missing from these utterances.

TABLE 3–1   Basic Word Combination Types and Examples

Combination Type	Example
Naming (that + thing)	that doggie; that ball
Recurrence (more + thing/person)	more water; more daddy; more go
Nonexistence (no + thing/person; thing/person + allgone)	no drink; no mommy; drink allgone
Person + action	mommy go; daddy run; doggie eat
Action + thing	hit ball; pet doggie; eat banana
Possession (person + thing)	my ball; daddy sock; mommy hair
Thing/person + location	drink there; mommy outside
Modifier + thing	big drink; diaper dirty
Person + action + thing	daddy hit ball; mommy eat apple
Person + action + location	mommy go outside; daddy eat there

The Relationship Between Age and Average Utterance Length   Research shows that there is a strong and significant correlation between a child's chronological age and mean length of utterance (MLU) in the early stages of language development (Miller & Chapman, 1981; Scarborough, Wyckoff, & Davidson, 1986). MLU counts words as well as bound morphemes (e.g., plurals, past tense *-ed, -ing*) because these word endings represent important linguistic acquisitions for which a child should be given credit. It is critical to remember that these utterance lengths are averages. Thus, a 2-year-old may have some one-word utterances, some two-word utterances, and some three-word productions that average out to two words. The relationship is especially powerful between ages 1 and 4 years. Basically, the relationship between the development of utterance length and chronological age is almost linear during this period and then begins to deteriorate after age 4 years. Thus, when a child is one year old, the utterance length is approximately one word on average, a 2-year-old has an average length of utterance of about two words, and when the child reaches the age of 3 years, the average length of utterance is about three words. It is generally accurate to state that age and mean length of utterance are highly related in the early stages of language development. At the end of the early word combination period, a child should have an average length of utterance of about two words and be working on the incorporation of function words and word endings into his utterances.

Summary of Early Communicative Development   By age 2-and-a-half years, the normal child should have all the building blocks of language in place (BACIS), have a vocabulary of 400–500 words, and be producing word combinations consisting of two to four words, with an average utterance length of about 2.5. The 3- to 5-year-old population as well as some older children with cognitive impairment may exhibit language abilities similar to those normally developing children exhibit in the nonverbal, single-word, or early multiword periods of language acquisition. This brief perspective can help orient classroom teachers to the types of language and prelanguage abilities that SLPs must evaluate in nonverbal to early multiword communicators. The following section deals with language development after age 2 years.

COMMUNICATIVE REFINEMENT AFTER THE EARLY MULTIWORD PERIOD: FIVE STAGES OF DEVELOPMENT

In 1973, Roger Brown published a landmark book describing five stages of language development. To sketch the refinement of the language system as children go beyond the age of 2 years, we follow Brown's stages and provide a general description of each. The beginning points of these stages are demarcated by mean length of utterance (MLU).

Stage I: Basic Roles and Relations in the Simple Sentence (MLU 1.75)   Thus far, we have discussed only this first of Brown's five stages: the development of early multiword utterances. By the time a child reaches the age of 20–24 months, she is constructing the early multiword combinations mentioned in the previous section. These basic relationships form the critical elements of simple sentences (e.g., "Mommy run outside"; "Jimmy eat sandwich"). Children embellish these basic roles and relations with other language elements they add in later stages.

Stage II: Modulations of Meaning in the Simple Sentence (MLU 2.25)   In Stage II, the child adds to the basic building blocks of the simple sentence by adding to utterances function words and word endings. Stage II acquisitions include function words such as *the, in, on, is* and word endings such as *-ing, -ed, -s.* Children develop other function words and word endings in Stage II; however, we do not attempt to provide an exhaustive review of this stage. It is enough to know that the child is filling in the gaps between the major words of sentences acquired in Stage I. Thus, a child in Stage I might say, "Mommy eat," but in Stage II he might say, "Mommy eating" and finally "Mommy is eating" near the end of Stage II. Children in Stage II are typically between 2 and 3 years of age.

Stage III: Modalities of the Simple Sentence (MLU 2.75)   In Stage III, children learn to transform basic sentence structures into different orders to make constructions such as questions and negative statements. For example, a child can make the statement "He is going" into a question by inverting certain elements ("Is he going?"). The ability to move sentence elements around and transpose them is critical to making more complex syntactic utterances. Children in this stage also develop modals such as *can, will, shall* and begin to use them in contractions such as *can't, don't, won't.* Children in Stage III are usually about 3 years old.

Stage IV: Embedding One Sentence into Another (MLU 3.50)   When a child reaches Stage IV (usually at about age 3.0 or 3.5 years), she learns to make complex and compound sentences by embedding clauses and phrases into other sentences. For instance, a child in an earlier stage may say two simple sentences to communicate a thought: "Mommy bought me a bike. I like to ride my bike." Embedding allows the child to construct a more adult-like sentence: "I like to eat the cookies that Mommy bakes."

Stage V: Coordination of Simple Sentences (MLU 4.0)   Stage V (typically achieved between the ages of 3.5 and 4.0 years) involves learning how to coordinate two sentences using conjunctions. As you know, there are many conjunctions such as *and, but, because, since, if, when.* Use of these conjunctions to join sentences allows a child to make more and more complex utterances.

As children traverse the five stages, they increase their ability to produce more complex sentences as well as process equally complex language spoken by others. By the time a child enters kindergarten, he is capable of producing and comprehending fairly sophisticated syntactic forms. But, as mentioned earlier, language development continues for the rest of a person's life, although at a much slower rate. People continue to learn new vocabulary throughout life. Their grammatical structure changes very slowly between the ages of 5 and 19 years and involves the use of more subordinate clauses and some other structures in sentences. Because these syntactic changes occur slowly, they can be detected only by sensitive measures such as the subordination index (Nippold, 1988). Summarizing this period, Nippold states:

> The research suggests that language development during the 9 through 19 age range unfolds in a slow and protracted manner, and that change becomes obvious only when sophisticated linguistic phenomena are analyzed and non-adjacent age groups (e.g., 9-year-olds, 12-year-olds) are compared. Document-ing language growth in older children and adolescents also requires that written forms of communication be scrutinized in addition to spoken forms. (Nippold, 1988, p. 3)

Upon school entrance, the acquisition of language takes on other dimensions that depend on a strong foundation in oral language development. For instance, other modalities (reading, writing), the use of figurative language (idioms, metaphors), and metalinguistic ability (analysis of language as an object of study as in spelling and language arts) are complex acquisitions for all children in the early years of education. As you will see in later chapters, children with a weak foundation in oral language development almost always have more difficulty with these later milestones in the use of their linguistic system for other purposes such as reading and writing (Catts & Kamhi, 2005).

DEVELOPMENT OF THE SPEECH SOUND SYSTEM

Children's ability to produce speech sounds, and to use those sounds to make words, develops over the first few years of life. Typically, children develop most of their speech sound system by the time they begin school. Children begin to produce speechlike sounds in infancy. We refer to these productions as "speechlike" because they occur before chil-dren begin to use words to communicate. These productions are not considered to be true speech sounds at this point.

Oller (2000) identified several stages of infant sound production prior to the use of true words. These stages are presented in **Table 3–2**. When reviewing Table 3–2, remem-ber that there is considerable overlap among the stages described and some variability in the ages associated with each stage. The production of strings of consonant–vowel syllables heard during Oller's canonical stage is generally referred to as **babbling**. Babbling is some-times divided into two stages. The early stage in known as *reduplicated babbling* and consists of utterances in which the same syllable is repeated (e.g., *mama, dada*). The later stage of babbling is sometimes referred to as *nonreduplicated* or *variegated babbling*. In this stage, the child produces strings of consonant–vowel productions that are not repeated (e.g., *patu, kami,* or *magati*) (Stoel-Gammon & Dunn, 1985; Pena-Brooks & Hegde, 2007). Nonreduplicated babbling often accompanies adult-like inflection patterns,

TABLE 3–2   Stages of Prelinguistic Vocalizations

Prelanguage Stage and Age	Speech Sound Activity
Phonation stage Birth to 2 month	Many "reflexive" vocalizations such as crying. Some nasal and vowel-like sounds are produced.
Primitive articulation stage 1 to 4 months	Some consonant–vowel (CV)-like sounds produced. Often these are back sounds such as k and g paired with the vowel oo. Because these utterances sound like the words "coo" and "goo" this stage is sometimes called the cooing stage.
Expansion stage 3 to 8 months	This is a period of vocal play. The infant begins to develop some control of the sound-producing mechanism and explores a variety of speechlike and non-speech-like sounds including grunts, squeals, yells, and raspberries. Vowels and closed sounds are combined in sequences of articulation that form primitive syllables. This is sometimes called marginal babbling.
Canonical stage 5 to 10 months	A significant milestone in development. The speech behaviors in this stage are generally referred to as babbling. The child produces well-timed, often repetitive patterns of consonant–vowel utterances that sound quite speechlike. Parents often mistake a sequence such as "mama" or "dada" for an attempt at naming and report that the child said his first words at 6 or 7 months. Although babbling represents a significant milestone in speech development, the strings of CV syllables produced during this period are not attempts at meaningful speech.

Source: Oller, 2000.

which causes these utterance to resemble true speech. Because of this, the nonreduplicated babbling stage was once referred to as the jargon stage.

At approximately 12 months of age, some (but not all) children produce utterances that they use consistently to refer to objects or people, but the utterances are not based on the adult form of any word. These utterances represent a transition between prelinguistic productions and true words and are therefore known as **transitional forms**. (Other terms, such as *proto-words, vocables*, and *phonetically consistent forms*, may also be used to describe these utterances.) One author's child demonstrated use of a transitional form. This child used the utterance "koo" to refer to yogurt. Whether he was being fed yogurt, saw it in the supermarket, or rubbed it in his hair, he always referred to it as "koo." This form does not appear to be a derivative of the adult word *yogurt*, but he used it consistently to refer to and request that item.

At about 12 to 18 months, children begin to produce their first true words. These first words are usually not accurate reproductions of the adult form and reflect the limitations of the child's developing phonological system. Early words are often single syllables, such as *up* or *bye*, or are reduplicated syllables, such as *dada* or *baba*. Words containing initial and final consonants such as *cake* or *hat* may also occur during this early period (Stoel-Gammon & Dunn, 1985).

The speech sounds that children can correctly produce during this early stage of meaningful speech are limited. Although children produce a wide range of sounds during the later stages of the prelinguistic period, they introduce these sounds into meaningful speech gradually. Several researchers have studied the age of acquisition of speech sounds in normally developing children. These studies have varied, sometimes widely, in the ages reported for acquisition of each phoneme. One reason for the variance among findings is the criteria used to determine when a sound had been acquired. For example, **Table 3–3** shows the results of three studies of sound acquisition. The earliest study by Templin (1957) reports the age when 75 percent of the children produced the sound correctly in initial, medial, and final position

TABLE 3–3   Ages at Which Children Acquire Phonemes: Results of Three Studies Using Different Criteria

Phoneme	Templin (1957)	Prather (1975)	Smit et al. (1990)	
			Females	**Males**
m	3	2	3	3
n	3	2	3:6	3
h	3	2	3	3
p	3	2	3	3
f	3	2.4	3:6 (I)	3:6 (I)
			5:6 (F)	5:6 (F)
w	3	2.8	3	3
y (*you*)	3.5	4	4	5
b	4	2.8	3	3
k	4	2.4	3:6	3:6
g	4	2.4	3:6	4
d	4	2.4	3	3:6
r	4	3.4	8	8
s	4.5	3	7 to 9	7 to 9
ch	4.5	3.8	6	7
sh	4.5	3.8	6	7
l	6	3.4	5 (I)	6 (I)
			6 (F)	7 (F)
t	6	2.8	4	3:6
v	6	4	5:6	5:6
th (*thin*)	6	4	6	8
z	7	4	7 to 9	7 to 9
j (*joe*)	7	4	6	7
th (*the*)	7	4	4:6	7

of words. Prather, Hedrick, and Kern (1975) report the age when 75 percent of the children studied used the sound correctly in only the initial and final positions. The data of Prather et al. indicate an earlier age of acquisition than that of Templin. Finally, Smit, Hand, Freilinger, Bernthal, and Bird (1990) report ages of acquisition based on 90 percent of the children studied producing the sound correctly. Smit et al. also report different ages for boys and girls. Many of the ages of acquisition reported by Smit et al. are later because the 90 percent criterion is more stringent and therefore more difficult to achieve.

Although they disagree on age of acquisition, most studies of speech sound development agree that children typically develop phonemes in a certain order (Wellman, Case, Mengert, & Bradbury, 1931; Poole, 1934; Templin, 1957; Sander, 1972; Prather et al., 1975; Smit et al., 1990). Stop consonants (*p, b, t, d, k,* and *g*) and nasals (*m, n,* and *ng*) develop early, while fricatives (*f, v, s, z, sh*) and semivowels (*l, r,* and *y*) develop later.

During the period from about 18 months to 4 years, children experience a tremendous growth in vocabulary. Many new words include speech sound, sound combinations, and syllable structures that are beyond the child's production ability at this point (e.g., later-developing sounds, consonant clusters, multisyllabic words). To use these new words, it appears that children apply several simplifying processes (Ingram, 1989). These **phonological processes** simplify the adult words in several ways. Some processes simplify the syllabic structure of a word (e.g., final consonant deletion changes *hat* to "ha"). Other processes substitute an early-developing class of sounds for a later-developing class (e.g., stopping allows *sun* to be produced as "tun"—a stop substituted for a fricative). A third category of processes changes the manner, place, or voice characteristics of one phoneme to be consistent with another phoneme in the word (e.g., velar assimilation changes *dog* to "gog"). Not all children demonstrate the same processes. Grunwell (1987) identifies the most common phonological processes in normal development. These processes, along with a brief description of each, are presented in **Table 3–4**.

Phonological processes are developmental devices that children usually suppress as their phonological skills improve. In normal development, children suppress most processes by the time they enter first grade. Stoel-Gammon and Dunn (1985) identify those phonological processes that are typically suppressed by 3 years and those that persist after age 3. A partial list of early- and later-suppressed processes is in **Table 3–5**.

Even those processes that persist after age 3 years are typically suppressed by the time a child enters first grade. One of the few processes that continues in some normally developing children beyond age 5 years is gliding of liquids (run → wun) (Grunwell, 1987; Pena-Brooks & Hegde, 2007).

By age 5 years, children have typically completed most of their phonological development. They still might need to master a few sounds in some positions or in some words. Yavas (1998) indicates that some children between the ages of 5 and 7 years have difficulty with longer words such as *thermometer* and *vegetable*. Yavas also suggests that children in this age group must learn to deal with changes in a root word when a morpheme is added. For example, the *i* in the word *decide* is pronounced differently in the word *decision*.

TABLE 3–4   The Most Common Phonological Processes Exhibited During Normal Development

Process	Description
Weak syllable deletion	In polysyllabic words, the unstressed syllable is deleted. (telephone → tephone)
Final consonant deletion	The final consonant of a word is deleted. (hat → ha)
Reduplication	Two-syllable words are produced by repeating the first syllable. (bottle → baba)
Harmony (this process is referred to as an "assimilation" by other authors)	The manner, place, or voice characteristics of one phoneme changes to be consistent with another phoneme in the word. (dog → gog [the initial *d* changed to be consistent with the final *g*])
Cluster reduction	Consonant clusters are reduced usually to a single phoneme. (stop → top)
Stopping	Continuant sounds (usually fricatives) are replaced by stops. (see → tee)
Fronting	Velar sounds such as k̲ and g are replaced by alveolar sounds such as t̲ and d̲. (go → do)
Gliding	Liquids such as r̲ and l̲ become glides such as w̲ and y̲. (run → wun)
Context-sensitive voicing	Voiceless consonants preceding vowels are voiced and voiced consonants at the end of words are produced as unvoiced. (toe → doe and red → ret)

Source: Data from Stoel-Gammon & Dunn (1985).

Note: The arrow symbol (→) should be read as "becomes" or "changes to."

TABLE 3–5   A Partial List of Early- and Later-Suppressed Processes

Processes That Disappear by Age 3 Years	Processes That Persist After Age 3 Years
Unstressed syllable deletion	Cluster reduction
Final consonant deletion	Gliding
Reduplication	Stopping
Velar fronting	Final consonant devoicing
Consonant assimilation	
Prevocalic voicing	

Source: Data from Grunwell (1987).

Perhaps you have noticed that most of the discussion to this point has been about consonants. Reports regarding the development of vowel sounds do not occur in the literature as often as do those addressing consonant development. Although there is a great deal of variability in vowel production, most studies suggest that children produce vowels reasonably accurately by age 3 years (Donegan, 2002).

Between the ages 4 and 7 years, most children master the production of the remaining sounds of their language. During this period, they also begin to produce correctly words with more complex sound structures such as multisyllable words and words that contain consonant clusters (Ingram, 1989).

PHONOLOGICAL AWARENESS

In addition to the ability to produce sounds and use those sounds to create words, children must develop another skill called **phonological awareness**. Stackhouse defines phonological awareness as "the ability to reflect on and manipulate the structure of an utterance (e.g., into words, syllables, sounds) as distinct from its meaning" (Stackhouse, 1997, p. 157). This definition identifies two aspects of phonological awareness: first, understanding that words are composed of smaller units, namely, syllables and phonemes (Catts, 1991); and second, the ability to manipulate those smaller units (Cunningham, 1990).

As discussed in Chapter 13, phonological awareness is not only related to expressive speech skills but also to reading and spelling ability. Phonological awareness is a developmental skill and therefore merits mention in the present chapter. Goldsworthy (1998) and Justice, Gillon, and Schuele (2009) reviewed the literature and describe the phonological awareness skills of children at various age levels. The following is a summary of their findings:

At age 2 years: Some children can detect rhyme inconsistently but at levels greater than chance. These children are able to select the word that does not rhyme from a group of three (*hat, cat, boy*). Tasks such as this are called rhyme oddity tasks.

At age 3 years: Presented with two words, many children can tell whether two words rhyme or not (rhyme detection). Some children can generate at least one word that rhymes with a target word. Many children this age can recite known rhymes such as "Jack and Jill." Many can identify a word in group of words that begins with a different sound (*mad, mop, cat*). Tasks such as the latter are referred to as alliteration oddity tasks. Sensitivity to alliteration generally lags behind sensitivity to rhyme.

At age 4 years: Children begin to exhibit awareness of syllabic distinction. For example, the word *baby* can be divided into "ba" and "by." About half of 4-year-olds can count the number of syllables in multisyllabic words.

At age 5 years: Most children can generate rhyme spontaneously during play or on demand in games. They exhibit general proficiency in rhyming detection tasks. Most 5-year-olds can count the number of syllables in multisyllabic words. Some children at this age can also count the number of phonemes in words. However, in terms of recognizing phonemes, it is more likely at age 5 years that children can separate the first sound of single-syllable words (onset) from the rest of the word (rime) that appears to be treated as a single unit. For example, children can separate the word *top* into t (onset) and op (rime) but not into t-o-p.

At age 6 years: Most children demonstrate the ability to identify phonemes as units comprising syllables. Many children can blend two to three sounds to make a word (e.g., c-a-t makes *cat*).

At age 7 years: Children begin to spell phonetically. They can segment three to four phonemes in words. At this age, many children can delete sounds from words (e.g., *moose* without the s is "moo").

As mentioned earlier, children who are delayed in the development of phonological awareness skills are at risk for speech, reading, and spelling problems. Speech-language pathologists, classroom teachers, and reading specialists should all work together to identify children who appear to have delayed phonological awareness.

HEARING ABILITY ACROSS THE LIFE SPAN

Although the ability of children to draw meaning from what they hear develops over time, the hearing mechanism itself is relatively mature at birth (Lasky & Willams, 2005). Speech-language professionals have known for some time that during the first few months of life infants can perceive differences between nonmeaningful speech sounds such as "ba" and "ga" (Eimas, Siqueland, Jusczyk, & Vigorito, 1971; Morse,1972; Eimas,1974). Those results were obtained by monitoring infants' sucking rate or heart rate in response to carefully monitored changes in sounds presented to them.

More recently, by introducing sound through the abdomen of an expectant mother and monitoring the response of the fetus, research demonstrates that the hearing mechanism appears to function even before birth. It has been reported that fetuses respond to sound as early as 19 weeks of gestation (Hepper & Shahidullah, 1994). Recent evidence demonstrates that fetuses at about 38 weeks of gestation can distinguish between their mother's voice and the voice of other women (Kisilevsky et al., 2003), and at about 33 to 37 weeks, they can distinguish nursery rhymes read repeatedly by their mothers from other rhymes (DeCasper, LeCanuet, Brusnel, Granier-Deferee, & Maugeais, 1994). As described in Chapter 10, speech-language professionals can now screen the hearing of newborn infants before they go home from the hospital and provide follow-up testing a short time later.

From a communication disorders perspective, however, SLPs may be more interested in what happens to hearing ability at the other end of the life cycle. As true of most body systems, the hearing mechanism and hearing ability tend to change as people grow older. The changes in the hearing mechanism that accompany aging reflect age-related changes in structure and function throughout the auditory system (Fire, 1995; McCarthy & Sapp, 2000). If you have ever noticed that older people often seem to have large ears, you are correct. Because of a loss of elasticity in the cartilage of the outer ear, the pinna may become larger and some changes in the dimensions of the external auditory canal may occur. Older people may also experience loss of elasticity of the muscles of the middle ear and arthritic middle ear joints (McCarthy & Sapp, 2000). However, the most frequent cause of age-related loss of hearing stems from atrophy and degeneration of the hair cells in the cochlea, changes in other cochlear structures, and the loss of neurons that conduct the auditory signal from the cochlea to the brain (Schuknecht, 1974; McCarthy & Sapp, 2000).

The term used to describe age-related hearing loss is **presbycusis**. Presbycusis typically results in a bilateral, symmetric, sensorineural hearing loss (Fire 1995; Willot, 1996). As discussed in Chapter 10, a sensorineural hearing loss typically affects some frequencies more than others. The result is that people with this type of hearing loss may hear only parts of a spoken message and therefore have difficulty understanding what is said. Older listeners also appear to have more difficulty discriminating speech in a background of noise (Schum, Matthews, & Lee, 1991; Wiley et al., 1998). Finally, because the inner ear structures also contribute to balance, older people may experience balance problems, leading to falls that are so common among older persons (Johnson, 2010).

CHANGES IN VOICE ACROSS THE LIFE SPAN

The larynx—and the voice that emanates from it—undergoes life cycle changes. At birth, the vocal folds are barely 3 mm long and produce vocalizations upward of 660 Hz (cycles per second). There are two major laryngeal growth periods with the first occurring during the first year of life. The vocal folds almost double in size, lengthening to approximately 5.5 mm. The pitch of the voice, or more accurately the fundamental frequency of vibration, lowers as the larynx grows, descends in neck position, and the folds lengthen and thicken (Zemlin, 1998). By first grade, age 6 years, the vocal folds are about 8 mm long, with no difference between males and females, and they produce a typical fundamental frequency of 240 Hz (Behrman, 2007).

The second major growth period occurs during puberty. Both males and females experience bodily changes during puberty, and the larynx is no exception. In fact, vocal changes can be quite dramatic in both sexes, but especially so in males. The term **vocal mutation** describes this period of change caused by hormonal influences. Change, of course, does not happen overnight but rather spans about 18 months of slow, progressive laryngeal cartilage growth and vocal fold muscle lengthening and thickening. At this stage in the laryngeal life cycle, male and female voices become noticeably different. By about age 17 years, the male vocal folds have reached a length of between 17 and 21 mm; the young adult male voice exhibits a fundamental frequency of approximately 115 Hz. In contrast, the young adult female voice averages 215 Hz with vocal folds that are typically between 11 and 17 mm long (Behrman, 2007).

The larynx, you will recall, consists of a cartilaginous structure that lies between the third and sixth cervical vertebrae. It descends with age, from birth to about age 17 years. The 2-cm-long soft, infant larynx grows to young adult proportions suitable to the person's body size and stature. The vertical dimension of the adult male larynx is approximately 7 cm, whereas the adult female length is approximately 5 cm long (this equals 2 inches).

The front-to-back and the side-to-side dimensions are both about 4 cm in the adult male and 3.5 cm in the adult female (Zemlin, 1998).

The normal aging process and certainly the cartilaginous, muscular, and epithelial tissue changes within the larynx affect voice. Understanding normal age-related voice changes is important for distinguishing pathological motor speech and vocal disorders.

With advancing age come changes in the respiratory system, which powers the voice. The tissues of the lungs lose elasticity. Accumulated effects of breathing pollution and smoking can affect the efficiency of the air sacs in the exchange of oxygen. Thoracic and abdominal muscles are the engine that expand and compress the lungs in the processes of inhalation and exhalation. With advancing age, the muscles may exhibit mass shrinkage and loss of flexibility. This increased stiffness consequently impedes smooth and efficient lung–thorax inflation and deflation. Aging also may alter lung volumes and capacities. In particular, older persons exhibit a decrease in vital capacity and a decrement in maximum expiratory flow (Linville, 2001). In essence, older adult speakers show a decline in the amount of air that they can move in and out of the respiratory system.

With aging comes calcification and ossification of the laryngeal cartilages. Degeneration of laryngeal joints, so important to vocal fold action, may be particularly affected. Intrinsic laryngeal muscles experience age-related atrophy. Shrinkage and loss of glandular efficiency may lead to dryness of the laryngeal epithelial tissues and, in turn, contribute to vocal fold stiffness. According to Linville (2001), such muscle and membranous tissue changes lead to a stiffer, less-compliant laryngeal mechanism, which often results in a 35-Hz elevation in the fundamental frequency of the voice of older adult men.

Although similar laryngeal changes occur in older adult women, other processes may be at work to create an opposite vocal result. After menopause and hormonal changes occur in the female body, the laryngeal tissues tend to thicken. Progressive thickening can even escalate after age 70 years. The older adult female voice tends to drop an average of 10–15 Hz (Linville, 2001).

Older voices, whether male or female, also tend to display changes in quality in a milieu of breathiness, harshness, and hoarseness. The atrophy of intrinsic laryngeal muscles seems to contribute to weakened vocal fold adduction or noticeable gaps in the glottal margin. The muscle and membranous tissue changes contribute to lack of stability and aperiodicity of both frequency and amplitude. This is detected by measures of jitter and shimmer, respectively (Linville, 2001).

LANGUAGE IN THE NORMAL AGING ADULT

In an otherwise healthy older adult, subtle changes in the language system occur. But it is quite incorrect to think that linguistic and cognitive declines, similar to the occurrence of dementia, are inevitable. Communication is a manifestation of cognition, and *cognition* is a general term that refers to both stored knowledge and the process of making and manipulating knowledge (Bayles & Tomoeda, 2007). Memory can retrieve, among other things, semantic concepts, lexical words, motor skills, and cognitive skills. It is best to view memory, cognition, and language as a fundamental triad.

After a lifetime of normal language abilities, the decline tends to occur so gradually as to be unnoticed for the most part. Occasional gaps in memory, euphemistically dubbed "senior moments," are a common and noticeable event. In normal aging, these events do not impede daily functioning. When tested in recall and sequential learning tasks, however, it is obvious that slight declines in the triad of language, cognition, and memory (especially episodic memory for recalling names) are occurring with the passage of time (Hume & Floyd, 2005). Processing and retrieval abilities seem slower with age.

With regard to semantic aspects of language, the older adult person generally maintains his or her level of performance. The command of vocabulary remains evident in conversations and even in working crossword puzzles. Vocabulary expansion remains possible throughout life. Learning new hobbies often affords individuals an opportunity to acquire novel words not previously used (e.g., a *jib* in sailing, a *mulligan* in golf, the words of a foreign language).

Researchers study semantic abilities by testing various word association tasks. Generally, older adults exhibit poorer performance than do younger adults in the number of associated words and in the time required to speak those words. Similar word tasks are known as word retrieval or word fluency measures, as encountered in many tests of aphasia. For example, a typical word retrieval task is to name as many animals that start with *b* as possible while a stopwatch collects a timed response. Slow semantic word recall suggests that, even in good health, the average older adult displays some central language inefficiency.

Researchers use various other methods to demonstrate slow word retrieval skills in older adults. Older adults experience lapses in word memory recall wherein the word is on the "tip of the tongue." Like anomia seen in persons with aphasia, the older person knows what she wishes to say and can often indicate the starting sound or a synonym. Regardless of age, all people experience the tip of the tongue phenomenon on occasion.

These various semantic delays may become evident in conversational speech and affect the person's rate of speech or lead to frequent disfluencies such as hesitations, interjections, revisions, or repetitions. These disfluencies seem related to semantic retrieval sluggishness that is linguistic and cognitive in nature rather than a stutter in motor fluency.

Syntactic skills in normal older adults appear to be intact with some exception of quality. There is a tendency for older adult speakers to use shorter utterances and fewer words per clause than younger adults do. Although length of utterance may be affected, there is no apparent lack of variety of sentence types (questions, statements, commands). It bears repeating that disfluencies in the form of uncertainty behavior (hesitations, interjections, sentence revisions) affect speech fluency and may be the result of slowed mental planning either at the syntactic or semantic level of language.

Other variables may affect the language characteristics and output of older adults. Whether they reside in a private home or in a retirement/institutional setting, older adults' maintenance of linguistic-cognitive skills seems to be influenced by stimulating activities rather than monotony. Social contacts stimulate conversation and thought, so older adults should remain engaged with a variety of people, shared activities, and hobbies. By staying engaged in the social milieu, older adults have a variety of topics to build communication around and need not fixate on health-related themes whereby medications and aches and pains dominate their semantic and syntactic expressive language.

Adult language changes over the life span are summarized in **Table 3–6**. The table reflects the writings of Bayles and Tomoeda (2007) and of Civil and Whitehouse (1991).

FLUENCY OVER THE LIFE SPAN

Apart from cognitive-linguistic word fluency (also called verbal fluency) measures (e.g., timed recall or animal categories or words that start with a target letter of the alphabet) and speech rate studies, few true studies of fluency over the life span exist. The fluency of individuals who do not stutter is often just assumed to be within normal limits and is infrequently researched. Much attention is paid to the early years of speech development so that speech-language professionals can better differentially diagnose children exhibiting stuttering-like disfluencies versus other disfluencies that are common and benign.

Stuttering affects people of all ages. Its onset tends to be in children who are between the ages of 2 and 5 years as they develop their language skills. Approximately 5 percent of all children stutter for some period in their life, and it lasts from a few weeks to several years. Most children outgrow stuttering, called **spontaneous remission**. Approximately 1 percent or fewer of the adult population stutters.

How stuttering is defined (often a hotly debated issue) is intertwined with the nature of fluency development. Clinicians and researchers use various definitions that compare data and normalcy across the life span. We ignore these complexities and simply address the fluency of nonstuttering (normal) speakers from childhood through adulthood.

TABLE 3–6   Summary of Normal Aging Effects on Language

Area	Change
Sensory system	Declines (e.g., hearing, vision)
Motor system	Declines (e.g., reaction time)
Memory	Mostly stable; episodic memory declines
Intelligence	Subtle decline (e.g., IQ)
Phonology	Stable
Syntax	Mostly stable; some reduced complexity
Vocabulary	Expands
Word retrieval	Declines in efficiency

The fluency of children who do not stutter has been well studied in the preschool population (Ambrose & Yairi, 1999; Pellowski & Conture, 2002). In general, 3- and 4-year-old children exhibit about 3–4 percent ordinary disfluencies in conversational speech (in contrast with 10 percent or so in children with stuttering who also display different types of disruptions).

Although adult fluency over the life span has received little research attention, Yairi and Clifton (1972) published a hallmark comparison of nonstuttering (normal-speaking) persons in three different age groups: preschool, high school, and older adults aged 69 to 87 years. Spontaneous speech was elicited from picture story telling. Manning and Shirkey (1980) reanalyzed the data in terms of interjections of sounds, syllables, words, and phrases; repetition of part words, whole words, and phrases; revisions or incomplete phrases; dysrhythmic phonations; and tense pauses. The preschool children averaged 7.65 disfluencies per 100 words spoken (more than 7 percent). High school seniors averaged 3.83 disfluencies (nearly 4 percent), and older adults averaged 6.29 per 100 words spoken (more than 6 percent). The overall impression is that fluency improves with age, but then reverses to nearly preschool levels with age. However, when analyzed by type of fluency disruption, despite the frequency count there is an alternate life span conclusion. Children display mostly repetitions whereas, proportionately, young adults and older adult speakers tend to display more interruptions and sentence revisions/incomplete phrases. This may suggest aging changes occur in the linguistic-cognitive realm as previously discussed.

Rosenfield and Nudelman (1991) conclude that fluent individuals develop disfluencies as part of the aging process. They further attribute these changes to delays in syntactic organization. As discussed earlier, other declines could account for these increased disfluencies such as slower motor speech planning. The reasons for increased disfluency with advanced age are not yet clear.

Terms to Know

Babbling	Presbycusis
Transitional forms	Vocal mutation
Phonological processes	Spontaneous remission
Phonological awareness	

Study Questions

1. Why should speech-language pathologists and other professionals have a knowledge of normal communication development?
2. What are the communicative changes that naturally occur in the elderly as they grow older?
3. Discuss the BACIS of language development.

Bibliography

Ambrose, N., & Yairi, E. (1999). Normative disfluency data for early childhood stuttering. *Journal of Speech, Language, and Hearing Research, 42*(4), 895–909.

Bayles, K., & Tomoeda, C. (2007). *Cognitive-communication disorders of dementia.* San Diego, CA: Plural.

Behrman, A. (2007). *Speech and voice science.* San Diego, CA: Plural.

Benedict, H. (1979). Early lexical development: Comprehension and production. *Journal of Child Language, 6,* 183–200.

Brown, R. (1958). *Words and things.* New York, NY: Macmillan.

Brown, R. (1973). *A first language: The early stages.* Cambridge, MA: Harvard University Press.

Catts, H. (1991). Early identification of reading disabilities. *Topics in Language Disorders, 12,* 1–16.

Catts, H., & Kamhi, A. (2005). *Language and reading disabilities.* Boston, MA: Allyn & Bacon.

Civil, R., & Whitehouse, P. (1991). Neurobiology of the aging communication system. In D. Ripich (Ed.), *Geriatric communication disorders* (pp. 5–20). Austin, TX: Pro-Ed.

Cunningham, A. (1990). Explicit versus implicit instruction in phonemic awareness. *Journal of Experimental Psychology, 50,* 429–444.

Curtiss, S., Fromkin, V., Krashen, S., Rigler, D., & Rigler, M. (1974). The linguistic development of Genie. *Language, 50,* 528–554.

DeCasper, A., LeCanuet, J., Brusnel, M., Granier-Deferee, C., & Maugeais, R. (1994). Fetal reaction to recurrent maternal speech. *Infant Behavior and Development, 17,* 159–164.

Donegan, P. (2002). Normal vowel development. In M. J. Ball & F. E. Gibbon (Eds.), *Vowel disorders.* Boston, MA: Butterworth-Heinemann.

Eimas, P. (1974). Linguistic processing of speech by young infants. In R. Schiefelbusch & L. Lloyd (Eds.), *Language perspectives-Acquisition, retardation, and intervention.* Baltimore: University Park Press.

Eimas, P., Siqueland, E., Jusczyk, P., & Vigorito, J. (1971). Speech perception in infants. *Science, 171,* 303–306.

Fire, K. (1995). Intervention with the elderly. In L. Wall (Ed.), *Hearing for the speech-language pathologist and health care professional.* Boston: Butterworth-Heinemann.

Goldsworthy, C. L. (1998). *Sourcebook of phonological awareness activities.* San Diego, CA: Singular.

Grunwell, P. (1987). *Clinical phonology* (2nd ed.). Baltimore, MD: Williams and Wilkins.

Hepper, P. & Shahidullah, S. (1994). Development of fetal hearing. *Archives of disease in childhood-fetal and neonatal edition, 71,* F81–F87.

Hume, L. & Floyd, S. (2005). Measures of working memory, sequence learning and speech reception in the elderly. *Journal of Speech, Language and Hearing Research, 48,* 224–235.

Ingram, D. (1989). *Phonological disability in children* (2nd ed.). San Diego, CA: Singular.

Johnson, C. (2010). *Aural rehabilitation: A contemporary issues approach.* Boston: Pearson.

Justice, L., Gillon, G., & Schuele, C. M. (2009). Phonological awareness: Description, assessment and intervention. In J. Bernthal, N. Bankson, & P. Flipsen (Eds.), *Articulation and Phonological Disorder: Speech sound disorders in children* (6th ed.). Boston: Allyn and Bacon.

Kisilevsky, B. S., Hains, S., Lee, K., Xie, X., Huang, H., Ye, H., Zhang, K., & Wang, Z. (2003). Effects of experience on fetal voice recognition. *Psychological Science, 14,* 220–224.

Lasky, R. & Willams, A. (2005). The development of the auditory system from conception to term. *Neoreviews, 6,* e141–e152.

Linville, S. E. (2001). *Vocal aging.* San Diego, CA: Singular.

Manning, W., & Shirkey, E. (1980). Fluency and the aging process. In D. Beasley & A. Davis (Eds.), *Aging: Communication processes and disorders* (pp. 175–189). New York, NY: Grune & Stratton.

McCarthy, P., & Sapp, J. (2000). Rehabilitative needs of the aging population. In J. Alpiner & P. McCarthy (Eds.), *Rehabilitative audiology: Children and adults* (3rd ed.). Philadelphia: Lippincott Williams & Wilkins.

McClean, J., & Snyder-McClean, L. (1978). *A transactional approach to early language training.* Columbus, OH: Merrill.

McCormick, L. (1984). Review of normal language acquisition. In L. McCormick & R. Schiefelbusch (Eds.), *Early language intervention.* Columbus, OH: Merrill.

Miller, J., & Chapman, R. (1981). The relation between age and mean length of utterance. *Journal of Speech and Hearing Research, 24,*154–161.

Morse, P. (1972). The discrimination of speech and non-speech stimuli in early infancy. *Journal of Exceptional Child Psychology, 14,* 477–492.

Nippold, M. (1988). *Later language development: Ages nine through nineteen.* Boston, MA: Little, Brown.

Oller, D. K. (2000). *The emergence of the speech capacity.* Mahwa, NJ: Lawrence Erlbaum Associates.

Owens, R. (2008). *Language development: An introduction.* Boston, MA: Allyn & Bacon.

Pellowski, M., & Conture, E. (2002). Characteristics of speech disfluencies and stuttering behaviors in 3- and 4-year-old children. *Journal of Speech, Language, and Hearing Research, 45*(1), 20–34.

Pena-Brooks, A. & Hegde, M. (2007). Assessment and treatment of articulation and phonological disorders in children, (2nd ed.). Austin, TX: Pro-ed.

Piaget, J. (1952). *The origins of intelligence in children.* New York, NY: International Universities Press.

Piaget, J. (1954). *The construction of reality in the child.* New York, NY: Basic Books.

Piaget, J. (1970). *Genetic epistemology.* New York, NY: Columbia University Press.

Poole, E. (1934). Genetic development of articulation of consonant sounds in speech. *Elementary English Review, 11,* 159–161.

Prather, E., Hedrick, D., & Kern, C. (1975). Articulation development in children aged two to four years. *Journal of Speech and Hearing Disorders, 40,* 179–191.

Rosenfield, D., & Nudelman, H. (1991). Fluency, disfluency and aging. In D. Ripich (Ed.), *Geriatric communication disorders* (pp. 227–238). Austin, TX: Pro-Ed.

Rutter, M. (1978). Diagnosis and definition of childhood autism. *Journal of Autism and Childhood Schizophrenia, 8,* 139–169.

Sander, E. (1972). When are speech sounds learned? *Journal of Speech and Hearing Disorders, 37,* 55–63.

Scarborough, H., Wyckoff, J., & Davidson, R. (1986). A reconsideration of the relation between age and mean utterance length. *Journal of Speech and Hearing Research, 29,* 394–399.

Schuknecht, H. (1974). *Pathology of the ear.* Cambridge, MA: Harvard University Press.

Schum, D., Matthews, L., & Lee, F. (1991). Actual and predicted word-recognition performance of elderly hearing-impaired listeners. *Journal of Speech and Hearing Research, 34,* 636–642.

Smit, A. B., Hand, L., Freilinger, J., Bernthal, J., & Bird, A. (1990). The Iowa articulation norms project and its Nebraska reduplication. *Journal of Speech and Hearing Disorders, 55,* 779–798.

Stackhouse, J. (1997). Phonological awareness: Connecting speech and literacy problems. In B. W. Hodson & M. L. Edwards (Eds.), *Perspectives in applied phonology.* Gaithersburg, MD: Aspen.

Stoel-Gammon, C., & Dunn, C. (1985). *Normal and disordered phonology in children.* Austin, TX: Pro-Ed.

Templin, M. (1957). *Certain language skills in children.* Minneapolis, MN: University of Minnesota Press.

Wellman, B., Case, I., Mengert, E., & Bradbury, D. (1931). *Speech sounds of young children, University of Iowa Studies in Child Welfare, 5.*

Wiley, T., Cruickshanks, K., Nondahl, D., Tweed, T., Klein, R., & Klein, B. (1998). Aging and word recognition in competing messages. *Journal of the American Academy of Audiology, 9,* 191–198.

Willot, J. (1996). Anatomic and physiologic aging: A behavioral neuroscience perspective. *Journal of the American Academy of Audiology, 7,* 141–151.

Yairi, E., & Clifton, N. (1972). Disfluent speech behavior of preschool children, high school seniors, and geriatric persons. *Journal of Speech and Hearing Research, 15,* 714–719.

Yavas, M. (1998). *Phonology development and disorders.* San Diego, CA: Singular.

Zemlin, W. R. (1998). *Speech and hearing science anatomy and physiology* (4th ed.). Boston, MA: Allyn & Bacon.

Chapter 4

SPEECH SOUND DISORDERS

NATURE OF THE PROBLEM

Speech is the process of producing sound patterns to communicate. The manner in which children develop those sound patterns is described in Chapter 3. This chapter discusses children who, for various reasons, have not mastered the sound patterns expected for children their age. Also, in the section titled "In Medical Settings," we identify challenges encountered by speech-language pathologists (SLPs) when working with children who have serious medical conditions that contribute to speech sound disorders. Finally, we discuss speech sound disorders, mostly in adults, that result from the surgical removal of all or portions of the tongue and other structures used to produce speech sounds.

DEVELOPMENTAL ASPECTS

To develop their speech sound system children must master two tasks. First, they must learn to produce the various sounds of their language. Second, they must develop a system of rules for organizing and using those sounds.

Children who have problems correctly producing sounds are sometimes described as having an **articulation** problem. Children who have not mastered the rules used to manage the sounds are described as having a **phonological disorder**. To illustrate these two types of problems, imagine a child who consistently produces the s sound as a th. This child would produce the sentence

"We went to see Aunt Sarah on Sunday"

as

"We went to thee Aunt Tharah on Thunday"

This child most likely demonstrates an articulation problem. He or she is unable to produce s and instead substitutes a th for every s sound. Now consider a child who produces the sentence

"My kitty cat climbs trees, and my dog Tiger does too"

as

"My kikky cak climbs trees, and my gog Kiger does too"

This child correctly produced the t in *trees* and *too* but not in *kitty, cat,* or *Tiger.* Also, the d is correctly produced in *does* but not in *dog.* Clearly, this problem represents more than an inability to correctly produce t and d sounds. There appears to be some pattern underlying this child's errors with regard to the production of t and d. This pattern of errors most likely reflects a phonological disorder.

The distinction between articulation and phonological disorders is not always as clear as it is in the preceding examples. Some authors choose to use the term *phonology* to refer to all aspects of the study of speech sound production. In this usage, phonology can be said to include both a motor aspect (articulation) and a cognitive-linguistic aspect that deals with the rules for sound usage (Stoel-Gammon & Dunn, 1985). To facilitate this discussion of individuals with problems in this area, we use the generic term *speech sound disorders* in this chapter.

Traditionally, speech sound disorders have been classified as one of three types: substitutions, distortions, or omissions.

Substitutions occur when one sound is substituted for another. For example, when a child says "tan" for *can* or "wed" for *red,* sound substitutions are evident.

Distortions occur when a child attempts the appropriate phoneme but fails to produce it accurately. The "slushy" s of Sylvester the Cat is an extreme example of a distortion.

Omissions signify that a phoneme is deleted, and nothing is produced in its place. The child who says "ha" for *hat* or "baball" for *baseball* is exhibiting an omission.

Errors that affect specific sounds or classes of sounds are sometimes given a specific name. The most common example of such an error is a **lisp.** A lisp affects **sibilant sounds.** Sibilants are s, sh, ch, and their voiced cognates. There are two common types of lisps. The **central lisp** occurs when the speaker produces the sibilant sound with the tongue between the teeth, resulting in a th-like sound. The child with a central lisp says "thun" for *sun* or "methy" for *messy.* A **lateral lisp** occurs when air is directed laterally around the side of the tongue rather than down the middle, resulting in air leakage between the tongue and the molars, producing a "slushy" s or sh sound.

Substitutions, distortions, and omissions can occur in three positions within a word. The first sound of a word is the **initial position,** the last sound is the **final position,** and anything between initial and final is the **medial position.** In the previous example, the child who said "Thunday" for *Sunday* demonstrates a th for s substitution in the initial position. Some authors describe the position of sounds in syllables rather than words. The nucleus of a syllable is a vowel and the word *vocalic* refers to a vowel sound. Thus, sounds at the beginning of a syllable preceding a vowel are identified as **prevocalic**. The h in *hat* and the s in *sun* are in the prevocalic position. Sounds at the end of syllables following the vowel are in the **postvocalic** position. The t in *hat* and the s in *gas* are in the postvocalic position. In some words, a consonant falls between two vowels and serves to end the first syllable and begin the second syllable. These consonants are said to be in the **intervocalic** position. The v in *shovel* and the k in *hiking* are in the intervocalic position.

The system of describing speech sound disorders according to substitutions, distortions, and omissions (SDO) works well for children who have few sounds in error, and when the errors reflect a motoric inability to produce the target sound correctly. In the case of the th for s substitution described earlier, you have a good idea about which sounds the child can and cannot produce. The other child in the example presents a different picture. The SDO system does not describe that child's errors as clearly as it does those of the first child. A better way to describe the second child's errors is to identify any underlying patterns or rules that might account for the errors. One type of pattern that might account for such errors is a phonological process. Phonological processes are discussed as part of normal development in Chapter 3. Some children fail to suppress these simplifying patterns at the expected age. If you examine the second speech sample closely (inconsistent use of t and d), you can see a pattern to the errors. When the alveolar sounds t or d are in a word that contains a velar sound (k or g), the t and d are produced as k or g. This is a fairly common phonological process known as velar assimilation.

PREVALENCE

Estimates of the prevalence of speech sound disorders in school-age children vary as a result of several factors including the diagnostic criteria employed by specific investigators. However, the National Institute on Deafness and Other Communication Disorders (NIDCD) estimates that 8–9 percent of young children exhibit speech sound disorders (NIDCD, 2009). Because the prevalence of this type of disorder is quite high, it is likely that most SLPs will encounter children with speech sound disorders at some point in their career.

It should be mentioned here that not all speech sound differences constitute a disorder. It is important to distinguish speech sound disorders from pronunciation errors, normal developmental differences, and dialectal differences.

Pronunciation errors generally affect only a few words and reflect an inappropriate selection of sounds by the speaker rather than an inability to produce sounds. For example, some people pronounce *Illinois* by including the s (actually a z sound) at the end of the word or refer to a photograph as a "pitcher" rather than a *picture*. Although these productions are not "correct," they do not represent a speech sound disorder. They reflect an inappropriate selection of sounds by the speaker. In most cases, when informed of the "correct" production, the person can alter the pronunciation (if he or she cares to do so).

Developmental differences reflect the fact that the speech sound system, like all aspects of language, does not burst forth in its fully developed form from the time a child begins to speak. Phonological development is a gradual process; what is "normal" for a 3-year-old preschooler may not be "normal" for a 6-year-old first-grader. For example, it is not unusual for a 3-year-old to say "top" for *stop* or "pin" for *spin*, but a first-grader who consistently deletes the s̲ from consonant clusters would be a candidate for speech intervention. To know what may be a problem, it is necessary to know what is typical for children at certain ages. Typical speech sound development is reviewed in Chapter 3.

Dialectal differences are linguistic variations that reflect, among other factors, historical, cultural, regional, and ethnic influences (Taylor, 1986). Dialectal differences are discussed in Chapter 7, but we point out here that individuals who are dialectal speakers may demonstrate speech sound differences that reflect their dialect and that are not considered disorders.

CAUSES OF SPEECH SOUND DISORDERS

Many people, including parents and teachers, often have questions about the cause of speech sound disorders. Are these children cognitively impaired? Do they have some physical disorder? Are they hearing impaired? Although these are all possibilities, in most cases, the answer to all of the preceding questions is no. In this section, we discuss some of the causes of speech sound disorders.

The causes of speech sound disorders can be divided into two broad categories. The first category, usually referred to as **organic disorders**, result from structural, physiologic, sensory, or neurologic deficits (Gordon-Brannan & Weiss, 2007). The second category of causative factors is not as apparent as the organic causes. It is not entirely clear what causes the problems in this second category, and the terms used to describe this category have changed over the years. Terms such as *functional articulation disorders, developmental phonological disorders*, and *disorders of unknown origin* have all been applied to this group of disorders (Bernthal, Bankson, & Flipson, 2009). In this chapter, we retain the label *functional disorders* and define these disorders as behaviors for which no known etiology could be pinpointed at the time of assessment (Davis, 2005).

ORGANIC FACTORS

Many organic conditions can affect the ability of children and adults to produce speech sounds correctly. Several of these conditions, including cleft palate, cerebral palsy, muscular dystrophy, and tracheostomy, are discussed in detail in Chapters 11 and 12. In the present chapter, we identify and briefly describe some additional organic causes of speech sound disorders.

Malocclusion refers to the misalignment of the teeth or an improper relationship between the upper and lower teeth. Terms such as *overbite, overjet, underbite*, and *openbite* are often used to describe different types of malocclusion. Those terms can be confusing and are often used differently by different people. Professionally, SLPs use the terms *distocclusion* or *Class II malocclusion* to refer to situations in which the top (maxillary) teeth protrude too far beyond the bottom (mandibular) teeth. The terms *mesiocclusion, prognathism,* or *Class III malocclusion* refer to situations in which the bottom teeth protrude beyond the upper teeth. Errors on the s and z sounds are often associated with malocclusion, but not all speakers with malocclusions experience problems with speech sound production. Missing teeth have also been associated with speech sound disorders (Snow, 1961; Bankson & Byrne, 1962); however, most children go through the transition from primary to permanent teeth with no serious disruption of speech sound production.

Structural deviations of the tongue can result in speech sound errors. **Macroglossia** is a condition in which the tongue is too large. **Microglossia** refers to a tongue that is too small. **Ankyloglossia**, or "tongue-tie," is a condition in which the flap of tissue that holds the tongue to the floor of the mouth (the lingual frenulum) is too short or attached too far forward. This limits the mobility of the tongue and affects the child's ability to produce tongue-tip sounds such as t, d, l, and r. This condition is not as common as many people seem to believe. The restriction must be quite severe to interfere with speech. Many infants appear to have a short frenulum at first, but after a few months of sucking and crying, the tongue becomes adequately mobile for speech. Most physicians now avoid the once common but mostly unnecessary practice of surgically "clipping" the frenulum in infants.

Another problem involving the tongue is **tongue thrust**. *Tongue thrust* refers to a swallowing pattern in which the tongue comes forward, pressing against the teeth and sometimes protruding between the teeth. Children with tongue thrust have a higher incidence of s and z errors than do other children, but not all children with tongue thrust exhibit speech problems (Bernthal et al., 2009).

Because most children learn their phonological system through hearing, **hearing impairment** can have an effect on accuracy of speech sound production. Factors such as the degree of hearing loss, the age at onset, and the type of hearing loss determine the effect of hearing loss on phonology. Hearing loss is discussed more fully in Chapter 10.

Damage to the central or peripheral nervous system can result in a weakening, paralysis, or loss of control over the muscles of the speech mechanism; the resulting speech problem is called **dysarthria**. Many conditions, including cerebral palsy, muscular dystrophy, tumors, traumatic brain injury, and diseases such as meningitis and encephalitis, can result in dysarthria. Dysarthria is characterized by slow, effortful speech and imprecise production of speech sounds. In this condition, the speech structures, including the tongue, lips, and soft palate, cannot move fast enough to keep up with the demands of connected speech or do not have the strength to achieve the appropriate place or shape to produce the sounds accurately.

Apraxia of speech describes a condition in which the ability to program and sequence the motor movements required for the production of speech sounds is impaired as a result of brain damage. The muscles are healthy and respond to the commands from the nervous system appropriately. The problem is that the commands are incorrect. Sound substitutions and **metathetic errors** (producing sounds in an incorrect order) are common. People usually acquire apraxia of speech as a result of injury or disease. In such situations, the person had normal speech until incurring the brain damage, and then lost some speech ability.

Some believe a condition known as **developmental apraxia of speech (DAS)** affects a child's ability to develop his speech sound system. DAS is a controversial diagnostic category. After reviewing the literature on DAS, Klein (1996) points out that there has never been total agreement on the signs and symptoms of DAS and some lists of signs and symptoms contradict others. Davis, Jakielski, and Marquardt (1998) provide a list that includes many of the most accepted characteristics of DAS. These characteristics include: (1) a limited number of phonemes, (2) frequent omission errors, (3) vowel errors, (4) inconsistent errors, (5) more errors on longer units of speech, (6) difficulty imitating words, (7) use of simple syllable shapes, (8) difficulty with voluntary oral movements, and (9) receptive skills better than expressive skills. The inconsistency of errors and the inability to imitate sounds and motor movements are just two of the factors that make children with DAS particularly challenging for SLPs.

There is a much higher incidence of phonological disorders among persons with cognitive impairments than among their nonimpaired peers. The type and extent of the phonology disorder appears to be related to the degree and cause of impairment. For example, Wilson (1966), in a study of individuals with developmental delays, reports that lower mental age is associated with a greater number of speech sound errors. He also reports that the speech of children with developmental delays who exhibit lower mental ages is characterized by omissions and the speech of those who exhibit higher mental ages is characterized by distortions. Dodd (1976) reports that the incidence of speech problems among children with Down syndrome is higher than among other children with similar degrees of developmental delay. Moran, Money, and Leonard (1984) report that adults with developmental delay exhibit many of the same phonological processes reported by Hodson and Paden (1981) to characterize unintelligible children of normal intelligence.

Because cognitive impairment affects both cognitive-linguistic and motor development, it is not surprising that there is a high incidence of phonological disorders among this population. We must point out that, within the range of normal intelligence, intellectual functioning is not an important factor in determining phonological ability (Powers, 1971; Bernthal et al., 2009).

FUNCTIONAL DISORDERS

The majority of speech sound disorders are not associated with organic conditions. In this chapter, we term these disorders functional and they are not as easy to account for as organic disorders. In most cases, the specific factor or factors that result in a particular speaker's speech sound disorder are impossible to determine. Many factors have been investigated as they relate to functional speech sound disorders. **Table 4–1** presents a

TABLE 4–1   Summary of Research on Selected Factors and Articulation Ability

Factor Investigated	Relationship to Articulation Proficiency
Intelligence	Within the normal range of intelligence, there is a slight positive relationship between intelligence and articulation; however, this is not an important consideration. Below the normal range of intelligence there is a high incidence of articulation disorders including the presence of phonological process disorders (Mackay & Hodson, 1982; Moran, Money, & Leonard, 1984; Shriberg & Widder, 1990; Bernthal et al., 2009).
Speech sound discrimination	Considerable evidence exists that children with speech sound disorders, as a group, perform more poorly on tests of speech sound discrimination than do children without such disorders. However, many individuals with articulation problems show no difficulty with speech sound discrimination (Shriberg, 1980; Gordon-Brannan & Weiss, 2007; Pena-Brooks & Hegde, 2007; Bernthal et al., 2009).
Motor skills	Although there is evidence that some children with speech sound disorders score lower than those with normal articulation on tests of rapid alternating speech movements (e.g., rapidly repeating the syllable *pu, tu, ku*), the nature of the relationship between motor skills and speech sound production is not clear (Shriberg, 1980; Gordon-Brannan & Weiss, 2007; Pena-Brooks & Hegde, 2007; Bernthal et al., 2009).
Socioeconomic level	There is some evidence that proportionally more children from low socioeconomic homes have poor speech sound production skills. However, this, by itself, does not appear to be a significant factor and such differences are often eliminated by the time a child enters school (Winitz, 1969; Shriberg, 1980; Pena-Brooks & Hegde, 2007; Bernthal et al., 2009).
Siblings	There is some evidence that first-born children, only children, and children with increased spacing between siblings have better speech sound production skill at some ages. Twins sometimes develop unique speech patterns (idioglossia) (Shriberg, 1980; Gordon-Brannan & Weiss, 2007; Pena-Brooks & Hegde, 2007; Bernthal et al., 2009).
Personality and adjustment	There is some evidence that children with speech sound disorders may have psychosocial difficulties, but the literature is contradictory and any relationship may be of little clinical relevance (Bloch & Goodstein, 1971; Shriberg, 1980; Shriberg & Kwiatkowski, 1994; Pena-Brooks & Hegde, 2007; Bernthal et al., 2009).

(continues)

TABLE 4–1   Summary of Research on Selected Factors and Articulation Ability (continued)

Factor Investigated	Relationship to Articulation Proficiency
Familial tendencies	Felsenfeld, McGue, and Broen (1995) report that children of parents with a history of phonological/language problems were more likely to require articulation treatment than were the children of parents with no history of phonological/language problems. However, the phonological errors exhibited by the children were not necessarily similar to those exhibited by the parents.
Language disorders	Many children with speech sound disorders, especially moderate to severe problems, also exhibit language problems (Ruscello, St. Louis, & Mason, 1991; Tyler, Lewis, Haskill & Tolbert, 2002; Gordon-Brannan & Weiss, 2007; Pena-Brooks & Hegde, 2007; Bernthal et al., 2009).
Phonological awareness	Many children with speech sound disorders perform more poorly on phonological awareness tasks than do age peers without speech sound disorders (Bird, Bishop, & Freeman, 1995; Cowan & Moran, 1997; Rvachew, Ohberg, Grawburg, & Heyuding, 2003; Gernand & Moran, 2007).

summary of research findings regarding some of these factors. It is important to keep in mind that most of the reported research is based on group data and the results may not apply to every child with a phonological disorder. A review of Table 4–1 reveals that most research demonstrates unclear relationships, weak relationships, or no relationship at all between speech sound disorders and factors many people have assumed play a large role in such disorders.

Despite years of research and an abundance of children with functional speech sound disorders, in most cases the specific cause of a functional speech sound disorder in any given child is unknown.

IN EDUCATIONAL SETTINGS

CASE EXAMPLES

To provide an appreciation of the range of speech sound disorders that SLPs might encounter in an educational setting, we present two hypothetical students, each representing one end of a continuum of severity. Mary and John are both in the first grade. They were referred by their teacher to the school SLP for a speech evaluation. To obtain a sample of their spontaneous speech, the SLP asks each child to talk about a picture of a rabbit. In response to the picture, Mary says:

"That is a wabbit, a bwown wabbit. Wabbits wun fast. They eat cawots."

The same picture elicits the following response from John:

"Da a bu wa. E wu pa. E ea ga. I no i pi."

(Translation: That's a bunny rabbit. He runs fast. He eats grass. His nose is pink.) Both Mary and John exhibit problems with their speech sound system. In Mary's case, the problem appears to be limited to the r sound. Although her problem is noticeable, most people would have little difficulty understanding her. John, on the other hand, appears to have a very limited speech sound system. He seems to be able to use only the earliest developing consonants (w, h, and some stop consonants). In addition to the sound errors, he appears to be able to produce only single-syllable words and the syllables are very simple consonant + vowel or just a vowel. These limitations on John's phonology make his speech unintelligible. Even when the listener knows that he is talking about a rabbit, it is almost impossible to understand what he is saying. A critical first step in improving speech sound disorders is to describe precisely the nature of the problem. This is the goal of an SLP when conducting a speech sound assessment.

ASSESSMENT OF SPEECH SOUND DISORDERS IN EDUCATIONAL SETTINGS

Screening Tests and Teacher Referrals Frequently, the first stage of assessment in an educational setting is a screening test. Screening tests are usually administered just prior to or shortly after the start of the school year. The purpose of a screening test is to determine which members of a group (e.g., all children entering kindergarten) are most likely to have a problem. Failing a screening test does not mean that the child has a disorder. It simply means that the child is a candidate for a more thorough evaluation. Screening tests must be quick and easy to administer and to score. Screening tests to assess speech sound production ability usually consist of a brief sample of connected speech obtained by asking the child to count, repeat words, name and/or describe pictures, or any other activity that provides the examiner with an opportunity to hear the subject produce a wide array of speech sounds.

In addition to such informal sampling, several published screening tests are available. The SLP may choose to use one of these published screening devices in place of, or in addition to, a less formal speech sampling technique. In most school settings, SLPs use the screening test to assess language development as well as speech sound production. In addition to being quick and easy to administer, screening tests must meet two other criteria. They must be able to identify a high percentage of children who have disorders (sensitivity), but must not fail too many children who do not have disorders (specificity). The SLP should monitor the screening procedure she uses to be sure it has high sensitivity and specificity. Good record keeping can be of help in this regard because many of the children screened may remain in the school system for years, allowing the SLP to follow them.

Another important method of identifying children with speech sound disorders is teacher referral. After a few years in the classroom, most teachers can easily identify students whose speech is markedly different from that of other students at a particular grade level. Teachers should refer to SLP students who are unintelligible or who have more or different speech sound errors than other children in class (not dialectal differences). When the SLP identifies either through screening or referral a child who might have a speech sound disorder, the SLP must obtain permission to evaluate from the parents and then give the child a diagnostic evaluation.

Standardized Diagnostic Tests   The objectives of a diagnostic evaluation include: (1) determining whether the child has a speech sound disorder, (2) determining the nature and extent of the disorder, and (3) suggesting methods that might be effective in remediating that disorder. To meet these objectives, the SLP has three basic types of standardized diagnostic tests available: **speech sound inventories**, **contextual tests**, and **pattern analyses**. Depending on the errors exhibited by the child, the SLP may choose to administer one, two, or all three of these assessments.

Speech Sound Inventories   A speech sound inventory is a test of each phoneme in the context of a word. Each consonant is generally tested in each word position (initial, medial, final) or in some tests in the initial and final position only. Consonant clusters are usually tested in at least the initial position. Some, but not all, inventories also test vowels. Speech sound inventories usually require a child to name pictures that contain one or more target phonemes. For example, examiners may use a picture of a foot to assess f̲ in the initial position and t̲ in the final position. Picture naming is preferable to reading because it allows the examiner to test students who cannot read and avoids possible confusion of a reading problem with a speech sound disorder. Having the child repeat words might be easier and faster than picture naming, but research indicates that spontaneous picture naming provides a more accurate sample of speech sound production ability (Snow & Milisen, 1954; Carter & Buck, 1958; Smith & Ainsworth, 1967; Kresheck & Sokolofsky, 1972). There are many published speech sound inventories. Following are some of the more commonly used:

> The *Goldman-Fristoe Test of Articulation (2nd ed.)* (Goldman & Fristoe, 2000), which provides color pictures to elicit single-word responses and a story retelling section to elicit a connected speech sample.
> The *Photo Articulation Test (3rd ed.)* (Lippke, Dickey, Selmar, & Soder, 1997), which uses photographs of objects to elicit single-word responses and a set of sequential photos to elicit a connected speech sample.
> The *Arizona Articulation Proficiency Scale (3rd ed.)* (Fudala, 2000), which provides a weighting of each sound to provide an intelligibility rating.

Speech sound inventories are quick and easy to administer. Many provide normative data that allow comparison of the subject's performance to that of an age peer group. Therefore, speech sound inventories are quite popular with most school-based SLPs who have large caseloads and a minimum of time available for diagnostic testing.

Although they provide some helpful information, speech sound inventories have certain disadvantages. Testing each phoneme once in each position of a word does not, in most cases, adequately define the child's ability to produce that sound. In many cases, the ability to produce a certain sound can be affected by the surrounding sounds, known as the **phonetic environment** or **phonetic context**. An example of the effect of phonetic context is in the word *statistics*. Many adult speakers, with no other speech sound disorders, have difficulty producing the second t and instead produce an st cluster, saying "stastistics." Speech sound inventories do not sample enough words to assess the effects of phonetic context on the sounds produced during the test. To assess such effects, an SLP may elect to use a contextual test.

Contextual Tests   The first widely used contextual test was the *Deep Test of Articulation* (McDonald, 1964). Subsequent tests employing a variety of phonetic contexts are sometimes referred to as deep type tests. In the original *Deep Test of Articulation*, a picture containing the target sound (a sound produced incorrectly in earlier testing) in the initial position is preceded by a series of 30 pictures ending with a different sound. For each picture pair, the student is instructed to say the two words together so that they sound like one big word. For example, if s is the target sound, a picture of "sun" would be preceded by pictures such as "cup," "tub," "kite," and so on. The child would then produce words such as "cupsun," "tubsun," and "kitesun." The procedure is then repeated with the target sound in the final position, for example, "house" followed by a series of words resulting in productions such as "housepipe," "housebell," and "housetie." When the test is complete, the examiner has a sample of the target sound as it is preceded and followed by many different phonemes. By using the *Deep Test*, the SLP frequently can identify one or more contexts in which the error sound is produced correctly. Although McDonald's test is the most widely known, there are other published deep type tests including *Clinical Probes of Articulation Consistency (C-PAC)* (Secord, 1981) and the *Contextual Test of Articulation* (Aase et al., 2000). Whether one of the published deep type tests are administered or not, the SLP will probably want to assess troublesome phonemes in several different contexts to determine the effect of phonetic context.

Pattern Analyses   Speech sound inventories and contextual tests reveal errors on individual sounds. Errors on multiple sounds may reflect an underlying pattern. Several types of patterns can account for errors on several sounds including distinctive feature patterns and patterns of phonological rules. However, the most common patterns used to account for multiple sound errors are phonological process. We discuss the concept of phonological processes in Chapter 3 as part of phonological development. Some children fail to suppress these normal processes at the expected age, or they exhibit unusual processes that are not part of normal development. If the SLP can identify one or more processes affecting a number of phonemes in the speech of a child, the intervention that follows will be much more efficient than working on each individual error sound.

   Two of the more frequently used tests of phonological process are the *Hodson Assessment of Phonological Patterns (HAPP-3)* (Hodson, 2004) and the *Kahn-Lewis Phonological Analysis-2*

(KLPA-2) (Kahn & Lewis, 2002). The *HAPP-3* employs spontaneous naming of objects, body parts, and colors to assess numerous processes and patterns. The *KLPA-2* uses the words from the sounds-in-words section of the *Goldman-Fristoe Test of Articulation* as its speech sample.

Combination Tests   Some recently developed tests are designed to allow the SLP to perform more than one kind of analysis. An example of this kind of test is the *Clinical Assessment of Articulation and Phonology (CAAP)* (Secord & Donohue, 2002), which includes an "Articulation Inventory" and two "Phonological Process Checklists."

Also popular, because of the large amount of data that can be provided in a small amount of time, are computer-based analyses such as the PROPH+ program of *Computerized Profiling* (Long, 2004). Once the child's utterances are typed, this program provides an analysis of several phonological processes plus a great deal of additional information about the child's phonological inventory, in a matter of seconds.

Type of Speech Sample   Speech sound inventories, contextual tests, and many of the published pattern analysis tests elicit speech one word at a time. Several studies have demonstrated that children exhibit more sound errors on words in connected speech than on those same words in isolation (Faircloth & Faircloth, 1970; DuBoise & Bernthal, 1978; Schmauch, Panagos, & Klich, 1978; Panagos, Quine, & Klich, 1979; Haynes, Haynes, & Jackson, 1982). Connected speech involves speaking in sentences. Sentences require the speaker to be concerned with tense constructions, subject–predicate agreement, and many other syntax considerations not involved in the production of single words. Therefore, connected speech is a more complex linguistic task than the production of isolated single words. As with most tasks, complexity increases the chance of error. Connected speech presents a more realistic assessment of a child's communication abilities than the somewhat artificial task of naming pictures. Because of this, SLPs should always supplement single-word responses obtained from standardized tests with a sample of the child's connected speech.

Although there are no hard and fast rules about how extensive a connected speech sample should be, an often cited minimum is 80 to 100 different words, which requires a total sample of about 200 to 250 words (Shriberg & Kwiatkowski, 1980). Obtaining such a connected speech sample can be challenging. Some children are shy with unfamiliar adults and speak only in one- or two-word utterances if at all. Even with a talkative child, it might take a very long time before he uses all the sounds in all of the contexts the examiner wishes to examine. Some children may avoid words containing sounds that are difficult for them to produce. Further complicating matters, when a child is unintelligible, it is difficult or impossible to determine the error patterns because the listener does not know what the child intended to say.

Faced with these problems, an SLP will often use some structured task to maintain control over the content in eliciting a connected speech sample. Having the child describe a picture is one way to elicit connected speech. By carefully selecting the pictures, the

SLP samples a variety of sounds in different contexts and has some idea of the topic. Another frequently used technique is story retelling. In this procedure, a child is shown pictures and told a story, and then is shown the pictures again and asked to repeat the story. This technique is used in published test instruments such as the Sounds-in-Sentences subtest of the *Goldman-Fristoe Test of Articulation-2.*

HOW TEACHERS CAN HELP IN ASSESSMENT

In educational settings, teachers can be an important source of diagnostic information. Next to parents, teachers have the most opportunity to observe their students' communicative behavior. Teachers can provide a great deal of assistance by answering the following questions:

1. With which sounds or words does the child seem to have difficulty?
2. Does the child ever produce any of the error sounds correctly?
3. Do you have trouble understanding the child?
4. Do other students have trouble understanding the child?
5. Are other students aware of the child's speech problem? How do they react?
6. How does the child get along with classmates?
7. Does the child talk as much as most students in the class?
8. Are the child's vocabulary and grammar appropriate for grade level?
9. How well does the child follow directions?
10. How is the child performing academically?

TREATMENT OF SPEECH SOUND DISORDERS IN EDUCATIONAL SETTINGS

When the assessment is completed, the SLP makes a recommendation to the eligibility committee. Children with speech and language problems are included on the caseloads of school-based SLPs only when those disorders negatively affect the student's education or limit participation in the educational program. In some school systems, children whose only problems are in the area of speech sound production may not be considered eligible for services; in other systems, they may. If the student is to receive treatment, the structure of the treatment sessions must be decided and a schedule must be worked out between the SLP and the teacher. Many children receive direct treatment in which they are removed from the classroom for a short period of time one or two days each week. During these away-from-class periods, the SLP works specifically on the child's speech sound skills either individually or in small groups of children with similar problems. Less frequently, speech sound improvement techniques may be incorporated into classroom and other educational activities in an indirect approach to treatment.

SLPs might employ many intervention techniques and procedures to remediate a speech sound disorder. Although it is not the purpose of this text to teach specific treatment techniques, we do wish to provide some description of the role of the SLP in remediating speech sound disorders in educational settings.

DIRECT TREATMENT TECHNIQUES

Throughout this chapter, we make the point that phonology problems occur on two different levels: a motor level, where the child is unable to correctly produce the sound, and a cognitive-linguistic level, where the child may be able to produce sounds but does not use them appropriately. Because there are two levels of phonological problems, there are two types of treatment to remediate those problems. Motor-based treatments are designed to teach the child to produce a target sound correctly; to transfer the correct production of that sound to all positions, contexts, linguistic units, and situations; and to maintain the correct production of that sound in habitual speech. Cognitive-linguistic approaches are designed to teach patterns that affect entire classes of sounds. The theory is that by selecting certain sounds (exemplars) that can be used to teach the new pattern, the pattern will generalize to untreated sounds, saving a considerable amount of treatment time. Sometimes children exhibit phonological problems on both levels. In such cases, SLPs might incorporate both motor-based and cognitive-linguistic approaches into the therapy program.

Motor-Based Treatment   Most motor-based treatment programs can be divided into three major stages: **establishment**, **generalization**, and **maintenance** (Bernthal et al., 2009). During the establishment phase, the child is taught to correctly produce the target sound or sounds in at least one context and to stabilize that correct production. During the generalization stage, correct production of the target sound(s) spreads to additional words, linguistic units, and situations. During maintenance, the student retains the correct production with decreasing support from the SLP. To illustrate some of the techniques that might be used in each of the three stages of a motor-based approach, we use an example, Mary, the hypothetical child with the w/r substitution described earlier in this chapter.

Establishment   Recall that Mary has difficulty with the r sound. During the establishment phase, Mary is taught to produce the r either in isolation or in a syllable such as "ro, ri, ray," and so forth. The specific techniques for teaching the sound will vary from child to child and from clinician to clinician. With young children, it is often helpful to give the target sound a name. For Mary, the r might be called the "growling tiger" sound. In other cases, f might be called the "angry kitty" sound or z the "buzzing bee" sound. In some cases, treatment might begin with **ear training** in which the student is taught to identify the sound when it is heard and to discriminate the correct production of the target sound from an incorrect production (Van Riper & Emerick, 1984). After ear training, the treatment shifts to production training. In production training, the student is first taught to produce the sound correctly. SLPs may use a number of techniques to achieve this first correct production. Sometimes the sound can be produced correctly in a particular phonetic context (word or syllable). In that case, it is a matter of expanding the contexts in which the sound can be produced correctly. If the sound is not correctly produced in any context, the child must be taught to produce the troublesome phoneme.

One technique frequently used to teach a sound is **auditory stimulation**. Normal-hearing children appear to learn the sound system of their language through hearing. There is a mechanism in every individual's brain that allows that person to produce sounds that are similar to those she hears. Sometimes this takes practice and may be easier for some children than for others. Many people who study foreign languages that contain phonemes not found in English know that it takes a great deal of practice before they can come close to producing correctly some German or French phonemes. For some children, the structured practice of trying to match the sound they hear results in correct production.

Another technique, **phonetic placement**, involves instructing the child where to place the articulators to produce the target sound correctly. Phonetic placement is often easier with visible sounds, such as th or f, when a mirror can be used to aid in proper placement. A third technique that can be used to teach a sound is **successive approximation**. In successive approximation, the child moves in small steps from a sound that he can produce correctly to the target sound. A child who can correctly produce the sh sound but cannot produce the s might be told to make the sh, and then gradually move the tongue closer and closer to the alveolar ridge until a correct s is produced. In Mary's case, an attempt might be made to achieve correct production of the r from the production of a closely related sound such as the l. When a sound is first produced correctly, it is often with much effort and inconsistency. The final stage of the establishment phase involves working toward an effortless and consistent production of the sound. It is only when the sound is produced in this manner that the child can move on to the generalization phase of therapy.

Generalization   Some SLPs refer to this phase as "transfer" or "carry-over." Regardless of the label, the goal of this phase is to enable the child to use the behavior learned in the establishment phase in all words and speaking situations.

Bernthal et al. (2009) describe five types of generalization that are of concern in articulation therapy. The first type of generalization is **position generalization**. Here, the student must generalize the correct production of the target sound from the position in which it was established (initial, medial, or final) to other positions in words. In the case of Mary, if she establishes the r sound in the initial position in a word such as *run*, she must now generalize that correct production to words such as *carrot* and *car*. The second type of generalization is **context generalization**. Here, clinicians are concerned with extending the correct production of a sound to all phonetic environments. If Mary can say r when it occurs with back vowels such as in the words *root, rope*, and *rot*, she must extend her production to front vowel contexts such as *read, rich*, and *ran*. She must also produce the sound in clusters such as *brown* and *price*. **Linguistic unit generalization** involves maintenance of the correct production of a sound or sound pattern in increasingly more complex utterances. Typically, the progression goes from isolation, to syllables, to words (if the sound is first established at the word level, isolation and syllables are omitted), to phrases and sentences, to connected speech. **Sound and feature generalization** is concerned with applying the skills learned with one sound to the correct production of similar sounds. In Mary's case, if she has been achieving success with the r in *run* and *car*, the clinician wants that ability to transfer to the slightly different er sound in *mother* and *early*. The last type of generalization to be discussed is **situation generalization**. The child must learn that "good speech" is expected in all speaking situations, not just in therapy or school, but on the playground, at home, at summer camp, and in all other speaking situations. Teachers and parents can provide a great deal of help in regard to situational generalization. However, the SLP should clearly define their role so that they are not expecting too much or placing inappropriate levels of pressure on the child for correct production.

Maintenance   The goal of the maintenance phase is for the newly acquired sound or pattern to be incorporated as a natural part of the child's everyday speech. Maintenance usually involves a reduction in the frequency of therapy sessions. The child may go from two sessions a week, to one session each week, to one every two weeks, and so on. Many of the activities used during maintenance are similar to those used during the generalization phase, but with less frequent reinforcement. Some SLPs use **negative practice** during the maintenance phase. In this technique, the child is asked to produce the error sound or sound pattern intentionally to sharpen the contrast between the "old" and "new" productions. Using negative practice, Mary might say, "I used to call a rabbit a wabbit, and I used to say bwown for brown. But I don't say that anymore."

Teachers and parents can probably expect consistently correct use of the target at this stage. When an error does occur, a raised eyebrow or a request to "Say that again, please," is usually sufficient stimulation to elicit a correct production. Because the SLP sees the child less frequently during this stage, feedback from teachers and parents is critical. Any apparent regression should be reported as soon as it is noted. Reports that the child is maintaining good speech are also important because they allow the SLP to determine which techniques have proven successful.

A Word About Oral-Motor Exercises   Recently, some SLPs have begun to employ oral-motor exercises to strengthen and/or improve muscle function before teaching specific sounds. Actually, this trend represents the most recent revival of a controversial approach to articulation disorders that goes back more than 50 years. The controversy revolves around the use of oral-motor training techniques even in cases where there is no obvious physical cause for the disorder. The assumption is that many so-called functional articulation/phonological disorders have underlying neuromuscular coordination or muscle strength problems as a contributing factor. These are not the severe motor problems exhibited by students with cerebral palsy or other clinically identifiable neuromuscular disorders or even those exhibited by children with the label of developmental apraxia of speech. Rather, these oral-motor problems are much more subtle and become noticeable only under the demands of complicated, coordinated activities such as those required for speech production.

Oral-motor techniques generally involve separating and simplifying the complex coordinated movements involved in speech production so that these simpler activities can be mastered before they are combined with other movements to produce speech. Clinicians use a wide variety of techniques to accomplish this purpose including flexibility and strength drills for individual articulators, sucking and blowing activities to facilitate coordination of oral and respiratory muscles, and sensory stimulation to improve the sensory abilities of the muscles of speech (Boshart, 2004). In some cases, the clinician presents these activities to the child as oral exercises or oral "gymnastics." Sometimes the SLP uses a variety of devices to shape, stimulate, and/or stabilize the various oral structures. SLPs may ask teachers of students enrolled in speech intervention programs using an oral-motor approach to help monitor homework assignments that require the children to "spear" Cheerios with their tongue, lick peanut butter from around their mouth, suck on straws that have the other end covered by a finger, blow horns or bubbles, or many other activities that involve the speech mechanism but not during speech activities.

Although many SLPs who use oral-motor techniques attribute excellent results to these activities, there is very little empirical evidence to support their use. Forrest (2002) reviews the existing literature that examines the use of oral-motor techniques in the treatment of articulation/phonological disorders. She concludes, "Based on currently available resources, oral-motor exercises cannot be considered to be a legitimate treatment protocol for children with phonological/articulatory disorders" (Forrest, 2002, p. 22). The use of such techniques remains a very controversial subject.

Cognitive-Linguistic Approaches　For children who exhibit problems of a cognitive-linguistic nature, the treatment program is somewhat different from that for children with a motor-based problem. In this case, the SLP would most likely target a pattern rather than a specific sound. The patterns most frequently targeted in such approaches are distinctive feature patterns or phonological processes (Stoel-Gammon, Stone-Goldman, & Glaspey, 2002). Stoel-Gammon and Dunn (1985) identify three characteristics of the approaches that we describe as cognitive-linguistic:

1. *These approaches are based on the systematic nature of phonology.* This means that no matter how unusual a child's phonology may be, it has some organization. The job of the SLP is to discover how the child's phonology is organized and reorganize it in a more typical fashion. That is one reason that patterns rather than individual sounds are targeted. For example, with the child who substitutes p̲ for f̲, b̲ for v̲, t̲ for s̲, and d̲ for z̲, rather than teach four different sounds, a cognitive-linguistic approach targets the elimination of the process known as stopping.
2. *These approaches use conceptual rather than motor activities.* Weiner and Bankson (1978) provide an excellent example of a conceptual approach. To eliminate the process of stopping on fricatives, they associated stop consonants with dripping water and fricatives

with flowing water, complete with pictures of a dripping and flowing faucet. The child was then taught to make flowing sounds in contrast to dripping sounds.

3. *These approaches have generalization as their ultimate goal.* By teaching the appropriate concept with a few phonemes, that concept will generalize to the entire class of phonemes. For example, an SLP might be able to get a child to make all fricatives "flowing" sounds, based on work with s and v.

In the case of the second hypothetical child described earlier, John, the SLP might want to teach him to eliminate or suppress the process of final consonant deletion. Just as the motor-based therapy began with ear training, the cognitive-linguistic approach might begin by teaching the student awareness of the pattern to be targeted through a process called **conceptualization** (Winitz, 1975; Weiner & Bankson, 1978). Conceptualization is a more cognitive process than auditory discrimination is. It is not enough that the child is able to hear the difference between *boat* and *bo* (discrimination); the child must recognize that *boat* has a sound on the end that makes it different from the word *bo*. Often, the student demonstrates understanding of the concept through some sorting task where pictures of words that end in a consonant are put in one pile and pictures of words that lack a final consonant are put in another pile. Words such as *bo* (possibly pictured as a bow) and *boat*, which differ in only one aspect, are called **minimal pairs**. Minimal pairs can be used to contrast a number of features. For example, *pie* and *bye* differ only in the voicing of the initial consonant. *See* and *tea* differ only in that *see* begins with a voiceless alveolar fricative and *tea* begins with a voiceless alveolar stop. Because the presence or absence of a feature changes the meaning of the word, minimal pairs constitute a powerful tool in the remediation of cognitive-linguistic phonology problems and can be applied to phonological disorders in several different ways (Barlow & Gierut, 2002).

Clinicians can use a minimal pairs technique in the production stage of John's therapy. Weiner (1981) provides an example of how minimal pairs might be applied to John's problem of final consonant deletion. In this approach, the SLP places five pictures of a boat and four pictures of a bow on a table in front of the child. The child is told that every time he says *boat*, the SLP will pick up a picture of boat. When the SLP has all five pictures, the child receives a star. Weiner reports very rapid success in establishing the presence of final consonants using this minimal pairs technique.

One problem that SLPs often encounter in cognitive-linguistic approaches is that, because a pattern rather than a specific sound is targeted, the early stages of treatment might require reinforcement of an incorrect sound. For example, if John, our final consonant deleter, learns to say *boat* and *seat* rather than "bo" and "see," the clinician would say, "Great!" But what if he says "gat" for *gas* and "bat" for *bath*? The SLP might say, "Great!" Teachers and parents might say, "Isn't it still wrong?" From a traditional motor-based view, it is just another error. However, in a cognitive-linguistic approach, SLPs are trying to establish the pattern of placing a final consonant at the end of words. John has established that pattern. John will work on getting the appropriate sound in the generalization stage of therapy.

HOW TEACHERS AND PARENTS CAN ASSIST IN DIRECT TREATMENT APPROACHES

We cannot make the point too strongly that the effectiveness of speech and language treatment is greatly enhanced by the active participation of parents and teachers. However, teachers clearly have their hands full with their required classroom work. Therefore, as Mowrer (1971) suggests, SLPs should ask classroom teachers to perform only activities that are compatible with normal classroom activities. As the SLP relates the goals and progress of the child, the teacher may be able to suggest classroom activities that fit into generalization goals for the student, and parents may be able to suggest times in the day when speech activities could be incorporated into their child's routines.

An effective means of communication between the SLP and teachers and parents is a **speech notebook**. This can be an inexpensive spiral notebook or even a folder with brads and pockets. The SLP can place speech goals, activities, exercises, progress charts, instructions, and comments in the notebook. Teachers and parents can check the notebook after each session or at the end of each week to find out what the child is doing in speech and how they can assist in the remediation program. Although specific activities must be determined on an individual basis for each student, the following represents a broad outline of the information that teachers and parents should have regarding students enrolled in therapy for speech sound disorders:

1. *Both teachers and parents should know the goals of the student's treatment program.* Which sound errors are being targeted? Is the child working on one sound or on a class of sounds such as voiceless consonants? Teachers and parents will probably be aware of long-term goals from the Individualized Education Program (IEP), but short-term goals may change frequently during a school year.
2. *Teachers and parents should be aware of progress toward the treatment goals.* What kind of speech production can be expected? Is the child working toward correct production via a sequence of closer and closer approximations of the target sound? Does a change in the sound a child substitutes for the target sound represent progress?
3. *Perhaps most important of all, both teachers and parents need to know how to help in achieving the speech goals.* Should they demand a certain level of performance? What kind of feedback should they provide to the SLP? How can everyday activities in school and at home be used to reinforce treatment and enhance the student's success? With regard to the latter question, Hoffman and Norris (2005) suggest that with some training parents can be taught to use shared book reading activities and to expand and recast children's utterances to support the SLP's work on specific sounds. Weiss, Gordon, and Lillywhite (1987) identify some activities teachers may perform to help the student generalize new skills from the treatment room to the classroom.
   a. Help the student carry out speech assignments. The assignments may involve repeating a word list, using "good speech" during a particular classroom activity, or demonstrating a newly learned ability to a variety of people. The assignments often are described in the student's speech notebook.

   b. Monitor the student's speech during certain activities. The SLP should keep the teacher informed as to what the student should and should not be able to do. The teacher may use the speech notebook to report to the SLP.

   c. Provide the SLP with classroom materials to be used during the treatment session. This allows for relevance of the speech activity; also, the classroom activities and speech activities reinforce each other.

   d. Monitor the student's error productions. Is the sound being used correctly in more words? Are other sounds improving? Is the improved production being maintained in all speaking situations?

   e. Reinforce correct sound productions when appropriate and remind the child to use the target sound or sound pattern. The SLP should clearly communicate to the teacher what feedback or correction technique should be used with the student. A student should never be made to feel embarrassed or "picked on."

INDIRECT TREATMENT OF SPEECH SOUND DISORDERS

The treatment methods just described all incorporate a very direct approach to remediation. Those methods target specific sounds or error patterns usually in a drill or drill-play format. SLPs focus their efforts on achieving a specified criteria at various levels of linguistic complexity (i.e., words, sentences, conversation). Recently, some authors suggest that intervention for speech sound disorders, especially those of a cognitive-linguistic nature, might in some cases be more effective using a less direct model. Because many of these less direct approaches to speech sound disorders incorporate realistic communication activities in natural language environments, the classroom becomes an important site for intervention. As a result, in these indirect approaches, the opportunity for interaction of the SLP and classroom teacher is much greater.

    Christensen and Luckett (1990) describe a procedure that combines the direct pullout-type approach with a less direct in-class approach, referred to as a **whole-class language experience**. In this approach, the SLP designs procedures that enrich the language skills of an entire classroom of children but that still allow for the targeting of specific skills for students with phonological disorders. Using this procedure, the SLP sees the child twice each week, once in a traditional session, and once as part of the whole-class language experience. The SLP targets specific skills for students with phonological problems in the traditional treatment session. Then, responses stressing that skill are incorporated into the weekly whole-class language experience. For example, a student who has difficulty producing the s̲ sound may work on s̲ in the initial position of words during a traditional pullout therapy session once each week. Later in the week, the student may be asked questions during the whole-class language experience that require the use of words containing s̲ in the initial position. Involvement of the classroom teacher in the whole-class language experience is critical. If the teacher clearly understands the goals and objectives for the child with phonological impairment, he or she will be better able to monitor the child's speech during other class activities. The teacher also may be able to help monitor the child's responses during the whole-class activity for IEP purposes. The teacher can be helpful to the SLP in terms of sharing knowledge of classroom management and working together with the SLP to develop whole-class activities that are consistent with the curriculum.

The term *indirect* may also be used to describe treatment techniques delivered in a traditional out-of-classroom setting in which speech sound errors are not directly targeted. Hoffman, Norris, and Monjure (1990) describe such a procedure in which phonological errors were not specifically targeted, but other language components, particularly syntax, were the primary focus. An interesting aspect of this study is that the subjects were two 4-year-old brothers from a set of identical triplets. The brothers exhibited delays in phonology as well as in other language components. One child was enrolled in an intervention program targeting his specific phonological disorder. The second child was enrolled in a whole language program that involved having the child retell stories to a puppet. In this whole language program, the child was encouraged through questions and modeling to make revisions, additions, and increases in sentence complexity. No particular attention was paid to the phonological errors of the second child. Results indicated that both children made about the same improvement in phonology, but the child enrolled in the whole language approach made greater improvement in expressive language. This study suggests that reorganization of language on one level, such as syntax, may result in reorganization at other levels, such as phonology.

Intervention programs for children with phonological disorders that do not direct at least some attention to phonology must, however, be viewed with caution. Fey et al. (1994) and Tyler and Sandoval (1994) both report carefully controlled experimental studies in which treatment directed primarily toward other aspects of language had negligible effects on phonology. Tyler (2002) indicates that a language-based approach is not appropriate for all children with phonological impairments, and when such an approach is chosen, the clinician must monitor progress closely to ensure its effectiveness. Of course, one of the ways in which an SLP could monitor progress in a language-based approach is through feedback from classroom teachers.

HOW TEACHERS CAN ASSIST IN INDIRECT TREATMENT APPROACHES

From the examples of indirect treatment programs discussed previously, you can see that meaningful language activities in a natural language environment are at the heart of such approaches. Because the classroom, playground, and cafeteria are common natural language environments for children, these situations provide ideal intervention opportunities. Some of the following opportunities for intervention involve the presence of the SLP, and some do not. Teachers can do the following to assist in treatment:

1. Inform the SLP of the topic, objectives, and materials used in class so that any intervention activities could be designed to fit with the teacher's lesson plan.
2. Provide suggestions to the SLP for classroom management. Remember that most SLPs are more accustomed to working with individuals or small groups. The skill of an

experienced teacher in classroom management could be very valuable to the success of indirect intervention programs.

3. Work with the SLP to understand the kinds of communication situations that will facilitate speech goals, and attempt to create such situations in the classroom and other settings.

4. Be flexible in planning activities (e.g., in classes with large number of students, the teacher may work with one group during a class period while the SLP works with another group that includes the student(s) with phonological problems).

5. Be able to monitor the child's speech so that the teacher can provide appropriate feedback and reinforcement when the SLP is not present, and so that the teacher can keep the SLP apprised of how well newly learned phonological skills are generalizing to the classroom setting.

IN MEDICAL SETTINGS

Many hospitals and medical centers operate outpatient or satellite clinics in which evaluation and treatment may be provided for the speech sound disorders described earlier. However, hospital-based SLPs may also be involved in the assessment and treatment of speech sound disorders experienced by medically complicated inpatients. Some of the conditions that might result in speech sound disorders in medical settings are covered in detail in other chapters in this text. For example, craniofacial anomalies including cleft palate are discussed in Chapter 11. Neurological problems such as apraxia and dysarthria are covered in Chapter 12. In the present chapter, we focus on two categories of patients who may exhibit speech sound disorders and require the services of a hospital-based SLP. These categories are medically fragile children and patients with structural deficits resulting from oral surgery.

MEDICALLY FRAGILE CHILDREN

The term *medically fragile children* is a broad one used to refer to children with chronic illnesses who require long-term intensive and specialized medical treatment. Children in this category display a wide range of diagnoses and conditions. Examples of the children in this category who might be encountered in a medical setting include the following:

- Those who are unable to breathe on their own and require ventilator support
- Children exposed to alcohol or drugs (e.g., infants with fetal alcohol syndrome or crack/cocaine exposure)
- Those with infectious or contagious diseases (e.g., hepatitis, sexually transmitted infections, HIV/AIDS)
- Those with specialized feeding problems requiring feeding tubes
- Children with chronic health problems such as seizure disorders
- Those who have received significant injuries as a result of accidents or physical assaults

In most cases, these children have multiple medical needs in addition to speech and language development. The effects on speech are particularly acute when these conditions occur during the developmental period for speech and language. In some cases, SLPs focus on language and voice problems exhibited by medically fragile children. However, many of these children are also at risk for speech sound disorders. For example, children who have had tracheostomies for any significant length of time have been reported to show articulation and phonological problems (Singer et al., 1989; Kertoy, Guest, Quart, & Lieh-Lai, 1999). Kertoy et al. report slow development of sound acquisition, vowel production, and distinction between voiced and voiceless stops for some children with a history of tracheostomy. They also report the excessive use of phonological processes among those children. The most common processes reported were stridency deletion, liquid deviation, and cluster reduction.

Assessment of Medically Fragile Children   The overall goals of assessment with medically fragile children are not all that different from early evaluations of any child. SLPs wish to determine how the child's speech sound production compares to normative data for children of similar age and determine the factors that might be causing the child to fall behind. There are, however, several factors that the SLP must consider when planning the assessment of medically fragile children (Bleile & Miller, 1994):

- Use of universal precautions with this population is critical for the protection of the patient, the clinician, and other patients with whom the clinician works. Wearing gloves and sometimes masks and gowns may be a standard procedure in some medical settings. Hand washing and cleaning of toys and materials after each use are critical steps to prevent the transmission of disease.
- Assess the alertness oxygenation of the child. Many children may be on medication or have conditions that cause their level of alertness to vary. Some with breathing or cardiac conditions may have varying levels of oxygen in their bloodstream.
- Avoid overstimulation, presenting too many items at one time, rapid movement, or speaking too loudly. This can be especially difficult for children with neurologic conditions causing hyperdistractability.
- Avoid excessive handling. Not only are some medically fragile children tethered to an array of instruments and tubes, but some may be sensitive to touch. The latter is especially true of children with severe burns or a condition known as allodynia, where simple touching can be painful.
- Ensure proper positioning. The SLP may have to physically position the child to establish eye contact or to accommodate physical limitations. Some children may even need to be cradled.
- Alleviate fears of procedures. Many medically fragile children have been through several, often painful, medical procedures. They often fear any stranger approaching them in a medical setting.

Treatment of speech sound disorders exhibited by medically fragile children, as with any at-risk population, should be proactive. That is, the clinician wishes to identify any potential problems as early as possible to prevent or minimize their effect (Bleile & Miller, 1994). To this end, Bleile and Miller (1994) describe four options for the treatment of speech sound disorders in this population.

- *No treatment:* This is typically only an option for children who are too medically fragile or dying.
- *Parent counseling:* This is essentially for children who are progressing normally and do not have major risk factors. An example of a child requiring this level of treatment might be an otherwise healthy but premature infant. Typically, periodic reevaluations of speech and language development are indicated.
- *Speech treatment without accompanying language treatment:* This option would be appropriate for a small number of children who had some impediment to speech production but who were developing language appropriately.
- *Combined speech and language treatment:* This is the most common situation, where treatment for speech sound development is included as part of an early language intervention program.

STRUCTURAL DEFICITS RESULTING FROM ORAL SURGERY

Cancerous growths on the tongue, the floor of the mouth, and/or the mandible often require surgical removal of all or part of those structures. This surgery can have a devastating effect on many aspects of the patient's life, including the ability to speak and swallow. As Leonard states: "It is difficult to imagine pathology that affects more functions critical to life and the quality of life than those that require ablation (removal) of oral and/or oropharyngeal structures" (Leonard, 1994, p. 74). In 2009, the Oral Cancer Foundation indicated that more than 30,000 people in the United States are diagnosed with oral or pharyngeal cancer each year, and there is some evidence that that number is increasing. The two most commonly cited causes of oral cancer are the use of tobacco and alcohol, and exposure to the human papillomavirus version 16 (HPV-16). Cancerous lesions can occur in many locations in the oral and pharyngeal area including the tonsils, tongue, floor of the mouth, the maxilla, and the mandible. Cancer may spread to include several of those structures. Treatment typically includes radiation, surgery, or both. In recent years, chemotherapy has also been included as an option for some patients (Casper & Colton, 1998; Matthews & Lampe, 2005). Surgery involves the removal of portions of those structures in which the cancer is present. Removal of portions of the maxilla and mandible affects speech as well as a person's physical appearance. However, the greatest effect on speech occurs as a result of the removal of all or part of the tongue, a procedure known as a **glossectomy**.

The effects of glossectomy on speech intelligibility vary according to several factors, including the location of the tumor, the amount of tissue removed, and the surgical procedure used. Additionally, there are individual differences in how well patients adapt to the altered structure, making it difficult to predict how surgery will affect the speech of a specific individual.

In cases where a very small lesion is removed, the surrounding tissue may simply be sutured together (primary closure) (Matthews & Lampe, 2005). When larger amounts of tissue are removed, the surgeon may choose to reconstruct portions of the tongue by means of one of several techniques such as skin grafts or moving a section of tissue with a blood supply (known as a flap) from areas within the oral structure (local flap) or outside the oral cavity, often from the forearm or chest (free flap), to replace the tissue removed in surgery (Casper & Colton, 1998; Matthews & Lampe, 2005; Thomas & Keith, 2005). Finally, in some patients, most or some of the tongue may be replaced by a prosthesis that, while lacking the flexibility of a human tongue, may replace some of the bulk to aid in speech and swallowing (Leonard & Gillis, 1982; Bredfeldt, 1992).

Recall that the production of consonant sounds involves altering the flow of air by bringing one articulator (often the tongue) into contact or approximation to another articulator (frequently the alveolar ridge or hard palate). Therefore, in addition to reconstructing the tongue, the ability to produce certain speech sounds may also be helped by lowering the palate. This is done by placing a specially made device called a palatal augmentation prosthesis (Leonard, 1994; Marunick & Tselios, 2004; Leeper, Gratton, Lapointe, & Armstrong, 2005). Palatal augmentation devices are usually constructed by a dental specialist known as a prosthodontist. The devices are specially made to fit each patient and constructed to provide maximum assistance for that patient with speech and swallowing. The underlying idea is that if the tongue cannot be raised adequately to contact the palate, the palate can be lowered so that the tongue may be more likely to contact the points of speech sound articulation.

The American Speech-Language-Hearing Association (1993) identifies the following specific tasks that an SLP may be required to perform when working with patients who have oral prostheses:

- Assess the patient's needs and appropriateness as a candidate for a prosthetic appliance
- Design features of the prosthesis for speech and/or swallowing facilitation
- Evaluate the effects of the prosthesis on speech and swallowing
- Teach the patient to care for the prosthesis
- Teach the patient to speak and swallow with the oral prosthesis
- Monitor effectiveness and use of the oral prosthesis

Assessment of Individuals with Glossectomy   Leonard (1994) provides three objectives of the assessment of individuals with partial or total glossectomy. Those objectives are identify those sounds that are in error, elaborate specifically the cause for the errors, and explore the possibilities for new or modified ways to produce the sounds in error.

To identify the sounds in error the SLP may use a formal speech sound inventory such as the *Goldman-Fristoe Test of Articulation-2* discussed earlier in this chapter. In addition to consonants, vowel production may also be affected by glossectomy. Therefore, the assessment should include vowel production tasks. Vowels are often assessed in an <u>h</u> vowel

<u>d</u> context such as *hid, heed, hide,* and so forth (Leonard, 1994). As with any assessment of speech sound production, the assessment of a glossectomy patient must include not only single-word utterances but multiword utterances and sentences. It is through these connected speech samples that the SLP can make judgments about the intelligibility of the patient's speech. Intelligibility may be assessed by means of formal or informal rating scales (Leonard, 1994; Casper & Colton, 1998; Leeper et al., 2005) or by tests designed to assess intelligibility among speakers with neurologic problems such as the *Assessment of Intelligibility of Dysarthric Speech* (Yorkston, Beukelman, and Traynor, 1984). This assessment instrument provides several measures including intelligibility for single words, intelligibility for sentences, rate of intelligible speech (number of intelligible words per minute), and a measure of communication efficiency. Sullivan, Gaebler, and Ball (2007) suggest that the intelligibility measures previously described should be supplemented by an assessment they refer to as "supplemented comprehension." This is a measure of the patient's intelligibility when the speaker employs additional strategies such as gesture, slow exaggerated articulation, and indicating the first letter of a word.

To help define the cause of the errors, an oral mechanism examination is performed. This enables the examiner to evaluate the amount and location of the tongue that has been removed and the range of motion and strength of the structure that remains. The SLP may model various tongue movements and have a mirror for the patient to see his or her attempts at imitating the clinician's movement. The clinician should assess the ability to raise the tongue as well as protrude and retract the tongue. Having the patient push against a tongue depressor may help to assess the strength of tongue movement. Several questions must be answered by the examiner concerning the nature of the sound errors made by the patient. Are sound errors made because the portion of the tongue that helps to form the sound is missing? Can the tongue no longer reach the typical place of articulation? Can the tongue not move quickly enough to move from sound to sound at a rate required for connected speech? It is also important to examine the patient's lips and teeth because some of the compensatory sounds to be taught later involve the use of these structures. Also, some types of palatal prostheses require teeth to anchor them.

Finally, the assessment should determine how the patient may develop alternative placements or different structures to make sounds that approach the sound the patient now omits or distorts. These alternative productions of sounds are called compensatory articulation. These decisions are based on the mobility of the remaining structures. For example, if the front of the tongue cannot reach the alveolar ridge for the production of <u>t</u> or <u>d</u>, can the middle portion reach the hard palate where a reasonable sound substitution might be produced? This information may also be valuable in constructing a palatal prostheses.

Treatment of Individuals with Glossectomy Treatment of speech sound disorders in patients with glossectomy centers around maximizing their ability to produce the sounds they are still able to produce and developing compensatory articulations for those that they are not able to produce. To meet these objectives, treatment frequently includes the following goals:

Increase the range and strength of motion. Surgery and radiation treatment may reduce muscle strength and limit the patient's ability to move whatever tongue structure remains. For purposes of speech and swallowing, SLPs want to be sure that the patient can move the remaining structure with as much range and strength as possible. This is often accomplished by various tongue exercises (for whatever parts of the tongue remain). These exercises involve protruding and retracting the tongue, raising the tip of the tongue (if the anterior portion is still present), and moving the tongue from side to side inside the mouth (Thomas & Keith, 2005). Once patients demonstrate that they can perform these exercises on their own, they should do them for short periods of time 5 to 10 times each day (Casper & Colton, 1998; Thomas & Keith, 2005).

Incorporate specific sound drills. In some cases, the patient may be able to produce some sounds with only slight distortion. These sounds may be produced correctly or near correctly with some increase in range of motion and/or strengthening of the tongue. For example, depending on which parts of the tongue have been removed, velar sounds such as k and g may be improved following range of motion and strengthening exercises involving lifting the back part of the tongue. Some modification of the placement or shaping of the remaining tongue may produce improved vowel production.

Develop compensatory articulations. For many patients, the ability to develop compensatory articulations may be the most important part of speech rehabilitation. The ability to develop compensations and the specific compensatory placements used vary from patient to patient and depend on the postsurgical oral structure. Also, to help develop compensatory articulations, the SLP should have some understanding of the acoustic aspects of speech sounds and how those acoustic cues are produced by the speech mechanism. For example, fricatives require air to be forced through a narrow opening, stops require that airflow to be completely stopped and then released. The task for the SLP and the glossectomy patient is to determine which structures are available to restrict or stop airflow as needed. In some cases, the pharynx may be used as an alternate place of articulation when the tongue is unable to reach the palate. The lips, teeth, and buccal cavity (cheeks) may be adapted to form anterior sounds when the anterior tongue is unable to achieve the typical placement for the production of front sounds (Skelly, Spector, Donaldson, Brodeur, & Paletta, 1971; Leonard, 1994; Furia et al., 2001). Often the compensatory articulations are perceived as closer to the intended target during connected speech than when produced in isolation. Furia et al. indicate, "The patient can learn to achieve new speech sound targets that approximate the acoustic characteristics of the original so closely that the listener will perceive them as the original" (Furia et al., 2001, p. 882).

Use contrastive drills. Having the patient produce words that differ in only one sound, either vowels (*pep, pip, pipe, peep,* etc.) or consonants (*face, pace, base, case,* etc.) while a listener attempts to identify the target word can help to sharpen the patient's articulatory precision (Leonard, 1994).

Slow the speaking rate. A slower speaking rate makes it easier for the patient to reach the articulatory targets and results in an easier perceptual task for the listener. This is true as long as the rate does not drop so low that the patient is essentially using a word-by-word production. Sullivan et al. (2007) suggest that if the rate falls below 100 words per minute, speech is no longer efficient.

Use inflection patterns and facial expressions to aid in communication. Factors such as pauses, pitch inflections, and even facial expressions are very helpful in communicating meaning in anyone's speech. A rising inflection at the end of an utterance suggests a question. Increasing the loudness and duration of important words is a way of verbally underlining the most important words in an utterance. Glossectomy patients should be encouraged to use these factors to their maximum to facilitate the expression of their intended meaning.

Consider augmentative/alternative communication. In some cases, the patient may be unable to develop effective oral communication following removal of significant portions of the oral speech mechanism. In such cases, the SLP may suggest the use of various alternative or augmentative communication devices. These devices may range from low-tech communication boards where the patient points to pictures to relatively sophisticated electronic communicators (Sullivan et al., 2007).

For those medical personnel who come in contact with glossectomy patients, especially in the period shortly after surgery, the next section discusses several suggestions that might help communication with these patients.

Suggestions for Medical Personnel Dealing with Glossectomy Patients Some of these suggestions are based on information provided by Casper and Colton (1998) and Thomas and Keith (2005).

1. Be sure that the patient has an alternate means of communication handy. A dry erase board or pad and pencil may suffice. If the patient is able to use them, electronic devices allowing text messaging may be helpful.
2. Assist the SLP by suggesting words or concepts to include on a communication chart or board.
3. Don't be put off by a patient who claps his hands or snaps his fingers to get your attention.
4. Reduce background noise such as televisions and radios when talking to the patient.
5. Watch the patient's facial expressions and body postures for additional cues to communicative intent.
6. Remember that intercom systems between the patient's room and the nurses' station may not be useful for glossectomy patients.
7. Be patient. Remember that the patient may be experiencing a great deal of fear, anger, and frustration, much of which is centered around the ability to communicate.

To use speech sounds to communicate effectively, speakers must be able to make precise and rapid movements of the speech structures to physically form the sounds of their language at just the right time and in the right order. Although this motor activity is challenging, it is not the only task that speakers must master for effective communication. On a cognitive-linguistic level, speakers must develop a systematic organization of speech sounds including rules that govern the use of those sounds in a particular language. Many physical conditions can result in speech sound disorders. However, in the majority of cases, the cause of these disorders is unknown. SLPs must describe the nature of the speech sound disorder and develop intervention techniques that are effective and efficient for a specific person in a specific situation. Whether speech sound disorders are encountered in an educational or medical setting, the SLP's tasks of assessing and treating speech sound disorders are facilitated by having a good working relationship with other professionals in those settings as well as the client's family.

Terms to Know

Articulation
Phonological disorder
Substitutions
Distortions
Omissions
Lisp
Sibilant sounds
Central lisp
Lateral lisp
Initial position
Final position
Medial position
Prevocalic
Postvocalic
Intervocalic
Organic disorders
Malocclusion
Macroglossia
Microglossia
Ankyloglossia
Tongue thrust
Hearing impairment
Dysarthria
Apraxia of speech
Metathetic errors

Developmental apraxia of speech (DAS)
Speech sound inventories
Contextual tests
Pattern analyses
Phonetic environment
Phonetic context
Establishment
Generalization
Maintenance
Ear training
Auditory stimulation
Phonetic placement
Successive approximation
Position generalization
Context generalization
Linguistic unit generalization
Sound and feature generalization
Situation generalization
Negative practice
Conceptualization
Minimal pairs
Speech notebook
Whole-class language experience
Glossectomy

Study Questions

1. Discuss the relationship between phonological disorders and each of the following:

   intelligence language development

   reading malocclusion

   spelling siblings

2. Briefly describe the differences between a speech sound inventory, a contextual test, and a pattern analysis.

3. Describe some differences in the way an SLP might treat motor-based and cognitive-linguistic speech sound disorders.

4. Briefly discuss how speech sound disorders might affect a student's academic performance in school.

5. Discuss specific activities that a classroom teacher and/or parent could use to assist in communication-centered treatment for a student with a phonological disorder.

6. Identify some of the unique challenges an SLP might encounter when providing services to medically fragile children.

Bibliography

Aase, D., Hovre, C., Krause, K., Schelfhout, S., Smith, J., & Carpenter, L. (2000). *Contextual Test of Articulation.* Eau Claire, WI: Thinking Publications.

American Speech-Language-Hearing Association. (1993). *Oral and oropharyngeal prostheses* [Guidelines, Knowledge and Skills]. Retrieved May 21, 2010, from http://www.asha.org/docs/html/PS1993-00100.html.

Bankson, N., & Byrne, M. (1962). The relationship between missing teeth and selected consonant sounds. *Journal of Speech and Hearing Disorders, 24,* 341–348.

Barlow, J., & Gierut, J. (2002). Minimal pair approaches to phonological remediation. *Seminars in Speech and Language, 23,* 57–68.

Bernthal, J., Bankson, N., and Flipsen, P. (2009). *Articulation and phonological disorders: Speech sound disorders in children. (6th ed.)* Boston, MA: Allyn & Bacon.

Bird, J., Bishop, D., & Freeman, N. (1995). Perception and awareness of phonemes in phonologically impaired children. *European Journal of Disorders of Communication, 27,* 289–311.

Bleile, K., & Miller, S. (1994). Toddlers with medical needs. In J. Bernthal & N. Bankson (Eds.), *Child phonology: Characteristics, assessment and intervention with special populations.* New York, NY: Thieme Medical Publishers.

Bloch, R., & Goodstein, L. (1971). Functional speech disorders and personality: A decade of research. *Journal of Speech and Hearing Disorders, 36,* 295–314.

Boshart, C. A. (2004). *Practical procedures to generate speech development* [Seminar series]. Temecula, CA: Speech Dynamics.

Bredfeldt, G. (1992). Tongue prosthesis for a total glossectomy patient. *Journal of Prosthodontics, 1,* 131–133.

Bryant, B., & Bryant, D. (1983). *Test of Articulation Performance-Diagnostic.* Austin, TX: Pro-Ed.

Carter, E. T., & Buck, M. W. (1958). Prognostic testing for functional articulation disorders among children in the first grade. *Journal of Speech and Hearing Disorders, 23,* 124–133.

Casper, J., & Colton, R. (1998). *Clinic manual for laryngectomy and head/neck cancer rehabilitation* (2nd ed.). San Diego, CA: Singular.

Christensen, S., & Luckett, C. (1990). Getting into the classroom and making it work. *Language Speech and Hearing Services in Schools, 21,* 110–113.

Cowan, W., & Moran, M. (1997). Phonological awareness skills in children with articulation disorders in kindergarten to third grade. *Journal of Children's Communication Development, 8,* 31–38.

Daniloff, R. G., & Moll, K. L. (1968). Coarticulation of lip rounding. *Journal of Speech and Hearing Research, 11,* 707–721.

Davis, B. L. (2005). Clinical diagnosis of developmental speech disorders. In A. Kamhiand & K. Pollock (Eds.), *Phonological disorders in children.* Baltimore, MD: Brookes.

Davis, B. L., Jakielski, K. J., & Marquardt, T. M. (1998). Developmental apraxia of speech: Determiners of differential diagnosis. *Clinical Linguistics and Phonetics, 12*(43), 25–45.

Dodd, B. (1976). A matched comparison of the phonological systems of mental age matched, normal, severely sub-normal, and Down's disorders. *British Journal of Communication Disorders, 11,* 27–42.

DuBoise, E., & Bernthal, J. (1978). A comparison of three methods for obtaining articulatory responses. *Journal of Speech and Hearing Disorders, 43,* 295–305.

Faircloth, M., & Faircloth, S. (1970). An analysis of the articulatory behavior of a speech-defective child in connected speech and in isolated-word responses. *Journal of Speech and Hearing Disorders, 35,* 51–61.

Felsenfeld, S., McGue, M., & Broen, P. (1995). Familial aggregation of phonological disorders: Results from a 28-year follow-up. *Journal of Speech and Hearing Research, 38,* 1091–1107.

Fey, M., Cleave, P., Ravida, A., Long, S., Dejmal, A., & Easton, D. (1994). Effects of grammar facilitation on the phonological performance of children with speech and language impairments. *Journal of Speech and Hearing Research, 37,* 594–607.

Flipsen, P., Bankson, N., & Bernthal, J. (2009). Classification and factors related to speech sound disorders. In J. Bernthal, W. Bankson, & P. Flipsen (Eds.), *Articulation and phonological disorders: Speech sound disorders in children* (6th ed.). Boston, MA: Allyn & Bacon.

Forrest, K. (2002). Are oral-motor exercises useful in the treatment of phonological/articulatory disorders? *Seminars in Speech and Language, 23,* 15–26.

Fudala, J. B. (2000). *Arizona Articulation Proficiency Scale* (3rd ed.). Los Angeles, CA: Western Psychological Services.

Furia, C., Kowalski, L., Latorre, M., Angelis, E., Martins, N., Barros, A., & Ribeiro, K. (2001). Speech intelligibility after glossectomy and speech rehabilitation. *Archives of Otolaryngology Head and Neck Surgery, 127,* 877–883.

Gernand, K., & Moran, M. (2007). Phonological awareness abilities of 6-year-old children with mild to moderate phonological impairments. *Communication Disorders Quarterly, 28*, 206–215.

Goldman, R., & Fristoe, M. (2000). *Goldman-Fristoe Test of Articulation* (2nd ed.). Circle Pines, MN: American Guidance Service.

Gordon-Brannan, M., & Weiss, C. (2007). *Clinical management of articulatory and phonological disorders* (3rd ed.). Philadelphia, PA: Lippincott Williams & Wilkins.

Haynes, W., Haynes, M., & Jackson, J. (1982). The effects of phonetic context and linguistic complexity on /s/ misarticulation in children. *Journal of Communication Disorders, 15*, 287–297.

Hodson, B. W. (2004). *Hodson assessment of phonological patterns* (3rd ed.). Austin, TX: Pro-Ed.

Hodson, B. W., & Paden, E. (1981). Phonological processes which characterize unintelligible and intelligible speech in early childhood. *Journal of Speech and Hearing Disorders, 46*, 369–373.

Hoffman, P., & Norris, J. (2005). Self-organization of a neuro-network. In A. Kamhi & K. Pollock (Eds.), *Phonological disorders in children: Clinical decision making in assessment and intervention.* Baltimore, MD: Brookes.

Hoffman, P., Norris, J., & Monjure, J. (1990). Comparison of process targeting and whole language treatments for phonologically delayed preschool children. *Language, Speech and Hearing Services in Schools, 21*, 102–109.

Kertoy, M. K., Guest, C., Quart, E., & Lieh-Lai, M. (1999). Speech and phonological characteristics of individual children with a history of tracheostomy. *Journal of Speech, Language and Hearing Research, 42*, 621–635.

Khan, L., & Lewis, N. (2002). *Khan-Lewis Phonological Analysis* (2nd ed.). Circle Pines, MN: American Guidance Service.

Klein, E. S. (1996). *Clinical phonology: Assessment and treatment of articulation disorders in children and adults.* San Diego, CA: Singular.

Kresheck, J., & Sokolofsky, G. (1972). Imitative and spontaneous articulatory assessment of four-year-old children. *Journal of Speech and Hearing Research, 15*, 729–732.

Leeper, H., Gratton, D., Lapointe, H., & Armstrong, E. (2005). Maxillofacial rehabilitation for oral cancer. In P. Doyle & R. Keith (Eds.), *Contemporary considerations in the treatment and rehabilitation of head and neck cancer: Voice speech and swallowing.* Austin, TX: Pro-Ed.

Leonard, R. J. (1994). Characteristics of speech in speakers with glossectomy and other oral/oropharyngeal ablation. In J. Bernthal & N. Bankson (Eds.), *Child phonology: Characteristics, assessment, and intervention with special populations.* New York, NY: Thieme Medical Publishers.

Leonard, R. J., & Gillis, R. E. (1982). Effects of a prosthetic tongue on vowel intelligibility and food management in a patient with total glossesctomy. *Journal of Speech and Hearing Disorders, 47*, 25–29.

Lippke, B., Dickey, S., Selmar, J., & Soder, A. (1997). *Photo Articulation Test* (3rd ed.). Austin, TX: Pro-Ed.

Long, S. (2004). *Computerized profiling.* Retrieved May 21, 2010, from http://www.computerizedprofiling.org

Mackay, L., & Hodson, B. (1982). Phonological process identification of misarticulation of mentally retarded children. *Journal of Communication Disorders, 12*, 243–250.

Marunick, M., & Tselios, N. (2004). The efficacy of palatal augmentation prostheses for speech and swallowing in patients undergoing glossectomy: A review of the literature. *Journal of Prosthetic Dentistry, 91*, 67–74.

Matthews, T. W. & Lampe, H. B. (2005). Treatment options in oral cancer. In P. Doyle & R. Keith (Eds.), *Contemporary considerations in the treatment and rehabilitation of head and neck cancer: Voice, speech and swallowing.* Austin, TX: Pro-Ed.

McDonald, E. T. (1964). *A deep test of articulation.* Pittsburgh, PA: Stanwix House.

Moran, M. J., Money, S., & Leonard, D. (1984). Phonological process analysis of the speech of mentally retarded adults. *American Journal of Mental Deficiency, 89*, 304–306.

Mowrer, D. (1971). Transfer of training in articulation therapy. *Journal of Speech and Hearing Disorders, 36*, 427–446.

National Institute on Deafness and Other Communication Disorders. (2009). Statistics on voice, speech, and language. Retrieved May 21, 2010, from http://www.nidcd.nih.gov/health/statistics/vsl.asp

Norris, J., & Hoffman, P. (1990). Language intervention within naturalistic environments. *Language Speech and Hearing Services in Schools, 21*, 72–84.

Panagos, J., Quine, H., & Klich, R. (1979). Syntactic and phonological influences in children's articulations. *Journal of Speech and Hearing Research, 22*, 841–848.

Pena-Brooks, A., & Hegde, M. N. (2007). *Assessment and treatment of articulation & phonological disorders in children* (2nd ed.). Austin, TX: Pro-Ed.

Powers, M. J. (1971). Clinical and educational procedures in functional disorders of articulation. In L. Travis (Ed.), *Handbook of speech pathology and audiology.* Englewood Cliffs, NJ: Prentice Hall.

Ruscello, D., St. Louis, K., & Mason, N. (1991). School-aged children with phonological disorders: Coexistence with other speech/language disorders. *Journal of Speech Language Hearing Research, 34*, 236–242.

Rvachew, S., Ohberg, A., Grawburg, M., & Heyuding, J. (2003). Phonological awareness and phonemic perception in 4-year-old children with delayed expressive phonology skills. *American Journal of Speech-Language Pathology, 12*, 463–471.

Schmauch, V., Panagos, J., & Klich, R. (1978). Syntax influences and accuracy of consonant production in language disordered children. *Journal of Communication Disorders, 11*, 315–323.

Secord, W. (1981). *C-PAC: Clinical probes of articulation consistency.* Columbus, OH: Merrill.

Secord, W., & Donohue, J. (2002). *Clinical assessment of articulation and phonology.* Greenville, SC: Super Duper Publications.

Shriberg, L. D. (1980). Developmental phonological disorders. In T. J. Hixon, L. D. Shriberg, & J. H. Saxman (Eds.), *Introduction to communication disorders*. Englewood Cliffs, NJ:, Prentice Hall, Inc.

Shriberg, L. D., & Kwiatkowski, J. (1980). *Natural process analysis*. New York, NY: Wiley.

Shriberg, L., & Kwiatkowski, J. (1994). Developmental phonological disorders I: A clinical profile. *Journal of Speech and Hearing Research, 37*, 1100–1126.

Shriberg, L. D., & Widder, C. (1990). Speech and prosody characteristics of adults with mental retardation. *Journal of Speech and Hearing Research, 33*, 627–653.

Singer, L., Kercsmar, C., Legris, G., Orlowski, J., Hill, B., & Doershunk, C. (1989). Developmental sequelae of long-term infant tracheostomy. *Developmental medicine and child neurology, 31*, 224–230.

Skelly, M., Spector, D., Donaldson, R., Brodeur, A., & Paletta, F. (1971). Compensatory physiologic phonetics for the glossectomee. *Journal of Speech and Hearing Disorders, 36*, 101–114.

Smith, M. W., & Ainsworth, S. (1967). The effect of three types of stimulation on articulatory responses of speech defective children. *Journal of Speech and Hearing Research, 10*, 333–338.

Snow, K. (1961). Articulation proficiency in relation to certain dental abnormalities. *Journal of Speech and Hearing Disorders, 26*, 209–212.

Snow, J., & Milisen, R. (1954). The influence of oral versus pictorial representation upon articulation testing results. *Journal of Speech and Hearing Disorders*, monograph supplement, 4, 29–36.

Stoel-Gammon, C., & Dunn, C. (1985). *Normal and disordered phonology in children*. Austin, TX: Pro-Ed.

Stoel-Gammon, C., Stone-Goldman, J., & Glaspey, A. (2002). Pattern-based approaches to phonological therapy. *Seminars in Speech and Language, 23*, 3–13.

Sullivan, M., Gaebler, C., & Ball, L. (2007). *Supporting persons with chronic communication limitations: Head and neck cancer*. Paper presented at the American Speech-Language-Hearing Association convention, Boston, MA.

Taylor, O. (1986). Language differences. In G. Shames & E. Wiig (Eds.), *Human communication disorders* (2nd ed.). Columbus, OH: Merrill.

Thomas, J., & Keith, R. (2005). *Looking forward: The speech and swallowing guidebook for people with cancer of the larynx or tongue* (4th ed.). New York, NY: Thieme.

Tyler, A. (2002). Language-based intervention for phonological disorders. *Seminars in Speech and Language, 23*, 69–81.

Tyler, A., Lewis, K., Haskill, A., & Tolbert, L. (2002). Efficacy and cross-domain effects of a morphosyntax and a phonology intervention. *Language Speech and Hearing Services in Schools, 33*, 52–66.

Tyler, A., & Sandoval, K. (1994). Preschoolers with phonological and language disorders: Treating different linguistic domains. *Language, Speech and Hearing Services in Schools, 25*, 215–234.

Van Riper, C., & Emerick, L. (1984). *Speech correction: An introduction to speech pathology and audiology* (7th ed.). Englewood Cliffs, NJ: Prentice Hall.

Weiner, F. (1981). Treatment of phonological disability using the method of meaningful minimal contrast: Two case studies. *Journal of Speech and Hearing Disorders, 46*, 97–103.

Weiner, F., & Bankson, N. (1978). Teaching features. *Language Speech and Hearing Services in the Schools, 9*, 29–34.

Weiner, F., & Ostrowski, A. (1979). Effects of listener uncertainty on articulation inconsistency. *Journal of Speech and Hearing Disorders, 44*, 487–493.

Wilson, F. (1966). Efficacy of speech therapy with educable mentally retarded children. *Journal of Speech and Hearing Research, 9*, 423–433.

Winitz, H. (1969). *Articulatory acquisition and behavior*. Englewood Cliffs, NJ: Prentice Hall.

Winitz, H. (1975). *From syllable to conversation*. Baltimore, MD: University Park Press.

Yorkston, K., Beukelman, D., & Traynor, C. (1984). *The assessment of intelligibility of dysarthric speech*. Austin, TX: Pro-Ed.

Chapter 5

CHILDREN WITH LIMITED LANGUAGE

EPISODE 5–1

Arnold Stephens is 3 years old and he cannot talk. You might assume that this would make his existence quite difficult, but actually, Arnold's life is fairly uncomplicated. He has no consistent playmates, gets the full attention of his parents, and is catered to around the clock. At noon, soup and sandwiches magically appeared on the kitchen table. At 3:00, it is "juice time" and mother opens the refrigerator and pours juice into his Mickey Mouse cup. Arnold rarely has to ask for anything . . . it is always there because his needs are anticipated. After all, he couldn't talk, although his parents desperately wanted him to. Mom and Dad often try to make Arnold talk by encouraging him to imitate. He watches these adults with fascination, and a certain sense of amusement, but he does not imitate. One time, the parents go too far and try to get Arnold to imitate saying the word *juice*. They say he can't have the drink unless he tries to say the word. Arnold throws a tantrum that registers about a 7 on the Richter scale, and the parents know never to do THAT again. As time goes by, the mother talks less and less to Arnold. After all, if no one answers, you tend to give up. Arnold's favorite activity is to play outside in the fenced backyard in his sandbox. One day on a talk show, Mrs. Stephens learned that the local public school system would be providing a preschool program for 3- to 5-year-old children with disabilities (including speech and language). She is elated that finally someone is going to do something about Arnold's problem.

EPISODE 5–2

Max Metcalf could only produce utterances consisting of a single word. This means that he can make simple requests quite efficiently. When he wants some milk, he could say "milk" and it would be provided. But when Max wants to explain something more complicated, he finds it quite difficult to communicate it in a few single words. For instance, one time his family was at the mall and Max wanted to go home. He did not have the words to explain this to his mother. Ultimately, he became so frustrated that he threw himself onto the carpet in the wide, central hallway of the mall and propelled himself around in a small circle, screaming like one of the Three Stooges used to do in the movies. Max's mom hates his tantrums, especially when they occur in public, so she scooped him up and the family terminated their shopping. The mother always feels guilty giving in to these behavioral displays, which are quite frequent both at home and in public, but sometimes it is the only way to make it through the day. The parents spend many hours arguing about Max and how to deal with his lack of communication and behavior problems because they are having a negative impact on both the child and the family.

EPISODE 5–3

Amanda Berringer has just taken a job at a children's hospital in a large urban area. One facet of her new position is providing services to children born with a variety of "high-risk" conditions. Such children enter the world with Down syndrome, fetal alcohol syndrome, craniofacial anomalies, cerebral palsy, exposure to prenatal toxins or trauma, abnormalities during the birth process such as oxygen deprivation, and many other conditions. One commonality among the conditions, however, is that research conclusively shows that these children are at risk for delayed or abnormal language development. Amanda knows that one clinical target that she needs to focus on with these cases is working with parents to facilitate communication development from birth until at least age 3 years or beyond.

EPISODE 5–4

Julie Christopher is a kindergarten teacher in the Highland Park Elementary School. This year she has Marcus Simmons in her class. Marcus had been diagnosed at age 3 years with cognitive impairment, and at age 5 years he had a limited vocabulary and spoke only in one- and two-word utterances. Julie and the SLP work together to facilitate Marcus's language development during regular classroom activities, and he also participates in treatment sessions outside the classroom. The specific language goals that were developed for Marcus include increasing vocabulary size and expanding one- and two-word utterances to three and four words in length. Julie is shown how to stimulate vocabulary during normal classroom activities such as art, music, circle time, and snack time. She is encouraged to frequently model vocabulary, expand shorter utterances into longer ones, and reinforce Marcus with additional attention when he produces longer verbalizations. The SLP periodically takes communication samples in the classroom to monitor progress and works with Marcus's mother to extend the treatment into the home environment.

GENERAL OVERVIEW OF LIMITED LANGUAGE DISORDERS: NATURE, CAUSATION, SYMPTOMS, AND RELATED PROBLEMS

Episode 1 illustrates several interesting aspects about some children with **limited language**. It could have just as easily been about a special education teacher who had a child in the classroom who did not talk or a kindergarten teacher who had a nonverbal child in the classroom for part of each day. The example could also have involved any number of medical professionals from physicians and nurses to physical and occupational therapists. The tendencies are the same: If a child does not talk, people often tend to address less language to that child and anticipate his or her needs. Those around such a child sometimes do these things because they know that the child cannot communicate effectively in gestures or words. This is especially true if the teacher is responsible for many other children in the same room, if a parent has several children in the family to care for, or if a medical professional is providing rehabilitation to groups of patients.

One important point to realize about children with limited language is that their problem often involves a number of participants. Parents, teachers, medical professionals, siblings, and peers become unwitting confederates and integral parts of the disorder. In the case of Arnold Stephens, he could not talk, and his parents learned to lower their expectations for communication. He could not ask for things, so people anticipated his needs and provided items before he even requested them. Life became a series of episodes that almost automatically unfolded without a real need to communicate. Soon, a comfortable medium was reached in which the child's life ran effectively without much communication. Does this mean that parents and professionals *caused* the child's language delay? Certainly not. The reactions of the parents and professionals are most likely the *result* of the child's language delay and not the cause. But these reactions do serve to *maintain* the problem.

Episode 2 illustrates another common scenario involving children with language disorders. In this situation, unlike the one with Arnold Stephens, life is *not* going along smoothly for the child and his parents. In fact, there is frustration, guilt, and behavior problems. Baltaxe (2001) reports that approximately 50 percent of children with communication disorders exhibit significant behavior problems. Some authorities attribute at least a portion of these difficulties to the communication disorder itself. When a child cannot communicate needs with gestures or language, acting out behaviorally is often quite effective, as illustrated in episode 2. Just as in episode 1, however, people in Max's environment are playing a role in his disorder by reinforcing tantrums as an effective method of communication. Fortunately, most studies generally support the finding that as children learn to communicate more effectively, behavior problems tend to decrease (Silverman, 1989).

Another curious aspect about dealing with children with limited language is that some parents and teachers may expect the speech-language pathologist (SLP) to remediate the problem single-handedly, shrouded in a small treatment room away from all legitimate needs to communicate in daily life. If the SLP does try to work with the child in isolation, situations that mimic real activities are constructed, and it is hoped that these artificial circumstances will generalize to the complex world of the classroom and home. An illogical and impossible task, you say? We agree!

The child with no language or limited language may not learn to communicate effectively unless at some point the treatment is conducted in the real world, with real people in legitimate interactions. Throughout the day, good language models must be provided and cues must be given at opportune times so that the child can produce target utterances. The child's life must be made a little more difficult by people failing to anticipate his needs and requiring the best communicative attempt the child is capable of producing during interactions. You can already see that we are going to push very hard in this chapter to make the case that *the child with limited language is part of a working system of people and events*. The implication of this is that assessment and treatment *must* include as much of the child's natural system as possible. This is not to say that individual treatment is not necessary because it certainly is in many cases. However, as we state in Chapter 1, at some point a team approach is necessary if the child has any hope of generalizing communication into natural environments. Teachers, medical professionals, and parents should *expect* the SLP to encourage their involvement in both assessment and treatment because of the vast amount of information they possess and the significant number of hours they spend with the child.

Episode 3 illustrates several important points. First, children who represent a wide variety of different conditions at birth will be at risk for a delay or disorder of language development. We know, for example, that a child born with fetal alcohol syndrome will have a high probability of struggling with the acquisition of language and communication abilities. This is especially true in the high-risk populations of children who begin their lives with poor nutrition, low birth weight, early respiratory distress, abusive home environments, or a wide variety of "syndromes" (Hubatch, Johnson, Kistler, Burns, & Moneka, 1985; Fox, Long, & Langlois, 1988; Paul, 2007). Research shows that even children born without a syndrome or identifiable condition such as Down syndrome can be at risk for language delay. For instance, children who are premature at birth are likely to acquire language slower than are full-term babies. Children born with respiratory distress who must be aided by a ventilator exhibit slower language acquisition than do peers who experienced no abnormalities in the birth process. It is interesting to note that language seems to be affected in a wide variety of congenital conditions. This is because language requires a host of cognitive, social, motoric, as well as linguistic abilities to develop normally, as we discussed in Chapter 3. Language is a complex ability that can be affected by so many different factors. Thus, it is not surprising that syndromes resulting in hearing impairment, motoric disorders, neurologic abnormalities, and cognitive difficulties *all* result in language delay. If anything is going to go awry in development, language is almost always at risk because of its complex nature that relies on so many subsystems in the human body. Thus, language is perhaps the most sensitive barometer of whether a child is developing normally. It is not unusual for severely involved children to be able to do gross motor behaviors and walk in a relatively normal fashion. Interruptions in more intricate skills such as fine motor ability and language development are signals that the child may have a developmental disorder. This is why language disorder is almost always a symptom of both serious conditions as well as those that are more subtle, such as learning disability.

A second implication of Episode 3 is that knowledge of the research on language development in children with conditions discovered at birth allows speech-language professionals the opportunity to engage in early intervention so that the impact of the disorder on communication development is minimized if possible. This is why Amanda will work with parents and families during the first year of life, even though this is a period in which even normally developing children are not producing much speech and language. Any proactive program that can be provided for high-risk children is much better than waiting for the children to fall behind.

Episode 4 shows that even though a child is chronologically beyond the preschool years, he can still be communicating using a limited language system. When such children reach school age, they are typically included in the "normal" classroom and are not isolated in remedial classes as was often done decades ago. Thus, limited language cases can be found in older children if their cognitive and linguistic limitations are severe enough, and professionals should not think of children who have limited language as exclusively in the preschool age group.

Chapter 3 establishes that language is the system of rules and symbols that humans use to communicate. It is rather like language is the music, and speech is the instrument that produces the song. Without the music, you would have just random notes played by the instrument. So, children must learn word meanings and how to combine words to make their needs known to others in the environment. In the space of only three to four years, a normal child must learn both the language and how to produce it intelligibly for communication. The typical child often receives little direct help in acquiring language, and sometimes even develops language despite a good deal of interference.

TWO MAJOR DIVISIONS OF LANGUAGE IMPAIRMENT

Child language disorders may be divided, for our purposes, into two major groups that represent children who are in two different phases of linguistic development. Dividing children by language level rather than by etiology or disorder makes understanding language impairment a bit easier and has been commonly done in textbooks on the subject (Paul, 2007; Haynes & Pindzola, 2007). The first group of children exhibits primitive communication most often seen in the beginning stages of language development. The communication of these children may range from exclusive use of gestures to the possible combination of two to three words in an utterance. Throughout this chapter, we refer to these children as having "limited language." Notice that we have not mentioned a child's chronological age as a requirement for having limited language. This is because a child, or an adult for that matter, can be communicating at this level regardless of age. A person with a severe cognitive impairment can be a single or early multiword communicator for an entire lifetime.

The second group of children with language disorders communicates in full sentences and may very well be capable of constructing utterances that are very long and complex. This population not only can use language for verbal communication but also in activities involving literacy skills such as reading, writing, and spelling. In the present text, we refer to this second group of children as "syntax-level" youngsters. These children may exhibit some more subtle disorders of language involving use of word endings (morphology), construction of certain complex sentences (syntax), and/or comprehension of elaborate utterances. These children often have difficulty making their language appropriate for the variety of changing social and educational circumstances in daily life (pragmatics). Most often their literacy skills such as reading and writing are affected as well by an underlying language disorder. The present chapter deals with children who have limited language, whereas youngsters talking at the sentence level are discussed in Chapter 6.

WHO ENCOUNTERS CHILDREN WITH LIMITED LANGUAGE?

As the title of this textbook indicates, professionals in medical/clinical settings as well as in educational environments see children with limited language abilities. In medical settings, speech-language pathologists, physical therapists, social workers, occupational therapists, physicians, and nurses routinely see these children from birth until they are seen by professionals in the educational system. No matter what kind of treatment is needed by a child, communication is always a vital part of the relationship between a clinician and a client. All members of the rehabilitation team should be aware of the communication goals of a particular child and incorporate these into all interactions in the medical/clinical setting. In many cases, children come to medical/clinical settings for outpatient treatment sessions until they have transitioned into the school system, and some continue to receive supplemental therapy in clinical settings even after they are enrolled on the caseload of the public school speech-language pathologist.

In the educational setting, teachers in regular as well as special education classrooms encounter children with limited language. Many people still think that school systems are not responsible for providing services for students with disabilities until they enter kindergarten. However, with the advent of **PL 99-457**, the U.S. public school systems are required to provide services for children with disabilities between the ages of 3 and 5 years. Many school systems have even taken responsibility for working with the birth to 3 years population even though they are not legally mandated to do so at the present time. Early childhood teachers and early childhood special educators have the primary responsibility for dealing with this population of children and perhaps will benefit the most from this particular chapter. As mentioned earlier, the bulk of the preschool children seen by the early childhood special education teacher will have language delays. Early childhood special education teachers need to know about the kinds of language impairments observed in the preschool population, about the speech-language pathologist's functions as a team member in assessment and treatment, and about the way(s) to make a contribution to the intervention process during day-to-day classroom interactions. This also applies to kindergarten teachers and those who teach "developmental kindergarten" or "prekindergarten" classes.

Those regular classroom teachers who are preparing to deal with "normally developing children" may be reading this and saying to themselves, "This doesn't apply to me." However, as we indicate in an earlier chapter, the current trend is toward more *inclusion* of children with disabilities in the normal classroom, not *exclusion*. The movement toward inclusion seems to be gaining momentum among professionals, and we should not expect it to diminish any time soon; on the contrary, we should anticipate *increased* integration of children with disabilities into classroom environments. The idea of incorporating children with disabilities into typical classrooms is consistently supported by legal decisions going back three decades. It is not unusual for a visitor to a "normal classroom" to see children with electronic communicators, wheelchairs, auditory trainers or a child with an aide to assist her in basic daily tasks. Some children in the regular classroom might have feeding or swallowing difficulties and those with serious respiratory problems may even be on ventilators. Teachers who conduct classes in music, physical education, or art will teach children with disabilities who are integrated into regular classrooms for all or part of their day. All of these regular education teachers, as mentioned in Chapter 1, *will* be asked to become part of the intervention team.

THE SYMPTOMS SEEN IN CHILDREN WITH LIMITED LANGUAGE

Children with limited language comprise three basic subgroups that are based on the length of utterance in their verbal communication. First, there are **nonverbal communicators** who, by definition, are not using verbal language. They may communicate with gestures or a combination of gesture and vocalization; however, they never say identifiable words. It should also be noted that the nonverbal child is not a child with an articulation disorder (see Chapter 4) who *has* language and is just unintelligible because of problems with sound production. Nonverbal children are nonverbal because they *have* no words. It is important to emphasize that these children may be *nonverbal*, but they are by no means *noncommunicative*. As stated earlier, they may be quite adept at communicating their needs through a combination of gestures and/or vocalizations. Many of these children understand some language but just cannot produce it.

The second subgroup of limited language children is those youngsters who speak primarily in one-word utterances. These are called **single-word communicators**, and they seem to be unable to produce word combinations. Thus, a single-word communicator may say "up" when trying to get the mother to lift him, "drink" when requesting a drink, or "horsie" when the car passes a pasture filled with horses. The parents of single-word communicators will attest to the fact that their child talks in one-word utterances. When asked if the child has ever produced a two-word combination, the parents will probably say "no." A child communicating at the single-word level is not necessarily using words produced verbally. The child can be on the single-word level if he is using some sort of alternative/augmentative communication device such as a communication board or electronic communicator. The point here is that most communications may be limited to the single-word level regardless of how the words are produced. We discuss **alternative/augmentative communication (AAC)** more fully in Chapter 12.

The third subgroup of children with limited language is **early multiword communicators**. They are called early multiword communicators because they are producing the most primitive and earliest-developing combinations of words that have been reported in the language development literature. For instance, an early multiword communicator may produce utterances such as "more milk," "daddy run," "mommy shoe," "juice allgone," "big doggie," "eat more cracker," "mommy fix car," "me drink more milk," "daddy garage." Note that some of these verbalizations are two words in length and some are three and four words long. Another item to notice is that most of the "little words" used in adult sentences such as *is*, *the*, *a*, and *in* are missing. Also omitted are word endings such as *-ing* and *-ed*. Just as children who use AAC devices can be at the single-word level as described previously, they can also be producing early multiword combinations. Thus, these utterances do not have to be produced verbally but can be produced by an AAC device.

As you can see, one way to characterize the primary "symptoms" seen in children with limited language is to describe the type of communication they produce. Note that we have not mentioned age, syndromes, or diagnostic labels here. A nonverbal client can be a preschooler, a school-age child, an adolescent, or even an adult. The same goes for single-word and early multiword level clients. Children representing all diagnostic labels (e.g., cognitive impairment, autism, Fragile X syndrome, hearing impairment) can be performing at any level of limited language described here. The task of the speech-language pathologist is to focus on and describe the communication of any child in assessment, and then move that child to the next higher level in treatment.

CHILDREN WITH LIMITED LANGUAGE WHO HAVE DIFFERENT "LABELS"

Some readers may be curious as to why we have not organized the language disorders section of this book by the type of disability a child represents. For example, we could have had a chapter on autism, one on cognitive impairment, and one on learning dis-abilities. One reason we did not organize the text in this manner is that the book is about communication disorders and not about the nature of these various conditions. There are some other important reasons as well. As most of you know, people in psychology and education have a history of "labeling" children as representing certain types of disorders. For instance, a child with an IQ below 70 may have formerly been labeled "mentally retarded." This term has fallen out of favor and is gradually being replaced by "cognitively impaired" or some other term, depending on geographical and professional preferences. There are many labels from which to choose, and interestingly many children have several of them (e.g., a single child could be labeled "cognitively impaired," "hearing impaired," "language delayed"). Also, professionals may not always agree on a particular label for a certain child. Unfortunately, labeling is not yet an exact science.

As we stated earlier, children with a variety of labels will have limited language. These children may or may not exhibit delays in domains other than communication such as motor skills, self-help abilities, social skills, or intelligence. In fact, a child with limited language may be perfectly normal in all of these abilities with communication as the primary developmental deficiency. These children are sometimes called **specifically language impaired (SLI)** (Watkins & Rice, 1994). Of course, language delay is seen in almost every type of condition affecting young children, including cognitive impairment, developmental delay, autism, hearing impairment, cleft palate, cerebral palsy, "high-risk" populations (resulting from respiratory distress or low birth weight), and other syndromes. The interesting point, however, is that there are no particular types of language symptoms associated with various con-genital or developmental conditions in children that significantly differentiate one group from another. In other words, there is no specific profile of language errors associated exclu-sively with a particular population. This in part is because of the heterogeneity of the disorders found in a particular diagnostic group. For example, children with autism can range from severely cognitively and linguistically involved to those children with complex language and literacy abilities. The diagnostic label of "autism" tells you very little in terms of what to expect with regard to language. Also, if you group children with different diagnostic labels by their language level (e.g., nonverbal, single-word, early multiword, syntax), you will prob-ably find that the types of language errors they make are similar whether they are children with autism, cognitive impairment, hearing impairment, learning disability, or specific language impairment. There certainly may be big differences in the way these groups respond to intervention or perhaps in the ways tests are administered to them, but the specific deficien-cies in communication are often far more similar than different. The implication here is that when the SLP evaluates a child the focus is on *communication ability, and the level of language development attained by the child,* as opposed to what label he or she has been given.

The other implication is that regardless of label, children who have language disorders are treated using the same basic set of techniques. So, when a teacher or medical profes-sional is trying to help a child with autism, cognitive impairment, or specific language impairment learn communication skills, she will use the same basic techniques for all of these children. The fact that you will not have to learn many different techniques to help children with communication disability in your clinic, classroom, or medical facility should be *good news* for SLPs, teachers, and medical professionals.

Here is a scenario involving autism that illustrates what we have been discussing. You are a first-grade teacher and a new child has transferred from another school system into your classroom. You have not yet met this new addition to your class, but your special education coordinator has received some paperwork from the child's old school system. According to the report, the student has been diagnosed with autism. In many cases, even though it may seem redundant, your school will want to reassess the child to determine whether he meets eligibility criteria for your school system and determine whether the former Individualized Education Program (IEP) goals are appropriate. Unfortunately, assessment methods and eligibility criteria vary considerably from state to state, and in some cases system to system. So, how helpful is the fact that the child has been diagnosed with autism?

1. *Do you know what to expect?* Actually, you do not know much at all if you look at the diagnosis. We have already stated that a child with autism can vary significantly in terms of cognitive, social, emotional, behavioral, and linguistic skills. If there ever was a disorder that exemplifies the **BACIS** of communication development, autism is very high on the list. Speech-language professionals know that children with autism vary considerably in cognitive ability, ranging from significant cognitive involvement to high-level children with Asperger syndrome who are capable of abstract thought, complex language, and literacy skills. Thus, the diagnosis of autism alone tells you nothing about the child's cognitive status. Socially, children with autism vary from those who will not even make eye contact with others to those who frequently demonstrate affection by hugging and enjoy the company of others. Some children with autism exhibit frequent negative emotion while others seem devoid of emotional reactions. Behavioral symptoms are highly variable in children with autism and can include self-stimulation, self-injury, obsession, insistence on sameness, vestibular stimulation (spinning), and many other manifestations. The particular pattern exhibited by an individual student, however, is highly variable across children. Many children with autism seem similar in some respects, yet each one is quite different. Regarding language symptoms, a child with autism can be communicating with gestures, single words, early word combinations, simple sentences, or complex sentences. Higher-level children with autism can read and write. So, what have the teacher and the SLP learned from the fact that this soon-to-be-arriving student has autism? The answer is very little. This student can come in talking and carrying his favorite reading book, or he could require assistance in every aspect of activities in the normal classroom.

2. *Does knowledge of the diagnosis help you to design your assessment?* The answer is probably not. It would be handy if there was a particular "test of autism" that focused on communication skill, but there is no such thing that is universally accepted. Basically, the IEP team will have to do assessments of this child and focus on individual areas of cognition,

social interaction, temperament, behavior, and language. We have already said that a child with autism can have differing strengths and concerns in all areas and there is no "profile" that you should expect. The SLP's assessment will focus on play, communicative intent, social interaction, analysis of language comprehension, inventory of phonology, gestural communication, and language production, among other things. The only way to find out how a child communicates is to focus on communication, not the label. So, when someone tells the SLP that a child has a particular condition, it always goes back to analyzing how the child communicates. That is highly similar whether the child has been diagnosed with autism, cognitive impairment, learning disabilities, hearing impairment, or any other syndrome. You have to inventory the strengths and limitations of expressive and receptive communication.

3. *Does knowledge of the diagnosis tell you which therapy technique to use?* This would only be true if there was a specific type of treatment that applied just to autism. Unfortunately, there is no single treatment that has been universally effective with children diagnosed as autistic. For example, you will see some children with autism in your classroom who are being treated by the SLP and school psychologist using highly behavioral techniques applied intensively to increase language and alter specific behaviors. On the other hand, some approaches focus on the BACIS of communication and incorporate most of the child's goals in play, social interaction, and functional communication. Finally, you will see other children with autism who are using some sort of nonverbal response mode such as sign language, communication boards, electronic communicators, and pictures to make their needs known. The point here is that the diagnosis of autism does not specify the type of treatment a child receives. What dictates the treatment mode is a thorough assessment, trial therapy to determine whether goals can be accomplished, and altering the treatment approach if the child is not making progress using a particular regime.

In summary, a focus on a general condition does not tell you much about the nature of the communication disorder you are likely to see and does not necessarily have implications for assessment or the type of treatment that will be prescribed. Certainly, a textbook describing the general nature of various conditions is a valuable resource for professionals. However, when considering communication disorders, it is more productive to focus on communication rather than symptoms affecting multiple domains of development.

GENERAL OVERVIEW OF THE ASSESSMENT PROCESS IN CASES OF LIMITED LANGUAGE (COMMON TO ALL SETTINGS)

EVALUATION OF CHILDREN WITH LIMITED LANGUAGE ABILITIES

A very important point to make at the outset of discussing assessment of a child with limited language is the necessity of a multidisciplinary evaluation. This is true in both medical and educational settings. In almost every case, the child with limited language is "high risk" for a wide variety of developmental disabilities. Because of the complexity in making a correct diagnosis, the involvement of a variety of professionals from audiology, speech-language pathology, medicine, education, psychology, special education, and a variety of other allied health disciplines is required. So, the first thing to understand about evaluation of the child with limited language is that no single professional should ever do it alone. This is not only against federal laws, but it is at best foolhardy, and at worst unethical.

When the speech-language pathologist is faced with a child who has limited language abilities, regardless of the youngster's chronological age, a primary consideration is always to ask the question *why*. If a child is 4 years old and should be speaking in four-word utterances but is still a nonverbal communicator, there must be some reason for this. If a child is 3 years old and still communicating in single-word utterances when the mean length of utterance should be near three words, the SLP must be curious about what has happened to the child. Unfortunately, you are not always able to answer the question of why a child has not developed normally with regard to communication. It is the ethical responsibility of the SLP, however, to at least examine potential reasons for the language delay. In examining these potential reasons for language impairment, you sometimes *do* find at least a partial explanation for the child's communication problem. But where would you look? What abilities would possibly be involved if a child's linguistic framework is inadequate, distorted, or nonexistent? As we have stated previously in Chapter 3, the linguistic framework is built on a foundation (BACIS), and it is possible that the language is impaired because of problems with these building blocks.

Thus, the SLP examines in detail, the *biological* bases of language, the *access* to a good language model, the *cognitive* abilities related to language, the presence of communicative *intent*, and the child's *social* behaviors. If any of these areas show a deficit, then you might begin to understand why a child has a language impairment. It is important for the teacher and medical professional to know that in the assessment of these building blocks of language, there are precious few standardized tests. The SLP must, therefore, rely on a combination of formal and informal assessment measures if information relevant to treatment is to be gathered. There is no "test" for access to a good language model, communicative intent, social behavior, or many cognitive and biological bases of language. Much of what the SLP will want to do involves observation of relevant play and interactions in natural settings such as the classroom and home. Research confirms that variables such as (1) language comprehension ability, (2) level of play development, (3) use of sounds in vocalizing, (4) evidence of an intent to regulate adult behavior/attention, and (5) use of communicative gestures in prelinguistic children are predictive of success in language development over a period of months (Calendrella & Wilcox, 2000). Thus, as a classroom teacher or medical professional, you should be aware that the SLP will appreciate spending a significant amount of observation time, and perhaps interaction time, in your setting to develop treatment goals for the child with limited language. Any cooperation that you can give in terms of allowing these observations and providing the SLP with the benefit of *your own* longstanding observations will be greatly appreciated. We briefly profile some assessment examples in each area in the following subsections.

BIOLOGICAL

The assessment of the biological prerequisites to language is very important and includes several areas.

1. *Sensory abilities:* One of the first things that the SLP requires in the evaluation of a child with limited language is an audiometric (hearing) evaluation. Federal law now mandates that infants be screened for hearing loss at birth, and it is usually the goal to provide intervention in the form of surgery or amplification by 6 months of age. It is very important to determine whether the child can hear adequately because hearing is *essential* to early language development. Also, performance in the assessment and treatment processes depends upon the child being able to hear language presented by the teachers, parents, and other team members. If the child does have a significant hearing loss, some sort of amplification (e.g., hearing aid, FM system) may be recommended. Certain children detected with hearing loss at birth may be candidates for a cochlear implant or other type of surgery to maximize their hearing ability. In this case, the teachers and medical professionals will want to become familiar with some information on types of hearing loss, surgical interventions, and amplification (see Chapter 10). Children with significant visual problems may need to be examined by an ophthalmologist and fitted with corrective lenses.

2. *Motor abilities and neurologic status:* If the child appears to have significant motor difficulties, it may be recommended that a neurologist be contacted for a consultation. A physical therapist may also be consulted regarding improvement of motor skills, and an occupational therapist may give input about adapting various objects (e.g., spoons, pencils, clothing) so that the child will have less difficulty in the activities of daily living. Chapter 12 deals with communication disorders that have specific neurologic causes.

3. *Anatomic structure:* In most cases, children with significant anatomic problems detected at birth will already have been treated surgically or with some sort of prosthetic device by the time a speech-language professional sees them in the school setting. In such cases, medical personnel such as surgeons, pediatricians, nurses, occupational therapists, speech-language pathologists, audiologists, psychologists, and dental professionals make up a team to deal with multiple areas of concern. For example, children born with clefts of the lip and palate are high risk for feeding difficulties, conductive hearing loss, language/speech delay and will undergo multiple surgical procedures before they reach the age of 5 years. In some cases, anatomic problems resulting in speech disorders may be caused by trauma such as in an accident and must be attended to if treatment of the communication impairment is to be successful. Chapter 11 discusses craniofacial anomalies and communication disorders. You can see that in the biological area, the SLP is interested in determining whether the mechanisms used for speech and language are operating at their highest level. Without adequate biological support, the language framework will not develop appropriately.

ACCESS TO A LANGUAGE MODEL

One of the most important aspects of learning language is the presence of a model or models that present examples of communication use in relevant situations. The child listens to these models and incorporates them into the developing language system. The major way that the SLP gains insight into the language model is to observe caretaker–child interaction. This may be done by placing the parent and child in a playroom and taking note of the types of communication modeled during play. Appendix 5–1 lists important social and linguistic characteristics of the language model presented to a child and is based on hundreds of studies of interactions of parents and normally developing children. In the school setting, the SLP is also interested in the language presented to the child by the teacher and others in the classroom setting. Often the SLP will ask to sit in the classroom and observe the child with language delay, the teacher, aides, and other children in the classroom to determine the frequency, type, and quality of interactions. Clinical observations and recent research show that some classroom environments are not particularly facilitative of interactions involving children with communication impairments. Specifically, Rhyner, Lehr, and Pudlas find the following:

> "Teachers did not provide a responsive classroom communicative environment for young developmentally delayed children in either child-directed or teacher-directed activities. In fact, the teachers often were either nonresponsive or responsive in a limited way to the children's attempts to initiate communicative interactions in both activities. There were few instances in which the teacher contingently responded to the child's communicative initiations in ways that led to maintenance of the interactions" (Rhyner, Lehr, & Pudlas. 1990, p. 95).

These results are especially interesting because the teachers involved in the research had stated that their specific intent during interactions was to "facilitate the children's communication and language learning." Prospective teachers reading the present book should not view this as an indictment of *all* teachers who deal with children with language impairment. Certainly, many teachers *do* provide good environments for communication development. The point here is that in most cases the SLP simply does not know what kind of classroom environment a particular child with language impairment is experiencing. We also realize that it is extremely difficult for teachers to remember the needs of one or two children with language impairments when there are 18 or so other children whose communication abilities are within normal limits. Most children in a classroom covet attention and verbal interaction. It is difficult for teachers to take the extra time needed to provide specialized stimulation to a child with a communication impairment.

An important part of the assessment process for children with limited language is a thorough evaluation of the classroom communication environment and an analysis of communicative demands of the curriculum. Teachers also vary considerably in their speech rate, language complexity, use of figurative language, and frequency of interaction with specific students. This observation lets the SLP know whether a particular child is exposed to the type of language models needed for development. If more or different types of models are required, the SLP can either (1) train the teachers/aides to provide such cues during normal interactions, or (2) arrange specific times for the SLP to enter the classroom and provide increased models during certain prescribed activities suggested through collaboration with the teacher.

There have not been as many investigations of interactions between medical professionals and language-learning children. However, it is often recommended that the child's environment be evaluated in terms of noise levels, opportunities for interaction, and the types of communications addressed to children in medical settings (Paul, 2007).

Another important provider of a language model is the parent. A routine part of assessing a child with a language disorder is to examine caretaker–child interaction strategies during free play and other activities (Haynes & Pindzola, 2007). A popular parent–child literacy activity is joint book reading, and the SLP may want to observe parents and children sharing books together to see the types of **language stimulation** provided by the parent (Kaderavek & Sulzby, 1998; Rabidoux & Macdonald, 2000).

The evaluation of language models available to the child with a language disorder is important in determining opportunities for language learning that currently exist. This assessment is also valuable in developing a treatment plan because part of the approach may involve training of parents, medical professionals, and education professionals to provide altered language models to facilitate learning. The SLP may see the child only for a limited time in treatment sessions, but teachers, parents, and medical professionals interact with the child throughout the day in the activities of daily living such as feeding, playing, dressing, and bathing. All of these activities are replete with opportunities to stimulate language development.

COGNITIVE ABILITY

As we stated previously, language rests on a cognitive base. Thus, children who are diagnosed as cognitively impaired are at risk for language delay. It is probable that the cognitive deficits are the cause of the language problem in such youngsters. If the child with a language delay is nonverbal, whether of normal or below normal intelligence, the SLP will attempt to examine the cognitive abilities most associated with language development. In many cases, standardized testing performed in a medical, clinical, or educational setting may have revealed cognitive deficits prior to the time the SLP evaluates the child.

If no prior assessment information exists, the SLP can use several ways to gain insight into a child's cognitive abilities associated with language. First, the SLP may simply want to watch the child play. We mentioned in an earlier chapter that children with cognitive deficits often play in a very primitive manner. For instance, they may throw, bang, or shake objects instead of using them appropriately. They may show little evidence of functional object use, object permanence, or means-end concepts. Thus, one level of cognitive assessment is to examine a child's free play and make some inferences about knowledge of concepts associated with language (Westby, 1980). This will most likely involve a visit by the SLP to the classroom or medical facility.

We emphasize here that although research shows certain cognitive abilities to be associated with language development, these abilities are not necessarily "prerequisite" to learning communication skills (National Joint Committee for the Communication Needs of Persons with Severe Disabilities, 2002). Often, cognitive goals are worked on concurrently with communication and children have been shown to benefit from such services (Brady & McLean, 2000; McCathren, 2000). On a general level, however, a child must have some basic understanding of objects, events, and relationships in the world before she can communicate about them.

INTENT TO COMMUNICATE

Without a reason to talk, a child will never develop language. SLPs will want to gather data on at least two important aspects. First, the SLP is interested in determining why the child does or does not make communicative attempts using gestures and/or vocal behaviors. You know that gestural communication develops prior to verbal communication and that there is a fairly predictable order to gestural development (Crais, Douglas, & Campbell, 2004). Most reasons for communication involve either (1) regulating the attention of other people (declarative communication), or (2) regulating the activity or behavior of other people (imperative communication). At the very least, the SLP will want to see whether the child regulates the attention and activity of others in natural situations and may also set up some particular situations in which the child might respond. For instance, the SLP would be greatly interested in finding out if the child asks for adult assistance (imperative) to accomplish some task in the classroom environment (e.g., pulls an adult to the shelf to obtain toy) or tries to direct adult attention (declarative) to a novel activity (e.g., points to a puddle of spilled paint and looks at the adult). If a child has these two types of intent to communicate he is well on the way to making progress in language treatment.

Interestingly, one of the earliest indicators of autism spectrum disorders is the absence of declarative communication (Haynes & Pindzola, 2007). Children with autism often regulate the behavior of adults through gestures and physical contact, but they may rarely use pointing, showing, and giving to regulate adult attention. This is one of the most promising diagnostic symptoms of autism and allows for early identification of the disorder even before age 2 years. The irony, of course, is that the average age of diagnosis of autism has been closer to 4 years of age. Hopefully, this will change with the current emphasis on early detection and intervention.

The second aspect the SLP wants to note about **communicative intent** is the *level* on which the intent is realized. For instance, a child can regulate adult attention in a totally nonverbal manner, simply by physically pulling the adult around. On the other hand, a child can pull an adult around and accompany the pulling with a vocalization. Finally, the child can regulate the adult behavior with words (*want, up*). Thus, the SLP gathers data on the types of communicative intents shown by the child with limited language and the levels on which these intents are demonstrated. SLPs do this using a variety of tasks and systems (Snyder, 1981; Coggins, Olswang, & Guthrie, 1987; Wetherby & Prizant, 1993, 2002). Brunson and Haynes (1991) and Rice, Sell, and Hadley (1990) provide concrete and practical examples of how SLPs can evaluate communication intent in a classroom context. Also included in the assessment of communicative intent is the influence of the environment on the child's reasons to talk. Does the child have *opportunities* to communicate, or does the teacher or medical staff anticipate all needs? Are peers or teachers talking for the child, eliminating the need to communicate? The SLP should do a careful analysis of the classroom, medical, and home environments.

SOCIAL ABILITIES

The SLP wants to determine whether the child possesses the social abilities mentioned in Chapter 3, namely, joint referencing, turn-taking, and the desire to interact with others. In an evaluation context, the SLP observes the child in play routines with peers and significant adults to find out whether the child has a preference for playing with others and focusing jointly on objects and activities. It is during these joint referencing routines that language can be stimulated by the SLP, teacher, medical professionals, and parents.

EVALUATION OF VERBAL/NONVERBAL COMMUNICATION

The beginning point for language assessment is the administration of a standardized test. The results of standardized testing allow the SLP to compare the child's performance to a normative sample of other children who took the test. In this way, the SLP can determine whether a child is performing significantly below the norm. Most standardized tests focus on language comprehension (pointing to pictures, performing actions when requested) and naming or describing pictures. Some tests require the child to perform examination tasks, and others use parents as informants because young children may not have the attentional abilities to take a test. Essentially, standardized tests determine whether a language problem exists, but they do not describe the nature of the disorder. Thus, it is important to follow an abnormal score on a standardized test with nonstandardized or descriptive procedures, such as language sampling. The language sample provides specific information on the types of language the child can produce and the kinds of errors the child makes.

Perhaps the easiest task the speech-language pathologist has with children with limited language is the assessment of their verbal communication. This, of course, is because they typically do not talk a great deal (especially if they are nonverbal), and there is little to actually assess. The greatest difficulty in assessing language productions of these children is to obtain a **representative language sample** of their communication. It is often the case that a child will talk more in the classroom and at home than in a testing situation when the SLP takes the child off to a small room and tries to talk one-on-one. Therefore, the classroom teacher should expect the SLP to ask permission to observe the child in the classroom setting, and the SLP may ask the parents about home visits. In the case of a nonverbal child, the SLP takes a complete inventory of gestures and vocalizations produced by the child. This can tell the SLP what sounds the child is capable of making even if she is not using real words. Research shows that some of the areas of BACIS are strong predictive variables for determining language growth in prelinguistic children. For instance, children who were assessed as having more sophisticated play (cognitive), clear communicative intent shown in gestures, good language comprehension, and the ability to make a variety of speech sounds have the best prognosis to develop language one year later (McCathren, Warren, & Yoder, 1996; Yoder, Warren, & McCathren, 1998; Calendrella & Wilcox, 2000). The SLP must ask teachers, medical professionals, and parents many questions regarding particular utterances they have heard the child produce in the classroom, medical, and home environments. There are some subtle differences in assessment of verbal productions depending on the child's level of language development. These are briefly discussed.

THE SINGLE-WORD CHILD

If the child is talking in single words, the SLP must gain insight into the number and types of words in the child's expressive vocabulary. It is unrealistic to expect that the SLP could possibly take such a large sample of language that every word the child knows would be captured. Probably the best way to obtain this type of information is to use the parents and professionals who have spent the most time with the child. In many cases, the SLP can ask these informants either to write down words the child says consistently or to complete a vocabulary checklist on which many words are listed that are often seen in the single-word period. Such checklists are typically arranged in categories such as foods, toys, people, and so forth. The teacher or parent simply checks the words or word approximations that the child typically produces in each environment. Similar information can also be gathered on language comprehension. Using informants in the single-word period has been shown to be quite valid and reliable in studies of this issue (Klee, Pearce, & Carson, 2000; Rescorla & Alley, 2001; Rescorla, Alley, & Christine, 2001; Fenson et al., 2003).

THE EARLY MULTIWORD CHILD

When the child begins to combine words, it becomes quite a bit more cumbersome to ask teachers and parents to remember the types of word combinations the child produces. Although these informants can easily recognize single words on a checklist that the child may have produced at a given time, there is much less reliability in asking parents and teachers to remember specific word combinations. This is not to say that parents and professionals should not be asked about word combinations because they often can reliably report specific utterances by the child in question (e.g., "I remember he said 'want book'").

Most SLPs rely to a larger extent on language sampling for the analysis of early multiword utterances. SLPs can take a language sample by visiting the classroom or clinical environment and taking notes on what the child says or by videotaping or audiotaping a play session and later transcribing the child's utterances.

Whatever the child's level of language development, the SLP must pinpoint the types of utterances the youngster can produce and compute the mean length of utterance (MLU) to select target therapy goals and monitor future progress. In Chapter 3, we provide a list of common multiword utterances that children produce. The SLP can take an inventory of the specific types of multiword utterances produced by the child to determine whether she has a good variety of word combinations.

GENERAL OVERVIEW OF DIRECT AND INDIRECT TREATMENT FOR CHILDREN WITH LIMITED LANGUAGE (COMMON TO ALL SETTINGS)

We want to emphasize three areas that deal with increasing the communication abilities in children with limited language. First, the types of treatment for these children vary on a continuum from structured to more child-directed. You can view this same continuum as "artificial" on one end and "naturalistic" on the other. Doing drillwork with a child in a small treatment room is artificial, and performing treatment tasks in the medical setting, home, or classroom during normal activities is regarded as more naturalistic.

A second area of importance involves the treatment targets selected by the SLP. Often, the SLP does not focus just on language, but also on some of the components (e.g., BACIS) that underlie linguistic acquisition. Thus, the SLP may be targeting biological, access to model, cognitive, intent, or social goals exclusively or in addition to the language objectives.

Finally, the mode of communication chosen for specific children may or may not involve exclusively using speech. The SLP may work with other team members and determine that it is unrealistic for certain children to express themselves using the speech mechanism as a result of motor, structural, cognitive, or other obstacles. In these cases, the child may have a gesture system, communication board, a picture exchange system for requesting things, or an electronic assistive (augmentative) device prescribed to use in communicative interchanges. We briefly expand on each of these three areas.

STRUCTURED VERSUS NATURALISTIC TREATMENT

As we mentioned, the SLP provides a continuum of services. On one end of the continuum is direct service provision in which the SLP takes the child out of the medical or classroom environment and performs drillwork activities calculated to increase the child's communicative ability. Basically, these sessions involve training the child to pay attention to language models and imitate words or word combinations to gradually encourage the child's spontaneous productions in more natural situations.

The number and length of sessions per week is determined jointly by members of the intervention team. The **structured treatment** format is best for teaching particular skills that may require massed practice, such as motor production of speech sounds or early establishment of imitative responses. This format is also used in cases of highly distractible children or those who may not benefit from treatment cues presented in more natural contexts. You can easily see that highly structured treatment is only a temporary method used at the beginning of some treatment plans. It is unlikely that the language trained in a drill procedure in an unnatural setting would generalize well to the natural environment. Thus, children receiving structured treatment must finally be dealt with using a more naturalistic approach. In most cases, the highly structured therapies in the school or medical setting are not exclusively used over long periods of time with a child. The SLP may also use a structured approach coupled with a more naturalistic classroom intervention approach. It would not be unusual, for example, for an SLP to see a child for individual structured treatment and again in the medical or classroom setting during more natural activities.

A variety of members of the intervention team conduct **naturalistic treatment** approaches to treatment of the child with limited language in the classroom, medical, and home environments. The SLP may want to come into the classroom or medical environment to conduct planned activities and provide language stimulation, models, and cues to facilitate language production in the child with limited language. On the other hand, the SLP may feel that the stimulation, models, and cues provided by the professional or parent are enough to result in adequate progress. In this case, the SLP acts mainly as a consultant and assists the professional in making routine classroom or clinical activities more easily facilitate language development for a particular child. The SLP can be active in periodically assessing the child's progress and acting as a resource for the medical or educational professional. For instance, the SLP might inform the professional that the goal has changed to include additional types of word combinations, or that a particular cue seems to work extremely well to elicit a correct response from a child. The SLP stays in close contact with the professional if a consultative/collaborative model is used.

Most naturalistic approaches to language have the following elements in common: (1) use of people, objects, and events in the natural environment; (2) modification of daily routines so that they are facilitative of language development; (3) provision of a greater number of opportunities for communication; (4) presenting many models of appropriate language in real situations using teachers, medical professionals, parents, and peers; and (5) presentation of specific cues to the child with limited language that are designed to elicit correct and more high-level language productions in real contexts. The keys, then, are *use of the natural environment, modification of daily routines, increased opportunity to communicate, provision of models in natural situations*, and *provision of specific cues the child can use to communicate at a higher level.*

There are many ways to provide increased opportunity in the environment. Appendix 5–1 illustrates seven principles that any parent or professional can easily incorporate into the daily routine. Appendix 5–2 provides 19 characteristics of a good language model for children with limited language. Any parent or professional who talks to children with language impairment should bear in mind that every interaction is a potential opportunity for the child to learn about the structure and use of language from a model. The more of these characteristics that can be incorporated, the greater the chance that the child with limited language will learn something about more advanced communication.

Appendix 5–3 and Appendix 5–4 illustrate two popular approaches to naturalistic language training that professionals can easily adapt to the home, clinical, or classroom environment. Decades of classroom research attest to the efficacy of the incidental teaching or milieu approach (Warren & Kaiser, 1986; Warren, Yoder, Gazdag, Kim, & Jones, 1993). There is no question that language treatment conducted in natural environments is effective with a wide variety of children representing different language levels and etiologies. There is also ample evidence that teachers can effectively learn and implement these principles in classroom environments (Warren, McQuarter, & Rogers-Warren, 1984).

Appendix 5–5 shows the most popular methods of stimulating language (providing models) that have been used with children with limited language. These techniques are applicable to the home, clinical, or classroom environments and can be used in a variety of activities. Finally, Appendix 5–6 illustrates the steps a professional or parent can go through to make *any* activity a language-learning experience for a child with limited language. The key is to *think language and communication* in every activity with these children. It is very easy to forget that a particular child has communication goals, especially when the medical professional or teacher has other children in the environment to deal with, and sometimes timing makes it impractical to provide extra stimulation to the child with limited language. However, if the professional or parent can incorporate communication and language into even half of the interactions with the child with limited language, it will go a long way toward creating progress in treatment, as well as progress in the classroom.

Judicious use of more advanced peers and aides also facilitates the language-learning process. The SLP can work with the child in activities the professional has planned that (1) demonstrate the language stimulation and cueing techniques, and (2) provide added practice for the child. Take time now to read Appendices A–F so that you will be familiar with how to provide opportunities for communication, give good language models, stimulate specific types of language, and create classroom activities that facilitate communication goals.

WORK ON THE BACIS OF LANGUAGE

We have made it clear in prior sections that the language framework will not develop normally without a strong BACIS. In some cases, a child with limited language may have to work on some of these building blocks in treatment along with language goals. Two foundation blocks that often are incorporated into treatment programs are cognitive and social skills. For instance, a child who lacks some of the cognitive abilities associated with language development may need some treatment designed to improve these concepts. A child may have primitive play behavior and not even understand the functional use of objects. Clearly, such a child will not talk about objects if he does not understand them to some degree. For example, a child will never say "push car" if all he ever does with cars is to chew on them or throw them. Some research shows that training of cognitive abilities (e.g., object permanence, means-end, functional object use) may facilitate the acquisition of language (Kahn, 1984).

Recall, however, that there is not strong support for viewing such cognitive attainments as *prerequisite* for language training (Brady & McLean, 2000; McCathren, 2000). SLPs can target cognitive and social skills concurrently with language goals. For example, a child with autism may lack social prerequisites or the intent to communicate. Such children often need assistance with eye contact, joint referencing, reciprocal play, turn–taking, and imitating adult models. An important point to make here is that teaching a child to play more appropriately and engage socially also facilitates the development of peer interactions, which are critical to learning language as well as many other skills. These examples all illustrate that the SLP may be involved in more than merely teaching language, but also in training the BACIS for language in some cases. Professionals and parents may incorporate activities in the classroom, clinic, or home environment dedicated to the advancement of various social, cognitive, intent, and language goals. Appendix 5–7 shows some routine things professionals can do to facilitate the social requisites for linguistic acquisition. Some suggestions for the cognitive area are in Appendix 5–8. It should be noted that most of these suggestions would benefit all children in a classroom, not only the child with limited language. Take some time to read these suggestions now.

VERBAL AND AUGMENTATIVE MODES IN TREATMENT

Most children with limited language can learn to talk. You must always remember, however, that language is the "music" and speech is the "instrument." A composer can write a beautiful song only to have it rendered dissonant by an untuned instrument. The major goal of the SLP is to facilitate *communication*, and this is not done exclusively through the speech mode. It is altogether possible for a child with language impairment to understand and even use the rules of language given the appropriate response mode. Communication using gestural or electronic assistance is called *augmentative/alternative communication (AAC)*. For instance, a child with cerebral palsy who has immense difficulty coordinating the speech mechanism may be able to communicate complex ideas using an electronic device with a keyboard or a pointing device. Much research has shown that many children with severe cognitive impairment or autism tend to be able to learn a sign language, picture communication system, or other augmentative systems more easily than speech (Silverman, 1989). Further, once an augmentative mode is introduced to a child, the research is clear that as communication increases, speech attempts increase, and negative aspects, such as behavior problems, decrease (Silverman, 1989). The bottom line is that the SLP wants the child to have *some* way to communicate at the earliest possible age.

Introduction of an augmentative system does not preclude working on speech and language at the same time, and research shows that children using augmentative devices usually use a combination of gesture, speech, and whatever system they have. Much research demonstrates that after an augmentative system is introduced, speech attempts tend to increase as opposed to decrease. Most clinicians agree that the earlier a system of functional communication is established, the better the potential outcome for the child. Chapter 12 discusses augmentative devices in more detail.

DETERMINING THE SUCCESS OF TREATMENT

Some people think of evaluation and treatment as two separate components of working with children with communication disorders. This, however, is an unfortunate misconception. Evaluation is an ongoing process that begins when a child is first diagnosed with a particular problem and ends when he or she is finally dismissed from treatment (Haynes & Pindzola, 2007). Evaluation and treatment must be intimately linked because SLPs must constantly gather assessment data to determine whether the child is making progress. With the advent of accountability and efficacy studies, SLPs and other professionals must not only be able to claim progress in their work, but they must also be able to *prove* it. Thus, the SLP who is working with a limited language case in the classroom environment will not only be designing treatment programs in collaboration with the teacher, but she will also build in methods of determining whether the therapy is successful.

In most cases, spontaneous interactions in the classroom are the best barometer of progress. For example, a 4-year-old child begins the year with an MLU of 1.0 in classroom activities. His treatment goals include increasing MLU with the typical types of early word combinations seen in normally developing children. The treatment involves the teacher modeling specific words and word combinations, expanding the child's one-word utterances into multiword combinations, and reinforcing attempts and multiword communications. Every month, the SLP takes a 30-minute sample of the child's utterances in the classroom during similar activities. She sits on the periphery of the room and writes down what the child says on a clipboard. As the five-month period progresses, the MLU data look like this:

First Sample: MLU = 1.0
Second Sample: MLU = 1.3
Third Sample: MLU = 1.9
Fourth Sample: MLU = 2.3
Fifth Sample: MLU = 2.4

Clearly, the child is increasing his utterance length under the treatment being provided by the SLP and teacher. The data show improvement on the goals stated on the child's IEP. The SLP can take many measurements to monitor progress, and as the treatment continues, the measurements change. For instance, in the child mentioned in the example, work may now be started on increasing the variety (number of different types) of his multiword utterances or introducing some function words to place between the multiword combinations. Whatever the new treatment goal, there must be a valid and reliable way of measuring it.

If the evaluation data show that the child is making progress, this is reinforcing to the SLP and teacher and impressive to parents and administrators. If the data show that the child is not progressing, this is a valuable cue to the SLP and teacher either to make alterations in the treatment approach so that progress *can* occur or to consider an alternative assessment method that allows documentation of growth. Nothing is sadder than to have continued an unsuccessful treatment program for the entire school year without any attempt at systematic modification of the approach. Every child should be able to make progress at *something*! Perhaps the treatment goals need to be less ambitious, the tasks simplified, the therapy more intensive, the stimuli more interesting, the reinforcer more reinforcing, or increases need to be made on parent involvement. None of these modifications would be attempted without accurate data on treatment progress to justify trying them. Teachers and parents should *expect and demand* from the SLP to see evaluation data on treatment progress. The common phrase "He's getting better" is no substitute for objective clinical documentation.

ASSESSMENT AND TREATMENT OF LIMITED LANGUAGE CASES IN MEDICAL/COMMUNITY CLINIC SETTINGS

As mentioned earlier, most children with limited language are often seen first by professionals in medical or community clinic settings. This is because hospitals engage in early identification efforts and medical or community clinics develop early intervention services. Although some school systems see children from birth to 3 years, many educational systems may not be heavily involved with children in this age range. The law states that the school system must provide services by age 3 years, and this is still the most common model in many states. Thus, teams of professionals in hospital settings, university clinics, and community clinics tend to be the early service providers for children with limited language, with the school systems in some states being notable exceptions.

Children with language disorders are identified in several ways. The first is prenatal identification. Children with certain syndromes (e.g., Down syndrome) may be discovered prenatally through the use of tests conducted during pregnancy coupled with knowledge of the genetic history of a family. If a child is identified with a disability prior to birth, the parents and the professional team can be prepared to begin intervention as soon as the child is born. It is not typical for the identification of a disability to be discovered prenatally, but it does occur. A second method of identification is discovery of the abnormality at the time of birth. If there are structural abnormalities or the child is born prematurely with low birth weight, the child has an increased risk for developmental delay or disorder. Again, identification at birth allows for early intervention.

A third way of identifying a child with disabilities is through referral by a parent or pediatrician who notices that the child is not developing normally. Many disorders are not observable at birth but manifest as the child matures and fails to achieve developmental milestones. Many types of cognitive impairment and autism are examples of impairments that do not become evident until the child has had time to develop and evidence developmental lags. The fourth method of identifying children with developmental disabilities is through state or local community efforts known as "child find" programs. Such programs widely publish developmental norms throughout the community and encourage parents and professionals to refer any child for evaluation who seems to be lagging in any domain of growth. For example, one criterion might be that most children should be speaking in single-word utterances by 12–18 months of age and walking somewhere between 12 and 15 months. If a child who is lagging in one or more developmental domains is evaluated and confirmed to be delayed, it is possible to begin intervention fairly early. Finally, many communities hold developmental screenings sponsored by the health department, clinics, or hospitals in the area. Such screenings can identify children who can be referred for evaluation and identified so that intervention can begin. In some cases, school systems participate in early detection programs and help to develop intervention plans.

Hospitals, children's hospitals, community clinics, and university clinics are usually the front line for providing identification, assessment, and intervention services for high-risk children between birth and 3 years. After age 3 years, the school system is more heavily involved in treatment because the child is preparing to enter the educational system. We focus in this section on some aspects of assessment and treatment services that are carried out in medical or community settings. We begin with inpatient services that start at birth and move on to outpatient services in which parents and their children come to a clinical or medical facility for therapy on a regular basis after the child is living at home.

Some infants are kept in the hospital for a period of time after they are born because they are too medically fragile to go home. These children may have difficulty breathing, be unstable in their vital signs, have trouble feeding, or need close medical supervision for one of a host of other reasons. Such children are usually kept in the neonatal intensive care unit (NICU) for close monitoring and treatment. Interestingly, 50 years ago high-risk children had only about a 50 percent survival rate. With advances in technology and medicine, more than 90 percent currently survive. However, with the increased survival rate comes a surge in the need for early intervention services because most of these children will exhibit lasting difficulties such as language delay, cognitive impairments, respiratory problems, cardiac abnormalities, intestinal disorders, and intracranial hemorrhages. It is estimated that 30–50 percent of premature infants are left with some sort of developmental delay (Rossetti, 2001). The good news, however, is that research has shown that early intervention is generally effective with these children (Bleile & Miller, 1993; Blair & Ramey, 1997; Burchinal, Campbell, Bryant, Wasik, & Rame, 1997).

The specific team members that could be part of an intervention team with high-risk infants could include, but is not limited to, the following: physicians, nurses, occupational therapists, physical therapists, social workers, psychologists, radiologists, audiologists, and speech-language pathologists. Other professionals are called in depending on the child's needs. For instance, we mentioned earlier that a child born with a cleft of the palate might need the services of plastic surgeons, pediatric dentists, and prosthodontists in addition to some of the professionals already mentioned. In Chapter 1, we indicate that the Individualized Family Service Plan (IFSP) includes treatment goals for children between birth and 3 years suggested from a multidisciplinary evaluation. Recall that the IFSP not only includes specific goals, but ways to measure them, a description of the frequency and intensity of treatment, and team responsibilities.

So, what does the SLP do on the intervention team dealing with high-risk infants? We are very general here because an entire text could be written about each area we mention. Generally, the SLP is involved in both assessment and treatment activities with neonatal cases. In assessment, the most important areas involve feeding, oral motor development, infant behavior, vocal behavior, evaluation of the home/hospital environment, assessment of family strengths/needs, and parent–child communication (Paul, 2007). We discuss each area briefly.

Many high-risk infants are born with feeding difficulties. Some of them must be fed through nonoral means such as various types of tubes. One of the many criteria used to determine whether a child should be released from the NICU is the child's ability to feed orally. The SLP is uniquely qualified to evaluate the infant's ability to swallow and ingest various types of foods and liquids. Often, team members cooperate on evaluating feeding, and professionals in occupational therapy and radiology play a major role. At any rate, the SLP usually performs a feeding assessment that helps other professionals on the team and the parents know the best way to provide nutrition for the child. As the child gets older, the SLP evaluates his abilities to deal with other textures and consistencies of food and develop chewing and swallowing maneuvers.

Infant behavior development is another area the SLP participates in evaluating. By *infant behavior* we mean reactions to external stimuli such as sound and light. The length of time an infant can tolerate interaction or stimulation is another target. Some infants are very sensitive to stimuli and develop "sensory defensiveness," which may persist until they are older. Infants provide cues that tell professionals and parents when they have had enough stimulation and these may be relatively subtle such as flushing, tensing, arching the back, and so forth. All members of the team must be aware of such signals to avoid pushing a child too far during intervention and parents need to know about them to make their interactions effective. Other aspects of infant behavior that the SLP is interested in are interactions with objects, development of imitation, use of joint referencing, turn-taking, eye contact, and the beginnings of play, but these are later developments in the first year of life. It never hurts, however, to watch for their emergence and to tell parents and professionals to encourage these behaviors.

Vocal development occurs on a predictable schedule (Proctor, 1989) and the SLP can be watching for the production of vowels, consonants, and different syllable shapes involving one syllable (e.g., *ba, wa, da, ma*) and multiple syllables (e.g., *baba, bada, mama*). Many of these vocal productions are first done by the child spontaneously, and some are first observed in imitation. It is important to remember that these are vocalizations, not verbalizations, which imply use of real words. Vocalizations are just the child exploring the vocal tract and attempting to coordinate phonation, respiration, and articulation by playing with sounds. Such productions are an important prelude to word production later on.

The notion of assessment has broadened to include an examination of the environments a child is a part of during development. Paul (2007) reports that noise levels produced by respirators, incubators, and monitors can not only disrupt sleep, but can possibly contribute to hearing loss. In addition to noise levels, if a child is in the hospital for an extended period of time, it is important to assess opportunities for interaction with parents and professionals. By evaluating these opportunities, the SLP can make suggestions to interaction partners whether they are parents, nurses, OTs, PTs, or other professionals. Such suggestions may include language stimulation, cognitive development, turn-taking, imitation, feeding, and other areas related to communication development. When the child is home, it is important to evaluate similar parameters of interaction opportunities so that the SLP can make suggestions regarding communication development. The SLP is interested in who interacts with the child, types of favorite activities, toys, and routines that could be used for language stimulation and cognitive development.

Federal laws specify that an assessment of a family's strengths and needs be conducted before developing an intervention program for a child between birth and 3 years. Obviously, with children so young, the focus cannot and should not be on the child in isolation. The child is part of an active environment that includes all members of the family. Members of a multidisciplinary team in cooperation with the parents should assess the family's strengths and needs. Some of the family's needs might be as simple as providing transportation for the child to a medical facility for treatments. Another need might be baby-sitting services for siblings while parents participate in the intervention process. Parents may qualify for financial assistance and could be aided in this effort by the social worker. Every family has strengths and needs, and the intervention process must begin with defining the things a family does well and the areas in which they might need some assistance. It is also important to involve the parents in all aspects of the assessment and the selection of treatment goals.

Parent–child communication is another important aspect to be evaluated by the SLP. This includes not only the type of language model presented by the parent, but the reciprocal communication between the infant and others. SLPs observe these behaviors by watching the parents and child during activities such as feeding, dressing, and play to determine whether there are opportunities for reciprocal exchanges, consistent language modeling, assisting the child with object manipulations, encouraging imitation, and providing reinforcement using natural consequences.

Regarding intervention, the SLP is engaged in many critical activities. Often, parents of high-risk children are overwhelmed by the number of professionals involved in their case and they may not fully understand the multifaceted intervention program. Thus, the SLP and other professionals take time to counsel parents and explain the process in which they are involved. Many parents experience increases in stress levels when faced with raising a child with special needs and all the attendant intervention activities. The intervention goals parallel the assessment targets mentioned previously. For example, the SLP is involved in helping the parent and child develop effective strategies for oral feeding and encouraging the development of play, social interaction, language, and cognitive abilities. These, as you might expect, are done through parent training. Early training might be done in the NICU or elsewhere in the medical facility while the child is an inpatient. Later training might be accomplished by parent–child visits to the medical facility for outpatient appointments or home visits by the SLP and other professionals. Most authorities agree that four areas are important in early intervention targeting communication development. These four areas overlap to some degree, as you will soon see. We address each area briefly.

One of the critical interaction behaviors parents must learn is to *take turns* with their child in reciprocal play and social communication. For example, early in development children do not behave intentionally. Much of their behavior is dictated by reflexes and responses to stimuli in the environment. They do not plan before performing a motor action or vocal behavior. Parents, however, must learn to treat these unintentional behaviors as intentional and respond to them in such a way that the child sees his behavior has an effect on others in the environment. If a child is shaking a rattle, the adult can shake a rattle in response, or say "shake" every time the child performs the action.

A second important interactive behavior for parents is to learn to imitate their child's vocal and motoric behaviors. If the child vocalizes a vowel sound (e.g., *ahhhhhhh*), the parent should imitate this vocalization. Just as mentioned, the vocalization may not have been intentional, but the child will soon learn that vocal behaviors have an effect on others in the environment when they imitate. The same goes for motor activities that do not involve vocalization.

The third critical behavior is the establishment of joint reference. We know from research that parents and children tend to follow each other's line of visual regard. They like to look at things together. Parents can help with establishing joint reference by holding objects for the child so that she can motorically explore the object. It is difficult for a child to both hold onto an object, stabilize it, and engage in sensorimotor exploration. Parents can facilitate looking at objects together by making it easier for the child. You want parents to follow the child's lead some of the time and become interested in what the child seems to prefer. On other occasions, the parent can introduce new objects to the child to promote joint referencing.

A final critical interactive strategy is the development of joint action routines with the child. These are activities that are repeated over and over that become predictable not only in their performance but in terms of the language that is used to accompany them. For example, games like peek-a-boo, gonna get you, or book sharing all carry with them a specific routine and common language used repeatedly. For example, parents tend to read the same books to children routinely and point to pictures while naming them. When caretakers put a cloth over the baby's head and say, "Where's Johnny?" they repeat this every time as a routine.

Many examples of activities and goals are illustrated in the appendices to this chapter. It should not be surprising that these activities and goals can be done in both medical/clinical environments as well as the educational setting.

ASSESSMENT AND TREATMENT OF LIMITED LANGUAGE CASES IN EDUCATIONAL SETTINGS

As mentioned in Chapter 1, speech-language pathologists in the school setting work as members of a team as mandated by federal law. Thus, a team approach is common to both medical and educational environments. In the educational setting, the team usually comprises of classroom teachers, special educators, psychologists, and SLPs. Just as in the medical setting, parents are a critical part of the assessment and intervention team. In Chapter 1, we indicate that school systems require a multidisciplinary evaluation of a student before any intervention goals can be developed. Chapter 1 also illustrates the central nature of the Individualized Education Program (IEP) for outlining treatment goals and measuring treatment progress.

In the educational setting, children with limited language are most frequently encountered in special education programs. These children most often present with cognitive delays, autism spectrum disorders, severe hearing impairment, and other less common conditions. Assessment includes preliteracy skills, literacy levels, classroom environment, curriculum requirements, and a battery of standardized tests focusing on intelligence and educational skills. Nonstandardized testing by the SLP includes everything in the general section presented earlier in this chapter. The school environment presents opportunities for the SLP to observe the child interacting in the classroom with both teachers and peers. Unlike the medical environment, with the exception of the NICU, the child is in the school setting for many continuous hours of the day. In early grades, the child is in the care of a small number of teachers and educational aides. The child also has play opportunities, lunch, art, and music in addition to academic and literacy instruction.

The unique nature of the school environment makes it an ideal setting for a consultative treatment model. That is, a child can receive individual therapy from the SLP as well as treatment activities conducted in the classroom, lunchroom, playground by either the SLP or educational personnel. The goals for language development are similar to those in the medical environment. One difference, however, is that the medical setting serves children at a much younger chronological age as compared to schools. The chapter appendices provide numerous suggestions for teachers and parents of children with limited language, and we do not reiterate them here. SLPs can easily incorporate these specific suggestions on providing a good language model, language stimulation, and activities for treatment into an academic or a home setting.

CONCLUSION

We began this chapter by indicating that children with limited language need to have treatment that extends beyond the therapy room and into the home, classroom, and clinic. If you reflect on all of the suggestions provided in the present chapter, you will find that *no* suggestion was made that would require a professional to do "special" activities with a child with limited language. All of our suggestions involve slight modification of interaction style, language models, and use of *existing* activities that the teacher or health professional has planned for use in their respective settings. This is the way it should be in a consultative approach to language treatment. We hope that most of you will have the opportunity to participate in the treatment of a child with limited language because what this youngster learns from you will make possible any further social or academic achievements. It is gratifying, indeed, to play such a pivotal role in the life of a child.

Terms to Know

Limited language	Specifically language impaired (SLI)
PL 99-457	BACIS
Nonverbal communicators	Language stimulation
Single-word communicators	Communicative intent
Alternative/augmentative communication (AAC)	Representative language sample
	Structured treatment
Early multiword communicators	Naturalistic treatment

Study Questions

1. Make a list of activities that preschool or kindergarten children perform in the classroom setting.
2. For each of the activities listed in item 1, rank order them in terms of the teacher's opportunity to stimulate language during performance of the task.
3. Discuss the positive and negative effects of the SLP assisting the teacher in conducting certain classroom activities to stimulate language.
4. Discuss the advantages and disadvantages of the SLP removing a child with language delay from the classroom for treatment.
5. How could the teacher and SLP work together to gain cooperation of a parent in treatment of a child with limited language?

Bibliography

Baltaxe, C. (2001). Emotional, behavioral, and other psychiatric disorders of childhood associated with communication disorders. In T. Layton, E. Crais, & L. Watson (Eds.), *Handbook of early language impairment in children: Nature*. Albany, NY: Delmar.

Blair, C., & Ramey, C. (1997). Early intervention for low birth weight infants and the path to second generation research. In M. J. Guralnick (Ed.), *The effectiveness of early intervention*. Baltimore, MD: Brookes.

Bleile, K., & Miller, S. (1993). Articulation and phonological disorders in toddlers with medical needs. In J. Bernthal (Ed.), *Articulatory and phonological disorders in special populations*. New York: Thieme.

Brady, N., & McLean, L. (2000). Emergent symbolic relations in speakers and nonspeakers. *Research in Developmental Disabilities, 21,* 197–214.

Brunson, K., & Haynes, W. (1991). Profiling teacher/child communication: Reliability of an alternating time sampling procedure. *Child Language Teaching & Therapy, 7,* 192–211.

Burchinal, M., Campbell, F., Bryant, D., Wasik, B., & Rame, C. (1997). Early intervention and mediating processes I, Cognitive performance of children of low income African-American families. *Child Development, 68,* 935–954.

Calandrella, A., & Wilcox, M. (2000). Predicting language outcomes for young prelinguistic children with developmental delay. *Journal of Speech, Language, and Hearing Research, 43,* 1061–1071.

Coggins, T., Olswang, L., & Guthrie, J. (1987). Assessing communicative intents in young children: Low structured observation or elicitation tasks? *Journal of Speech and Hearing Disorders, 52,* 44–49.

Crais, E., Douglas, D., & Campbell, C. (2004). The intersection of the development of gestures and intentionality. *Journal of Speech, Language and Hearing Research, 47,* 678–694.

Fenson, L., Dale, P., Reznick, S., Thal, D., Bates, E., Hartung, J., Pethick, S., & Reilly, J. (2003). *MacArthur-Bates Communicative Development Inventories.* Baltimore, MD: Brookes.

Fox. L., Long, S., & Langlois, A. (1988). Patterns of language comprehension deficit in abused and neglected children. *Journal of Speech and Hearing Disorders, 53,* 239–244.

Hart, B., & Rogers-Warren, A. (1978). A milieu approach to teaching language. In R. Schiefelbusch (Ed.), *Language intervention strategies.* Baltimore, MD: University Park Press.

Haynes, W., & Pindzola, R. (2007). *Diagnosis and evaluation in speech pathology.* Boston, MA: Allyn & Bacon.

Hubatch, L., Johnson, C., Kistler, D., Burns, W., & Moneka, W. (1985). Early language abilities of high-risk infants. *Journal of Speech and Hearing Disorders, 50,* 195–206.

Kaderavek, J., & Sulzby, E. (1998). Parent–child joint book reading: An observational protocol for young children. *American Journal of Speech-Language Pathology, 8*(3), 261–272.

Kahn, J. (1984). Cognitive training and initial use of referential speech. *Topics in Language Disorders, 5,* 14–28.

Klee, T., Pearce, K., & Carson, D. (2000). Improving the positive predictive value of screening for developmental language disorder. *Journal of Speech, Language and Hearing Research, 43,* 821–833.

Lucas, E. (1980). *Semantic and pragmatic language disorders.* Rockville, MD: Aspen.

McCathren, R. (2000). Teacher-implemented prelinguistic communication intervention. *Focus on Autism and Other Developmental Disabilities, 15*(1), 21–29.

McCathren, R., Warren, S., & Yoder, P. (1996). Prelinguistic predictors of later language development. In K. Cole, P. Dale, & S. Thal (Eds.), *Assessment of communication and language.* Baltimore, MD: Brookes.

National Joint Committee for the Communication Needs of Persons with Severe Disabilities. (2002). *American Speech-Language-Hearing Association Technical Report IV.* Rockville, MD: American Speech-Language-Hearing Association, 59–68.

Owens, R. (2007). *Language development: An introduction.* Needham Heights, MA: Allyn & Bacon.

Paul, R. (2007). *Language disorders from infancy through adolescence: Assessment and intervention* (3rd ed.). St. Louis, MO: Mosby.

Proctor, A. (1989). Stages of normal noncry vocal development in infancy: A protocol for assessment. *Topics in Language Disorders, 10*(1), 26–42.

Rabidoux, P., & Macdonald, J. (2000). An interactive taxonomy of mothers and children during storybook interactions. *American Journal of Speech-Language Pathology, 9,* 331–344.

Rescorla, L., & Alley, A. (2001). Validation of the language development survey (LDS): A parent report tool for identifying language delay in toddlers. *Journal of Speech, Language and Hearing Research, 44,* 434–445.

Rescorla, L., Alley, A., & Christine, J. (2001). Word frequencies in toddlers' lexicons. *Journal of Speech, Language and Hearing Research, 44,* 598–609.

Rhyner, P., Lehr, D., & Pudlas, K. (1990). An analysis of teacher responsiveness to communicative initiations of preschool children with handicaps. *Language, Speech & Hearing Services in Schools, 21*(2), 91–97.

Rice, M., Sell, M., & Hadley, P. (1990). The social interactive coding system (SICS): An on-line, clinically relevant descriptive tool. *Language, Speech & Hearing Services in Schools, 21*(1), 2–14.

Rossetti, L. (2001). *Communication intervention: Birth to three* (2nd ed.). San Diego, CA: Singular.

Silverman, F. (1989). *Communication for the speechless.* Englewood Cliffs, NJ: Prentice Hall.

Snyder, L. (1981). Assessing communicative abilities in the sensorimotor period: Content and context. *Topics in Language Disorders, 1,* 31–46.

Warren, S., & Kaiser, A. (1986). Incidental language teaching: A critical review. *Journal of Speech & Hearing Disorders, 51,* 291–299.

Warren, S., McQuarter, R., & Rogers-Warren, A. (1984). The effects of mands and models on the speech of unresponsive language delayed preschool children. *Journal of Speech and Hearing Disorders, 49,* 43–52.

Warren, S., Yoder, P., Gazdag, G., Kim, K., & Jones, H. (1993). Facilitating prelinguistic communication skills in young children with developmental delay. *Journal of Speech and Hearing Research, 36,* 83–97.

Watkins, R., & Rice, M. (1994). *Specific language impairment in children.* Baltimore, MD: Brookes.

Westby, C. (1980). Assessment of cognitive and language abilities through play. *Language, Speech and Hearing Services in Schools, 11,* 154–168.

Wetherby, A., & Prizant, B. (1993). *Communication and symbolic behavior scales.* Chicago, IL: Riverside.

Wetherby, A., & Prizant, B. (2002). *Communication and symbolic behavior scales: Developmental profile.* Baltimore, MD: Brookes.

Yoder, P., Warren, S., & McCathren, R. (1998). Determining spoken language prognosis in children with developmental disabilities. *American Journal of Speech-Language Pathology, 7,* 77–87.

Appendix 5-1

CREATING COMMUNICATIVE OPPORTUNITIES

Whatever the level of communication of the child with language impairment (gesture, single word, word combinations), one of the most important parts of therapy is giving him the opportunity to communicate. Creating opportunity for the child with language impairment involves providing him with many chances to use language appropriately. The ideal setting for facilitating a child's use of language is the natural environment (e.g., home, classroom, medical/clinical environment). Following are some specific ways to create communicative opportunities.

1. *Do not anticipate the child's needs.* Expect the child to perform necessary tasks independently rather than doing them for her. Do not anticipate the child's needs; wait for her to verbalize a request. For example, if the child knows you will automatically provide juice and cookies at snack time, she will not verbalize a request for these. When snack time comes, do not give the child refreshments until she asks for them (or tries to). If you see the child struggling with a jar lid screwed on too tightly, do not quickly offer assistance. Wait for the child to ask for your help.

2. *Withhold access to objects and events.* Withholding the child's participation in a desired task or withholding a desired object provides the opportunity for more language use. The child with language disorder should not get a chance to participate or obtain an object until a verbal, vocal, or gestural attempt is made. For example, you might say, "Who wants to play ball?" Withhold the child's participation in this task until he responds to you.

3. *Use sabotage.* Set up a situation in which the child needs to ask for your assistance. This can be done by providing objects that do not work correctly or omitting a familiar step in a routine activity.

4. *Use cues that provide opportunities to elaborate.* Make open-ended statements and ask questions that require more than single-word answers (Lucas, 1980).
   Examples: "What do you want?" "Ask Mike to play with us." "Tell me about that." "Tell me more."

5. *Let the child speak for herself.* When a child is not a good communicator, parents and teachers sometimes let a sibling or friend talk for her. This reduces the opportunities for communication and should not be encouraged.

6. *Use pause time.* Use pause time when interacting with the child. After asking a question or making a statement, do not immediately provide an answer or reply for the child. Wait for the child to respond. Open-ended utterances such as, "Who wants to help? Who can tell me? What do you want?" followed by a pause are ideal ways to provide language opportunities because these leave an opening for the child to respond verbally.

7. *Limit your talking time.* Reduce your utterances when interacting with the child. By reducing your utterances, you are providing more opportunities for the child to initiate and use language.

CHARACTERISTICS OF A GOOD LANGUAGE MODEL AND INTERACTION

1. *Encourage and respond to communication.* Whenever possible, talk to the child about things that are happening at that moment. Whenever possible, answer the child's verbalizations with what you think is an appropriate response at the child's level. You can also imitate the child's speech and try to have her imitate you.

2. *Alternate your emphasis between directing the child and following his lead.* Do not always direct the child by trying to get him to talk about and pay attention to things *you* are interested in. About 50 percent of the time talk about and pay attention to the things that *the child* is interested in.

3. *Always talk about objects that are present and events that are currently happening.* Do not talk about things in another room or things that have happened in the past or will happen in the future. Language is learned first in talking about objects in the here and now.

4. *Reduce your sentence length.* Your sentence length should be one or two steps ahead of the child. If the child is nonverbal, you can use one- to three-word utterances. If the child is at the one- to two-word stage, you should use three- to five-word utterances.

5. *Reduce your sentence complexity.* Do not use complex sentences. Simplify your sentences and when possible avoid connecting two thoughts together or using a lot of modifiers.

6. *Paraphrase and repeat a lot.* Repeat your sentences a few times in a conversation with the child. Sometimes, say the same statement in a few different ways (e.g., "Want a cookie? Want one? Does Johnny want a cookie? Want it?").

7. *Exaggerate your intonation and put stress on important words.* Emphasize important words and concepts by the way you say words. For example, "This is a *big* ball."

8. *Use simple, concrete vocabulary.* Do not use big words for things. For instance, call a car "car," not "Chevrolet."

9. *Use "broad-based" words.* Choose words that can be used over and over again for many objects and events. For instance, *go* can be used for cars, people, walking, running, swinging, and so forth. On the other hand *spin* can be used only for objects that twirl.

10. *Stimulate the language forms that are the next ones the child will develop.* Use language models that are "one step ahead" of the child's. For example, if the child uses mostly one-word utterances, you should model two- to three-word utterances.

11. *Talk at eye level with the child.* Speaking to your child at her eye level may mean kneeling, sitting on the floor, or sitting across the table. Such a position not only secures the child's attention but also helps the child understand the meaning of the message from your facial expression and eyes.

12. *Create communication opportunities.* Encourage the child to become more mature by urging him to do more activities independently. Do not anticipate the child's wishes. The child has fewer reasons to talk if needs are fulfilled before there is an opportunity to use language. You might even arrange situations so that the child must use language to get a desired object, food, information, and such.

13. *Avoid "baby talk."* Permit the child to grow up. Avoid using baby talk when talking to the child. If the child hears baby talk, she will talk baby talk.

14. *Do not talk too much.* Try to avoid overwhelming the child by providing so many verbal models that there is no time left for him to respond or contribute to the conversation. It is acceptable and even desirable for periods of silence to occur in conversation. This gives the child the opportunity to initiate new utterances.

15. *Avoid too many questions and commands.* Model good conversation and language, but do not *command it.* Avoid commands and asking too many questions such as: "Say this," "What's this?"

16. *Demonstrate your expectations.* Show the child that you expect her to communicate. For example, after you provide a model, pause and show the child that you expect a response. Do this by maintaining eye contact and looking at the child expectantly.

17. *Try to figure out what the child means.* Interpret the child's utterances as meaningful. When the child attempts to communicate, interpret the utterances as important and communicative.

18. *Show enthusiasm. Be enthusiastic.* Let your face and voice show the child that what you are doing is interesting and fun. Let the child actively participate. Language is best learned while doing.

19. *Slow down and pause.* Reduce your rate of talking and use natural pauses to highlight the main idea of your utterances.

Appendix 5-3

SUGGESTIONS BY LUCAS FOR NATURALISTIC LANGUAGE TREATMENT

Several overriding aspects that Lucas (1980) emphasizes are (1) the treatment must not be dominated by the adult (should be child-directed), and (2) the child will benefit most by observing peer models performing legitimate speech acts. The suggestions are in several areas.

1. *Providing opportunity:* This can be done in several ways. First, the adult should *stop anticipating the child's needs.* A number of studies recommend incorporating *pause time* into interactions with these children. One group of researchers found that teachers in a preschool handicapped class frequently provided materials, treats, and opportunities for activities before the children had the opportunity to make a verbal request. When these researchers asked teachers to *wait 5 seconds* before providing things, the children's rate of spontaneous verbal responses increased dramatically. One key to establishing opportunity for speech acts is to make as many problems as possible for the child to solve verbally (Lucas, 1980, p. 213): taped together scissors, plugged glue bottles, empty or dried-up pens, broken pencil leads, coat sleeves turned inside-out by the morning aide when the children aren't watching, not enough chairs, not enough snacks, cups with holes in the bottom, missing toys, flat balls, short jump ropes, missing colors or paints, not enough paper, no tacks for hanging pictures, tables with missing legs, water faucets turned off tightly, baseballs without bats or bats without baseballs, and so forth. The problem-solving tasks require more than the performance of speech acts; the tasks necessitate better attending to the environmental cues and thus more discrimination and sorting of the features that lead to knowledge development.

     Opportunity is important in classroom environments and in home situations as well!

2. *Models:* The child needs to see and hear other children using language to accomplish various purposes. The more variety in models the better in terms of varying the forms (gimme *x*, I want the *x*, can I have the *x*?, want *x*, etc.).

3. *Direct cues or prompts:* For some children, the opportunity and a chance to see models is not enough. Speech-language professionals and caretakers can use a variety of cueing systems in language training. The adult should provide the cue that gives the *least amount of information first.* Lucas gives examples like, "If you want the ball, you can get it from me," "You can ask me for the ball," and so on.

4. *Utterance act imitation:* This should be a last resort, to imitate an utterance after the clinician. The one saving grace of this procedure is that the imitation takes place *in context*; it is at least done in a real communication situation.

Picture the preceding four steps as part of a continuum. Some children respond by developing communication skills only when you provide opportunity. Others need many models to finally develop. Others require prompts and imitations. The point here is that the treatment is being done in the natural environment, and the clinician is not being intrusive.

INCIDENTAL TEACHING SUGGESTIONS

Incidental teaching (Hart & Rogers-Warren, 1978) is sometimes called the "milieu" approach but has more recently been referred to as incidental teaching. An increasing amount of research on this type of intervention has been conducted, and it has been shown to be effective with a variety of types of language cases. It is also adaptable in that the SLP can use it for nonverbal, single-word cases, and early multiword cases.

The basic model assumes that language is taught in functional ways. The training is carried out in the place where the child spends the most time (classroom, home). All waking hours are infested with training opportunities. The settings can be arranged to learn language and reinforcers are natural consequences of communication acts.

1. *Arranging the environment:* You must have a variety of attractive materials and activities (child should be the judge, not the clinician). Certain materials should be accessible to the child, while other materials can be obtained only on request. The adult mediates the materials and you make this a *rule* (that all materials must be asked for). If a child doesn't ask, put your hand over his and say, "You need to ask for that."
2. *Building rate:* You respond to the child's highest level of communication (gestural, vocal, verbal, single-word, early multiword). Thus, any level child or a mixture of children can be incorporated into this type of treatment. The teacher's response should be immediate, consistent, and strong when a child makes a request (that is, give the child what is asked for, attend to what she wants you to look at). Note that a child must be able to initiate requests at some level, be able to imitate, and the environment must be controlled.

3. *Building requesting:* A version of the specific procedure is as follows:
   a. Focus attention on child when he initiates.
   b. Allow time for the child to make a request at his level.
   c. If the child can't request, ask a question: "What is this?"
   d. If response is incorrect, provide a model of the language expected from the child (want ball). Listen for a correct imitation or approximation.
   e. Confirm the behavior of the child ("OK, you can have the ball.").
4. *Building commenting:* A version of the specific procedure is as follows:
   a. Teacher focuses full attention on the child who initiates a statement.
   b. Adult confirms and repeats all or some of what the child says . . . take a guess if you don't understand (e.g., "That IS a big horsie").
   c. Adult can model a statement in appropriate context if child is not talking and thus can hope for imitation.

LANGUAGE STIMULATION TECHNIQUES

The following techniques give a child an example of a higher level of language complexity than she is presently using. The techniques can be administered while the child plays or in response to a verbal turn in a conversation.

A. SELF-TALK

Verbalize what *you* are seeing, hearing, doing, and/or feeling. This type of speech is useful for children who are reluctant to interact because it provides some model of speaking while making no demands on the child.

Examples: "I am washing my hands."
"The water is warm."
"I dropped the soap."

B. PARALLEL TALK

Talk about what *the child* sees, hears, does, and feels. The adult producing utterances that are related to what the child is experiencing demonstrates possible utterances the child may say.

Examples: "You're petting the dog."
"Johnny is pushing the car."
"That feels hot."

C. EXPANSIONS

Take the child's utterance and expand it into a closer approximation of a grammatically correct utterance. This shows the child that you are interested and listening to what he says. Young children are likely to imitate expansions of their own utterances.

Examples: The child might say, "eat." The adult would say: "Eat banana."
The child might say, "baby sleep." The adult would say: "The baby is sleeping."
The child might say, "want ball." The adult would say: "You want the ball."

D. EXPATIATION

Take the child's utterance, expand it, and add something new to the child's meaning. Make sure to keep your expatiations in a simple sentence format.

Examples: The child might say, "want milk." The adult would say: "The milk is cold."
The child might say, "eat." The adult would say: "Eat more cereal."

E. BUILDUPS AND BREAKDOWNS

The adult takes the child's utterance, expands it, breaks it down into sentence components, and then builds it up again using all components that were modeled.

Examples: Child: "Baby sleep."
Adult: "Yeah, the *baby* is *sleeping.*" (breakdown) "*Sleeping* in the *bed.*" (breakdown) "The *baby* is *sleeping* in the *bed.*" (buildup)
Child: "Baby sleep bed."

F. RECAST SENTENCES

This is a specific type of expansion where the language model does not change the child's meaning but only adds grammatical information. For example, if the child says, "The doll is sick," the language model may respond by saying, "She is sick." In this example, the adult has shown the child how pronouns can be used to substitute for nouns.

Appendix 5-6

INCORPORATION OF LANGUAGE GOALS IN CLASSROOM AND HOME ACTIVITIES

The speech-language pathologist does not necessarily want teachers or parents to do specific language activities in the classroom or the home. Typical home and classroom activities can be adapted to include language goals. For instance, in the classroom, teachers can use the following activities easily for language development: snack time, music time, motor skills, play time, story time, nap time, arts and crafts, show and tell, and so on.

In the home environment, parents can use the following activities easily for language development: bath time, mealtimes, dressing, changing, play time, traveling, playing outside, helping, preparing for bed, book reading, and so forth.

Medical environments offer feeding time, bath time, changing, play time, physical therapy activities, occupational therapy activities, and others.

Thus, special activities do not need to be devised for language training; language can be easily incorporated into the classroom and home daily routines. Incorporating language into the daily routine requires only that the parent or teacher think about these daily activities in a particular way. The following steps may be helpful.

1. Decide on a normal daily activity that you are willing to use for language training.
2. Remind yourself of the child's specific language goal. For example: producing single words, producing certain word combinations, initiating more utterances, use of prepositions.
3. Mentally rehearse steps in the activity and consider the objects and actions involved in the activity.
4. Pinpoint where the specific language goal can be included in an activity step, object, or action. For example, during bath time, the target might be action + object utterances. The parent will stimulate action + object and encourage the child to produce

action + object utterances. The activity allows for some of the following action + object utterances: turn water, splash water, drink water, push boat, wash face, wash hair, throw soap, dry hair, pull drain. Other specific parent bath routines may provide additional opportunities for action + object combinations. What are some classroom activities that could be used to stimulate action + object word combinations?

5. Recycle steps 1–4 in other activities throughout the day.

If parents or teachers simply think of routine activities in terms of language, the daily routine is saturated with opportunities to stimulate and encourage language use.

SOCIAL ASPECTS RELATED TO COMMUNICATION

Social interaction is the basis of communication. Before children can communicate, they must first have the desire to interact socially with others; they express this desire through many different social behaviors. The child's communication does not necessarily require the use of verbal language, but the acquisition of language is associated with the development of these social behaviors. These behaviors are discussed in the following sections.

JOINT REFERENCING

Joint referencing refers to both the adult and the child focusing their attention on the same thing at the same time. It is important for the adult to allow the child to direct attention about half of the time. Encourage the child's direction of joint referencing. Encourage the child to become interested in objects and events focused on by the adult. For example, when looking at a book together, name the pictures the child is looking at. Show the child how a toy works, but be sure she is looking at it and sharing reference on it while you demonstrate. When talking together, if the child says "car," do not begin talking about crayons; share something about the car with her such as, "Yes, the car is red."

ENCOURAGE SOCIAL PLAY

You should encourage the child to participate in activities that include other children. The child's social behavior improves when playing with others because he learns to cooperate, participate, and share and also to respect other people's feelings. Because communication is social, encouraging the child to participate in social play stimulates his communication behaviors. Parents and teachers should discourage isolated play in children with language delays.

ELIMINATE ANTISOCIAL BEHAVIOR

You should try to eliminate any antisocial behaviors the child might have (e.g., biting, spitting, hitting, kicking). These behaviors decrease the child's opportunity for social interaction and communication.

TURN-TAKING

Develop routines or games that contain pauses for the child to respond. The child's turn does not necessarily have to be verbal; a gaze, facial expression, body movement, or vocalization can fill the child's turn. This teaches the child to wait for another person's action and to take her own turn in response. It also teaches the child to assume responsibility for her turn. You can encourage the development of this skill by playing games such as peekaboo or rolling a ball back and forth with the child.

GAMES/RITUALS

Establish games and rituals with the child that have assigned roles and predictable events (who does what and what comes next). Repeat them over and over again so that the child becomes familiar with the games and language associated with them. Choose a few common games such as: give-and-take (objects), peekaboo, horsie, Pat-a-Cake, bye-bye, roll a ball back and forth, build and knock down blocks, no-no, point and name, put on/ take off, open/shut, joint book reading, question/answer, verbal imitation.

Appendix
5–8

COGNITIVE SKILLS RELATED TO LANGUAGE DEVELOPMENT

Research in language development shows that certain concepts relate to a child's ability to communicate. These important concepts are learned from frequent interactions with people, objects, and events in the environment. There is recent support in the literature for encouraging children with language impairment to learn these communication-related concepts. The activities described in this appendix can facilitate the development of these concepts in the classroom and home environments. Teachers and parents should think of specific activities that can foster these concepts. Throughout these activities, teachers and parents should talk about important aspects of these events.

CATEGORIZATION

Children should learn to put similar things in categories. For example, children should eventually be able to group objects by shape, color, size, and class (foods, transportation, and animals). Practice in pointing out similarities and differences among objects facilitates this skill.

MEANS-END

The concept of means-end has to do with the child knowing how to make things happen. For instance, a toy that is out of reach (end) can be obtained by using a large stick (means). If a child does not know how to turn on the television (end), mother (means) can be used to achieve this. Ultimately, speech is used as a means to acquire a variety of ends (attention, objects, and such), and a basic understanding of this concept is essential to good communication.

USING OBJECTS APPROPRIATELY

A child needs to know what an object is and what to do with it before he can talk about it. Show the child how to use objects correctly. Do not allow him to throw objects, bang them, or put them in his mouth.

CONCEPTS OF OBJECTS

A child needs to be able to hold a picture of something in her mind. If a child is playing with a toy and it suddenly rolls under the couch, the child should realize that the toy still exists but cannot be seen. If a child does not have this skill, play games such as hide-and-seek. Leave part of the object showing so that the child can see it; then, gradually hide the whole object and see if the child can find it.

IMMEDIATE IMITATION

A child needs to be able to imitate things you do right after you do them. Do things with the child that would be easy for her to imitate. Games such as Pat-a-Cake and peekaboo are good to keep a child's attention and teach this skill.

DELAYED IMITATION

A child also needs to be able to imitate things you do at a later time. Perform different activities with the child such as putting a puzzle together or putting rings on a stick. See that the child can later play these games without a model.

SYMBOLIC (PRETEND) PLAY

A child needs to be able to use pretend play. One of the earliest kinds of pretending is using one's own body in play (pretending to eat, sleep). Later, see if the child can pretend to feed a doll or pretend to be talking to someone on the phone. If a child is able to do these activities, see if he can pretend without having appropriate objects to help (e.g., use a block of wood as a car). Finally, a child can pretend with no objects at all. This could include pretending to be a cowboy by using the fingers for a gun or pretending to drive a car with no steering wheel.

COMBINING TWO OR MORE OBJECTS IN PLAY

See if the child can combine objects in play. For example, see if the child can put a doll in a toy car or hammer pegs in a pegboard.

SEPARATING AND COMBINING OBJECTS

A child needs to be able to take things apart such as stacked rings, blocks, or nesting cups. A child usually can take things apart before she can put them together. A child then needs to be able to put these things together again.

Chapter 6

SCHOOL-AGE AND ADOLESCENT LANGUAGE DISORDERS

EPISODE 6–1

Answer given by an 8-year-old with a pragmatics disorder:

SLP: And tell me what your favorite toy is, Calvin.

Calvin: An orange because a motorcycle doesn't have doors.

An adolescent explains a basic process (Chappell, 1985, p. 226):

Well . . . to fix a tire . . . or your wheel . . . you gotta take the tire off. You gotta lift up . . . you jack up the car and use this thing . . . its square metal wrench . . . to loosen the bolts . . . you know the nuts . . . then you take the wheel off the axes. First you ask the guy at the garage if he will fix the tire. You lock up the car so it won't . . . you put the car in gear so it stays put.

BACKGROUND INFORMATION

The preceding examples are the utterances of a child and adolescent who have trouble expressing themselves. Often, their sentences are well formed from a grammatical point of view, but the students struggle to make themselves understood and they frustrate their listeners. They have trouble finding the right words to explain even the simplest events. They do not tell their story in the correct order and/or leave out important elements of their explanation. They have difficulty in staying on a conversational topic. Often, these students pass language tests and screenings given by the speech-language pathologist (SLP), but their problems are quite evident to the people who interact with them frequently in conversations or classroom work. Students who have conversational abilities like those just mentioned most often have trouble with other language skills such as reading and writing. They may have difficulty following directions and comprehending concepts taught in the classroom. This chapter is about such students who have trouble with the more subtle aspects of language and, as a result, may have academic problems as well.

When children are first learning to talk, the importance of language in their lives is relatively simple to understand. In essence, very young children use language for two major purposes: (1) speaking to others in their environment, and (2) listening and understanding others in their environment. When a child enters school, however, the importance of language becomes quite a bit more complex. In addition to speaking and listening, children are taught to use language for purposes of reading and writing. Lay persons often consider these later skills taught in school to be radically different from the language used in speaking and listening; however, *all* of these operations involve the use of the basic language rules that are learned in the preschool years. That is, a student must have a basic grasp of the rules of language to be able to read, write, speak, and listen because all of these skills have these basic rules in common.

Recall from Chapter 3 that speakers must master a number of components of language to achieve linguistic competence. We mention these areas again, just to refresh your memory. **Semantics** are the rules for word meaning that are associated with vocabulary. Thus, a child is applying semantic rules whenever she selects a word and places it in an utterance. Children with small vocabularies have underdeveloped semantic systems. **Syntax** refers to rules that speakers use to combine words into the variety of types of sentences in a language. There are "legal" ways to string words together (e.g., "The boy hit the ball") and there are also unacceptable ways of doing this (e.g., "boy the ball hit the"). Children who leave out words in a sentence (e.g., "My car in garage") or misuse words in a sentence (e.g., "Her is my sister") are said to have problems with syntax. **Morphology** refers to the attachment of certain endings to words to refine and add additional meaning (e.g., "cat*s*," "runn*ing*," "Mary*'s* car," "walk*ed*"). Children who omit these endings from words (e.g., "Yesterday I walk") or misuse them (e.g., "He gotted the bike") are said to have morphological problems. **Phonology**, or the sound system of a language, also has rules for sound selection and combination. Children who misuse sounds in systematic ways (e.g., "tat" for "cat") are said to have phonological problems. Children who misarticulate often have difficulties in other linguistic domains such as semantics, syntax, and morphology. **Pragmatics** refers to the rules for the use of language in a particular communicative context. The context can take into account different types of listeners (adults, children, those with cognitive impairments, those who are deaf, socially prestigious persons, the principal, a teacher) to whom speakers talk differently because of their various characteristics or positions. The context also can take into account the physical arrangement in which the communication takes place. For instance, a person can point to a chair and say, "I like this one," and not have to use the word *chair*. If, however, a chair is not present in the communicative context, the speaker would have to use the word *chair* and probably also spend some time describing the type of chair he likes the best.

Another pragmatic area concerns the rules speakers use to carry on conversations and involves how to introduce, maintain, and change different topics of conversation and take turns with a conversational partner. Pragmatics also includes the ability to generate an utterance that is clear (not ambiguous) and that is presented in a well-ordered sequence so that the listener has no trouble understanding the contribution to the conversation. If someone tries to give directions to another person on how to fix something and the directions are unclear or the steps are out of order, a pragmatic failure has occurred. The sentences may be well formed from semantic, syntactic, and morphological points of view, but if they do not communicate accurately, a pragmatic problem exists. The area of pragmatics is quite complex, but it is enough to say that it concerns the use of language in real communication situations that take into account the context, the clarity, and the accuracy of the message generated.

One basic message of this section is that the language rules a child learns before age 5 years underlie all functions in which linguistic symbols are used, including speaking, listening, reading, and writing (Catts & Kamhi, 2005). The implication of this is that if a child has a difficulty with language, *all* of the language-dependent functions could be affected. That is, a child who makes errors in spoken language also may make mistakes in written language or have trouble reading and understanding the spoken utterances of others. It is common for lay persons not to see the intimate relationships among the language activities of reading, writing, speaking, and listening, as if all of these are separate skills. In reality, there is a common bond among all of these functions, and it depends on a thorough understanding and facility with language. These issues are addressed more fully in Chapter 14.

A second aspect emphasized earlier is the fact that language comprises a number of components that speakers must learn and use together to be competent language users. The implication is that a language disorder can occur in one or all of these component areas. That is, a language disorder can have a variety of "faces." One student may have obvious problems with omission or misuse of words in sentences. Another may have all of the language elements correct but, because of sequencing problems and an inability to take into account the listener's perspective, simply cannot describe how to get downtown. Thus, the "territory" to be covered when talking about older students and their disorders of language includes all the components of language and all of the potential uses of language between early elementary school years and adolescence.

SYMPTOMS REPORTED IN STUDENTS WITH LANGUAGE PROBLEMS

It has often been said that, as students with language impairments get older, their problems become more subtle in nature. In fact, it is not unusual for a student with language impairment to be "rediagnosed" several times during school. For instance, a child may begin with a preschool language delay and enter kindergarten with the remnants of this disorder. Hopefully, this child is enrolled in language treatment, and the SLP eliminates all major residual symptoms of the problem. When the student begins learning to read, she may have difficulty and be diagnosed as exhibiting a reading problem (Catts, Fey, Zhang, & Tomblin, 2001). Later, as the content of the academic program becomes more complex, the student may be diagnosed as having a specific learning disability. It is altogether possible that most of the student's problems may represent a broad, underlying difficulty with learning language and using it effectively to solve problems, even though the student may *speak* clearly. Thus, the high-risk groups for language disorder in older children are as follows:

1. Students with a history of late talking or language delay as preschoolers (Johnson et al., 1999; Rescorla, 2002)
2. Students who score low on standardized reading tests or struggle with learning to read (Catts, 1997)
3. Students diagnosed with language-based learning disabilities
4. Students who are struggling academically

It is important for both medical and educational professionals to know that language disorder appears to persist in more than half of children diagnosed in the preschool years with linguistic impairment. When they enter school and must learn more complex syntax/vocabulary and linguistically based literacy skills such as reading and writing, their weakness in the area of language once again manifests. We discuss this in greater detail in Chapter 14. For now, it is enough to say that high-risk children seen in medical/clinical settings with limited language are at age 3 years eligible to receive services from the public school system. Speech-language professionals always hope for a smooth transition from the medical/clinical setting to the educational system. Hopefully, the medical/clinical team provides all information regarding assessment and treatment to the educational team.

Table 6–1 lists some linguistic symptoms reported in the literature by researchers and clinicians who work with older students diagnosed as language-impaired and/or learning-disabled. Some of these behaviors also may be found in academically low-achieving students who are ineligible for special education services. If teachers note students from the high-risk categories mentioned in this chapter who exhibit some of these symptoms, they can make a referral to the SLP. Note that the behaviors cross *all* areas of language (semantics, syntax, and pragmatics); that they can manifest in speaking, reading, or writing; and that they can be present in production *or* comprehension of language. The list is certainly *not* all-inclusive and should not be viewed as exhaustive.

SETTING AND THE OLDER CHILD WITH LANGUAGE DISORDERS

Although the present text is designed to discuss disorders in the context of medical/clinical and educational settings, speech professionals deal with some specific impairments disproportionately across environments. For example, speech professionals deal with adults who experience strokes exclusively in medical/clinical settings and not in the public school system. Similarly, high-risk neonates are seen in medical/clinical settings and not typically

TABLE 6–1 Common Symptoms of Language Disorder in Older Students

Semantics

- Word-finding/retrieval deficits
- Use of a large number of words in an attempt to explain a concept because the student cannot remember the name (circumlocutions)
- Overuse of limited vocabulary
- Difficulty recalling names of items in categories (e.g., animals, foods)
- Difficulty retrieving verbal opposites
- Small vocabulary
- Use of words lacking specificity (e.g., *thing, junk, stuff*)
- Inappropriate use of words (selection of wrong word)
- Difficulty defining words
- Less comprehension of complex words
- Failure to grasp double word meanings (e.g., *can, file*)

Syntax/Morphology

- Use of grammatically incorrect sentence structures
- Simple, as opposed to complex, sentences
- Less comprehension of complex grammatical structures
- Prolonged pauses while constructing sentences
- Semantically empty placeholders (e.g., filled pauses, *uh, er, um*)
- Use of many stereotyped phrases that do not require much language skill
- Use of "starters" (e.g., "you know")

Pragmatics

- Use of redundant expressions and information the listener has already heard
- Use of nonspecific vocabulary (e.g., *thing, stuff*) and the listener cannot tell from prior conversation or physical context what is referred to
- Less skill in giving explanations clearly to a listener (lack of detail)
- Less skill in explaining something in a proper sequence
- Less conversational control in terms of introducing, maintaining, and changing topics (may get off track in conversation and introduce new topics awkwardly)
- Rare use of clarification questions (e.g., "I don't understand," "You did what?")
- Difficulty shifting conversational style in different social situations (e.g., peer vs. teacher; child vs. adult)
- Difficulty grasping the main idea of a story or lecture (preoccupation with irrelevant details)
- Trouble making inferences from material not explicitly stated (e.g., "Sally went outside. She had to put up her umbrella." Inference: It is raining)
- Difficulties comprehending and using slang
- Difficulties in deriving meaning from vocal inflection and prosodic cues (e.g., sarcasm)

in a school environment. Most adults with communication disorders are seen in medical/clinical settings. Conversely, school-based SLPs predominantly see most school-age children. Sometimes, supplemental treatment provided by medical/clinical settings is elected by parents to augment therapy from the educational system. Thus, the population of school-age children with language disorders is seen, predominantly, in the school environment. The treatment in the public school system is free of charge, and the language therapy can more easily be coordinated with the student's educational program. Thus, in this chapter we do not discuss medical/clinical settings but focus on the school environment.

One important point that should not be lost is that language disorder ranges on a continuum from preschool children with limited language to older children who have difficulty with more complex language and literacy skills. In most cases, they are the same children who have simply grown older and manifest a different form of language disorder. Thus, the children who were treated in the medical/clinical setting at a younger age transition into the educational system between 3 and 5 years of age.

ASSESSMENT ISSUES

One of the most important aspects in dealing with older students with language disorders is the initial detection of these youngsters. An equally critical process involves the thorough evaluation of their language-based competencies. This section generally describes these processes.

THE IMPORTANCE OF TEACHER REFERRAL

In most school systems, the SLP does not engage in screening large numbers of older students for communication problems. If a student is observed experiencing a communication difficulty, the classroom teacher is often the first one to note its occurrence. It is relatively obvious when a student has a problem with articulation, stuttering, severe hoarseness, or some language problem where an element of language is omitted or clearly misused. On the other hand, it is sometimes quite difficult for teachers to discriminate the more subtle disorders of pragmatics and metalinguistics that plague the older student with a language disorder. Also, it is not always clear that the academic problems exhibited by a particular student may have a partial basis in a subtle language difficulty. What the teacher sees is a student who is performing poorly on an academic level, and it may not seem that a referral to the SLP is indicated. We suggest that teachers make *routine referrals* for a language screening and/or evaluation for the following students:

1. Any student who experiences sustained academic problems (consistent below-average grades, retention in a grade)
2. Students who have been diagnosed as learning disabled and who are experiencing academic difficulty

3. Students who exhibit obvious problems with reading (either orally or reading comprehension)
4. Any student who appears to have trouble with communication in spoken language.

More specifically, the teacher should watch for the following symptoms:

- Inability to explain something clearly and concisely
- Problems with sequencing information appropriately
- Problems staying on the topic of conversation
- Problems understanding and/or giving directions
- Evidence of retrials, hesitations, filled pauses, and such
- Word-finding problems
- Inappropriate use of words
- Grammatically incorrect sentence structures

It is *only* through teacher referral that these students will be detected in most school systems, so the importance of this role of the classroom teacher cannot be overemphasized. Many SLPs conduct brief in-service training presentations to school faculty on the symptoms that indicate the appropriate referral for screening or evaluation (McKinley & Larson, 1985).

The identification of a student with a language impairment is simplified in cases where the child was discovered in the early preschool years and received services in community medical/clinical settings. In such instances, the student enters the school system with a complete file summarizing his assessment and treatment history.

EVALUATION

If a student is referred to the SLP for testing, the SLP needs to explore several areas; these can be tapped by both formal and informal assessment techniques. **Formal testing** refers to standardized examinations that have been given to large groups of normally developing students that provide norms for performance on the measure. Through formal testing, SLPs can determine how the student is performing compared to same-age peers in areas of language comprehension and production. There are literally hundreds of standardized tests of language ability, and providing all the names and references for these examinations is beyond the scope of this text. It is enough to say that a large variety of formal tests exists for evaluating all aspects of language ability, and the SLP uses these for part of the assessment. Specific tests used by SLPs vary with their background, training, and professional preferences, thus the examinations might change from one school system to another. No doubt, the SLP will consult with the classroom teacher and other school personnel regarding the types of tests that have been used in a student's evaluation, the results, interpretation, and classroom application of the findings.

The use of **informal evaluation** tasks is another way to gain insight into a student's language and communication ability. Many authorities suggest that using informal, descriptive methods in evaluation actually provides more information that is directly relevant to treatment and academic performance (Haynes & Pindzola, 2007; Paul, 2007).

Because the biggest concern of the SLP is language and communication, most of the formal test instruments and nonstandardized evaluation tasks focus on a number of areas. As mentioned earlier, language can be divided into components of semantics, syntax, morphology, phonology, and pragmatics. All of these components are used in both input (language comprehension) and output (language production). Thus, for a thorough evaluation, the SLP should test the student's facility with vocabulary, sentence structure, word endings, and the use of language in various contexts. For instance, standardized tests and informal tasks can be directed toward assessing the student's understanding of semantic elements (vocabulary) as well as the ability to produce or retrieve words given a specific cue. Syntax ability is tapped by having a student follow directions that vary in their grammatical complexity (syntactic comprehension). The production of syntax is evaluated by having the student engage in conversation or description tasks, and then taking an inventory of the sentence types constructed and any grammatical errors produced by the student. Morphological ability in comprehension is assessed in a similar manner through asking a student to point to pictures illustrating a particular word ending (e.g., asking the student, "Point to a picture of cats" when one picture contains only one cat and the other has two). Production of morphemes can be evaluated best by noting morphological errors in spontaneous conversation (e.g., "I goes to the store") and the use of other specific elicitation tasks. Phonological ability can be evaluated through a variety of articulation tests (see Chapter 4). Finally, because there are no widely accepted standardized tests of pragmatics, these skills are best assessed in spontaneous conversation using a series of specific tasks that require the student to carefully describe pictures or provide particular information to a listener. Another popular task is to have the student produce a narrative about a favorite book, movie, or event such as a vacation. Students with pragmatic disorders often produce narratives that have sequence problems, shorter length, less syntactic complexity, less story grammar elements, and more problems taking into account the listener's perspective (Haynes & Pindzola, 2007). Pragmatic disorders are often associated with social difficulties in children with language impairment (Fujiki, Brinton, & Todd, 1996; Fujiki, Brinton, Isaacson, & Summers, 2001). This again illustrates how the SLP should extend assessment beyond formal testing and determine environmental effects of the communication disorder using teachers and peers as informants. After the evaluation, the SLP should know whether the student is performing within normal limits in all areas of language and in the use of language to solve problems.

Because reading and writing are language-based activities (Catts & Kamhi, 2005), these areas represent another assessment concern for the SLP. Apel states, "Speech-language pathologists should assess and facilitate reading and writing skills, in addition to oral language skills, if they have been identified as areas of concern" (Apel, 1999, p. 229). The SLP cannot only assess specific skills such as decoding, spelling, reading, and writing, but can integrate these into treatment activities (Graham & Harris, 1999; Masterson & Crede, 1999; Apel & Swank, 1999).

A final assessment area involves the student's environment. The SLP may be interested in visiting the student's classroom(s) to gain an idea about the teaching styles that she encounters in different classes. The SLP needs to determine whether aspects of a teacher's presentation (e.g., speech rate, use of complex or figurative language) could interfere with the processing of information by a student with language impairment. The SLP also needs to determine what types of teaching aids (e.g., media, study guides, outlines) different teachers use. Such aids are very helpful to all students in the class, but especially to students with language impairment. The curriculum is also a target of evaluation by the SLP. She can ask about textbooks and the order of teaching material in a particular class. Many SLPs have incorporated "portfolio evaluation" into their assessment of students with language problems (Kratcoski, 1998). Thus, samples of a student's written work, classroom tests, and projects can be incorporated into the assessment. Many times linguistic problems surface across the different modalities of reading, writing, and speaking and use of portfolio materials can provide a broader evaluation of a student's language ability. In this way, the SLP also finds out what kinds of subject matter the student should be able to talk about and explain. Often, the treatment sessions center on academic subjects and classroom work.

DIRECT AND INDIRECT TREATMENT FOR STUDENTS WITH LANGUAGE IMPAIRMENT

Note that many of the ideas that follow are not merely "suggestions." Children with disabilities such as language impairment are protected under several federal laws that *require* teachers and school systems to make appropriate accommodations in the classroom (see Chapter 1 for further details). Adjustments such as extended time on exams, permission to tape record lectures, use of books on tape, use of FM amplification systems, preferential seating, and many other accommodations are reasonable and appropriate for students with disabilities. It is a sad commentary that some students receive their first classroom accommodations when they begin their university careers and learn about their rights when they report to the office for students with disabilities their first week of college. We can only speculate about the quality of learning that could have occurred if such students had received appropriate classroom accommodations in elementary, junior, and senior high school.

When dealing with school-age children with language disorders, SLPs generally draw treatment goals from a number of areas (Schwartz & McKinley, 1984; McKinley & Larson, 1985; Miller, 1989; Larson, McKinley, & Boley, 1993; Wallach & Butler, 1994; Lord-Larson & McKinley, 1995).

1. *Academic organization:* Students with language disorders often have difficulty with time management, study skills, and the ability to perform critical thinking activities. These difficulties are compounded if the student has Attention Deficit Disorder (ADD) or a learning disability on top of the difficulties with language. The SLP in concert with other professionals can work with the student on these academic organization issues

and develop strategies that allow the student to succeed in the school culture. Often, teachers do not perceive the need or make the time to work on academic organization with students who have language disorders. Whereas the SLP can do this, others must recommend it as a valid need/goal. The SLP can integrate these goals into the treatment plan, but this may justify and necessitate time and resources to accomplish these additional objectives.

2. *Listening/comprehension:* As mentioned previously, students with language disorders often have difficulty comprehending classroom language because of the interaction of their language disorder with the complexities of teacher utterances. If the student has difficulty comprehending instructions, academic information, or even social interaction language, the student will experience communication failure that has academic as well as social consequences. Thus, the SLP often has listening/comprehension goals for the student with language disorders.

3. *Oral language production:* Table 6–1 lists a number of symptoms of language disorder in older students. Some of the most frequent language production goals include maintaining a conversational topic, taking into account the listener's perspective, providing adequate detail, and putting information in a correct sequence. Some of these students also need assistance in producing more syntactically complex utterances and correcting errors in sentence formulation.

4. *Written language/reading:* As noted earlier, language-based activities such as speaking, writing, reading, and spelling are most often affected as a group in a student with a language disorder. The SLP often incorporates reading and writing goals into the language work and uses written language as stimulus in treatment (Fleming & Forester, 1997).

FOUR GENERAL GUIDELINES IN DESIGNING TREATMENT

No matter which mode of treatment is used (direct or indirect), the SLP should consider four guidelines for the conduct of language therapy with older students:

1. *Teach strategies, not just memorization.* Older students tend to require strategies for academic, social, and communicative success, rather than learning a series of rote behaviors for each difficult situation they encounter. That is, these students need to learn methods to increase their organization, comprehension, memory, test-taking skills, oral communication, and reading/writing abilities that apply to a broad range of circumstances. SLPs do not just want to help the student get through only one problem situation. The notion of strategy implies that students learn ways of dealing successfully with a variety of circumstances that are similar. For example, teaching a study skill for a certain type of information is applicable on other occasions when the student must learn similar material. Teaching a social interaction strategy (stay on the conversational topic) is applicable to all of the student's conversations.

2. *Design activities appropriate to age/cognitive level.* This guideline should be obvious; however, sometimes SLPs overlook it. Dealing with teenagers or preteen students is a slippery endeavor. Sometimes a teacher or clinician may forget that certain materials that have been designed for younger children may not be appropriate for older students. By the same token, SLPs should not use materials that are significantly above the student's level of performance.

3. *Make activities relevant.* It is especially important when dealing with older students that they see the relevance of treatment activities. Topics such as getting a driver's license, dating, getting a part-time job, improving study skills, politics, and world history may be great topics to use in language treatment because students can then generalize the language training to other important situations. It is a great waste of time for the SLP to center treatment sessions around talking about "what we did on the weekend" and exclude academic and social issues. One of the most important facets of language treatment is to include "survival language." Survival language is the type of communication people use to be successful in everyday life. When SLPs teach a student language they can use in a job interview, how to take accurate telephone messages, or how to tell a story/joke, they are providing training in basic life skills. If speech professionals focus on teaching vocabulary associated with specific survival areas such as cooking, transportation, label warnings, and health issues, they can increase the student's ability to communicate more easily about activities of daily living. This is much more important than teaching arbitrary vocabulary words that may not contribute to the student's ultimate success in society.

4. *Look for the triple payoff.* SLPs must consider any language treatment activity in light of whether it has a triple payoff in communication, social, and academic areas. It is easy to design an activity to enhance a student's language abilities (e.g., using more complex sentences). It is more difficult to make that activity communicatively, socially, and academically relevant. For example, the SLP can work on production of more complex sentences while talking about the federal government, which is the topic of concern in the student's political science class. Talking about how the government is organized is just as easy as talking about what the student did at the beach last summer, and it has an academic payoff. If the SLP uses the student's textbook as a springboard for conversations about classroom material, there is an academic as well as a communication payoff. If the SLP works on production of more complex sentences while teaching the student to produce oral narratives, the student's ability to tell personal experiences and humorous stories will be enhanced. This constitutes a social payoff. Ideally, the SLP should seek activities that have this triple payoff and not just work on communication.

Lasky provides some of the most useful suggestions we have found for classroom teachers and SLPs who deal with students with language learning disabilities (Lasky, 1985). The suggestions fall into several areas and are discussed next.

THE INFORMATION TO BE COMMUNICATED

Although it is not recommended that the SLP perform tutoring of classroom material, the SLP can certainly use some academic content to teach strategies that apply across classes. For example, in teaching a student a strategy for how to retrieve new vocabulary, the SLP could use words particular to a certain class to illustrate the concept. This is certainly preferable to teaching a retrieval strategy using vocabulary that is unrelated to the student's academic work. Some specific suggestions about modifying information follow:

1. Let the SLP check comprehension and expression of specific concepts taught in the classroom (social studies, science, reading, and so on). In this way, the student's educators can determine whether the student really understands and can explain concepts learned in class. The teacher does not have time to routinely check the understanding or speaking facility of individual students until it is time for a test. This, of course, is too late for a student with language learning problems.

2. If there are new vocabulary words associated with a chapter, the teacher and SLP could put these in a handout to emphasize their importance. As part of a larger process to teach vocabulary-learning strategies, the SLP could work directly on tasks that require the student to explain or comprehend these new vocabulary items.

3. If the student has difficulty comprehending complex sentences, the SLP could explain new classroom concepts in simpler grammatical sentences and then gradually increase the syntactic complexity when she talks about the new concept. Thus, the student may be better able to grasp the material in classroom presentations when the teacher is likely to use more complex language.

4. Again, as part of an overall program to increase vocabulary size, the SLP can teach new semantic concepts in advance of the teacher's classroom presentation. This could enhance the student's ability to understand the material when it is presented later by the teacher.

5. If there are specific tasks that involve use of metalinguistic ability, complex language, or nonliteral meanings (e.g., figurative language), the SLP could drill the student on these types of skills prior to or concurrently with their use in the classroom.

MODIFYING THE PRESENTATION

Lasky indicates that another important aspect of helping students with language disabilities is to present material in such a way as to facilitate comprehension (Lasky, 1985, p. 119).

Clinicians and teachers need to work as a team not only to present contextual cues but also to help the child recognize *when* contextual cues are presented. Types of contextual cues include (1) stating the topic to be discussed; (2) providing specific verbal instructions to guide the listener; (3) supplying a prepared outline; (4) using slides, charts, pictures, graphs, diagrams, or a film; and (5) presenting directed questions. These cues trigger listeners' expectations, help focus their attention on critical points, and aid listeners in anticipating information, seeing relationships, and organizing and remembering information.

Other suggestions for modifying the presentation involve the following.

1. *Redundancy:* The more the teacher can repeat a particular concept in a number of different ways, the greater the chance that the student will understand it. This aid is not just important or helpful for students with language learning disabilities, but for everyone in the class.
2. *Slower rate:* Many investigations show that children and adults with language impairments are more likely to comprehend utterances that are presented at slower speech rates. Teachers who have students with language impairments in their classes should try to use a slower rate, especially when explaining important and abstract concepts.
3. *Tape recording:* Students with language disorders and learning problems can also be encouraged to tape record lectures so that they can listen to them as often as needed at home to fill in gaps in class notes.

MODIFYING THE ENVIRONMENT

A potential problem for students with language disabilities in the classroom is paying attention. Many studies show this population to exhibit attentional difficulties. The classroom is especially susceptible to ambient noise and distractions from a variety of sources. Some studies show that, although most classrooms have varying degrees of environmental noise (e.g., traffic, hallway noise, sounds from fans), the conversations of others provide the most distracting type of noise (Lasky & Tobin, 1973). This is especially true if the student with language impairment is listening to a small number of talkers seated nearby as opposed to large numbers of talkers in, for instance, a lunchroom (Miller, 1947). When students with language impairment listen to small numbers of talkers, they hear certain words and phrases, and this is more distracting than listening to a large group of talkers, where particular parts of the conversation cannot be deciphered.

At any rate, the teacher must be aware that both environmental noise and classroom talking/whispering can and do affect the attention of students with language impairment. Perhaps preferential seating in the front of the room can enhance listening and be coupled with cautions to the class members against talking when they should be listening. Also, teachers can make available study carrels or isolated work areas for use by these students to enhance their attention and concentration on assignments.

MODIFYING THE RESPONSE

Sometimes when teaching a particular concept, speech professionals tend to demand responses from students for relatively shallow activities that require little processing of information. For instance, having students imitate, point to pictures, or memorize lists of information may not truly help them to "learn" the essence of the concept or how it may be applied in a variety of contexts. Some students with language impairment may have more difficulty memorizing material if they do not see how it applies in meaningful contexts. The SLP and teacher can work with such students on meaningful application of material that may facilitate understanding and memory instead of using shallower and less meaningful response modes.

Teachers might consider allowing students who have particular difficulty with written language use of a computer for written assignments. Computers add the advantages of spell-checking, thesauruses, and word prediction software that could be valuable to the student with a language disorder. When a student's writing is very poor, perhaps the student can read his book report that the rest of the class is writing into a tape recorder as a reasonable alternative. Teachers and SLPs, of course, must decide this on an individual basis for each student and assignment.

MODIFYING LEARNING STRATEGIES

Students develop strategies for processing information in the early elementary school years, and then modify these strategies as they change grade levels and as teacher expectations change over time (Naus & Halasz, 1979). Several researchers have pointed out that students with language impairments are not as adept as normally achieving students are at developing specific strategies for organizing material and devising overt methods for learning it (Kavale, 1980; Schworm & Abelseth, 1981; Lasky, 1985).

Among the typical strategies normally achieving children use are verbal mediation, rehearsal, paraphrasing, visual imagery, analysis of key ideas, networking, and use of systematic retrieval strategies (Lasky, 1985). Research shows that these strategies can be overtly taught to students, and this training is effective, retained over long periods of time, and generalized to different situations (Kestner & Borkowski, 1979). The teacher and SLP could actively teach the student with a language disability to use specific strategies to enhance the understanding, recognition, recall, and application of concepts taught in the classroom.

Whereas normally developing students evidently need little overt assistance in developing study skills and learning strategies, the student with a language learning disability may not spontaneously generate such abilities. Direct teaching helps such students understand material and demonstrate knowledge on tests and examinations. The teacher and SLP no doubt need to experiment with a variety of methods for each student with language impairments to determine the optimal strategies that student can use to learn particular material presented in the classroom. In an ideal scenario, the particular learning style of the student with language impairments is matched with a teacher having a compatible teaching style. Although this is not always feasible, it is possible to consider such a match when there is flexibility in deciding to which classroom to assign a student with language impairment.

WHICH TYPE OF TREATMENT FORMAT IS BEST?

The suggestions discussed earlier imply that the classroom teacher and SLP work together in facilitating the linguistic, communicative, and academic performance of the student with language impairment. Some of this work can be accomplished through individual sessions with the SLP, but much work can be done with these students in groups. In fact, for the majority of students many authorities recommend group treatment in preference to individual treatment (McKinley & Larson, 1985; Simon, 1987). Many strategies for learning, memory, and retrieval that benefit most students with language impairments can be taught and practiced in group work. Even listening skills, study skills, organizational skills, and strategies for more effective expression can be taught in a group environment. McKinley and Larson also recommend the following, especially for adolescents with language disorders (McKinley & Larson, 1985, p. 8).

1. *Using existing time modules:* Removing students from classes twice a week for 20 minutes is token service and can cause serious disruption academically and socially.
2. *Using supportive labels for services:* "Speech therapy" and "language therapy" may be poor labels for adolescents with language disorders trying to appear similar to their peers. Better labels might be "individualized language skills" or "oral communication strategies."
3. *Recognizing students' efforts:* Offering language intervention as a course for credit (e.g., one fourth credit per semester) is more appropriate than not offering any credit at all. Students invest at least as much time and energy working on their communication skills as they do on other skills taught as courses for credit.
4. *Using group settings:* Intervention with adolescents requires much more grouping of students into classes than does intervention with younger students. Students need to be grouped to facilitate interaction because a major goal for many adolescents with language disorders is appropriate and effective communication (i.e., pragmatic skills).

Many SLPs in elementary grades conduct group units in communication for English classes or other related subjects (Simon, 1987). Such group (class) instruction can benefit large numbers of students, often without the formal process of Individualized Education Program (IEP) writing, unending meetings, or the reams of paperwork required to formally add the child to the SLP's caseload. The students receive additional services focusing on communication skills, study skills, and "playing the school game," and they are not singled out as "disordered." Although most students can benefit greatly from such group sessions, some require the individual attention of the SLP to work on specific language disorders and would be formally evaluated and added to the caseload. The most current recommendations suggest that the SLP offer a variety of treatment options for the older student with language impairment (Larson et al., 1993).

The child with language impairment may also benefit from additional tutoring, both within and outside of the school setting; some students enjoy peer tutoring, if it proves practical and effective. Finally, there is a need to recognize that a child with a language disorder may never fully develop a normal ability to deal with linguistic material in reading, writing, speaking, or listening. These children can especially benefit from career testing and vocational counseling early in their secondary school years. They need to know which types of jobs require complex language and communication skills. In fact, federal law requires school systems to provide a transition plan for students with disabilities by age 14 years or earlier, if appropriate (Prendeville & Ross-Allen, 2002). If university training is required, they need to be directed to campuses that offer services for students with language and learning disabilities.

A large group of students who struggle in the academic setting could benefit from the combined assistance of the classroom teacher and the speech-language pathologist. Through a true collaborative effort, teachers and SLPs can save these students from "falling between the cracks" of the educational system and give them a better chance to succeed academically.

Terms to Know

Semantics	Pragmatics
Syntax	Formal testing
Morphology	Informal evaluation
Phonology	

Study Questions

1. Record yourself giving instructions to an imaginary class on how to do a specific assignment. Play back the tape and analyze the complexity, rate, and disfluency in your instructions. Note your use of figurative language. How would you change these instructions if you had a chance to do them again? How do you think a child with language learning problems would understand the instructions?

2. Pretend you are a teacher. Make up a specific lesson plan to teach a simple academic concept. Assume that you have two children with language disorders in your class and indicate how you would teach the lesson differently because they are in the class in terms of visual aids, handouts, explanations, questioning, and class discussion.

Bibliography

Apel, K. (1999). An introduction to assessment and intervention with older students with language-learning impairments: Bridges from research to clinical practice. *Language, Speech and Hearing Services in Schools, 30*, 228–230.

Apel, K., & Swank, L. (1999). Second chances: Improving decoding skills in the older student. *Language, Speech and Hearing Services in Schools, 30*, 231–242.

Catts, H. (1997). The early identification of language-based reading disabilities. *Language, Speech and Hearing Services in Schools, 28*, 86–89.

Catts, H., Fey, M., Zhang, X., & Tomblin, B. (2001). Estimating the risk of future reading difficulties in kindergarten children: A research based model and its clinical implications. *Language, Speech and Hearing Services in Schools, 32*, 38–50.

Catts, H., & Kamhi, A. (2005). *Language and reading disabilities.* Boston, MA: Allyn & Bacon.

Chappell, G. (1985). Description and assessment of language disabilities of junior high school students. In C. Simon (Ed.), *Communication skills and classroom success: Assessment of language-learning disabled students.* San Diego, CA: College-Hill.

Fleming, J., & Forester, B. (1997). Infusing language enhancement into the reading curriculum for disadvantaged adolescents. *Language, Speech and Hearing Services in Schools, 28*(2), 177–180.

Fujiki, M., Brinton, B., Isaacson, T., & Summers, C. (2001). Social behaviors of children with language impairment on the playground: A pilot study. *Language, Speech and Hearing Services in Schools, 32*(2), 101–113.

Fujiki, M., Brinton, B., & Todd, C. (1996). Social skills of children with specific language impairment. *Language, Speech and Hearing Services in Schools, 27*, 195–202.

Graham, S., & Harris, K. (1999). Assessment and intervention in overcoming writing difficulties: An illustration from the self regulated strategy development model. *Language, Speech and Hearing Services in Schools, 30*, 255–264.

Haynes, W., & Pindzola, R. (2007). *Diagnosis and evaluation in speech pathology.* Needham Heights, MA: Allyn & Bacon.

Johnson, C., Beitchman, J., Young, A., Escobar, M., Atkinson, L., Wilson, B., Brownlie, E., Douglas, L., Taback, N., Lam, I., & Wong, M. (1999). Fourteen-year follow-up of children with and without speech/language impairments: Speech/language stability and outcomes. *Journal of Speech, Language and Hearing Research, 42*, 744–768.

Kavale, K. (1980). Learning disability and cultural economic disadvantage: The case for a relationship. *Learning Disability Quarterly, 3*, 97–112.

Kestner, J., & Borkowski, J. (1979). Children's maintenance and generalization of an interrogative learning strategy. *Child Development, 50*, 485–494.

Kratcoski, A. (1998). Guidelines for using portfolios in assessment and evaluation. *Language, Speech and Hearing Services in Schools, 29*, 3–10.

Larson, V., & McKinley, N. (1995). *Language disorders in older students.* Eau Claire, WI: Thinking Publications.

Larson, V., McKinley, N., & Boley, D. (1993). Service delivery models for adolescents with language disorders. *Language, Speech & Hearing Services in Schools, 24*, 36–42.

Lasky, E. (1985). Comprehending and processing of information in clinic and classroom. In C. Simon (Ed.), *Communication skills and classroom success: Therapy methodologies for language learning disabled students.* San Diego, CA: College-Hill.

Lasky, E., & Tobin, H. (1973). Linguistic and nonlinguistic competing message efforts. *Journal of Learning Disabilities, 6*, 243–250.

Lord-Larson, V. & McKinley, N. (1995). *Language Disorders in Older Students: Preadolescents and Adolescents*. Eau Claire, WI: Thinking Publications.

Masterson, J., & Crede, L. (1999). Learning to spell: Implications for assessment and intervention. *Language, Speech and Hearing Services in Schools, 30*, 243–254.

McKinley, N., & Larson, V. (1985). Neglected language-disordered adolescent: A delivery model. *Language, Speech and Hearing Services in Schools, 16*, 2–15.

Miller, G. (1947). The masking of speech. *Psychological Bulletin, 44*, 105–129.

Miller, L. (1989). Classroom based intervention. *Language, Speech and Hearing Services in Schools, 20*(2), 153–169.

Naus, M., & Halasz, F. (1979). Developmental perspectives on cognitive processing and semantic memory structure. In L. Cermak & F. Craik (Eds.), *Levels of Processing in Human Memory*. Hillsdale, NJ: Lawrence Erlbaum Associates.

Paul, R. (2007). *Language disorders from infancy through adolescence: Assessment and intervention* (3rd ed.). St. Louis, MO: Mosby.

Prendeville, J., & Ross-Allen, J. (2002). The transition process in the early years: Enhancing speech-language pathologist's perspectives. *Language, Speech and Hearing Services in Schools, 33*, 130–136.

Rescorla, L. (2002). Language and reading outcomes to age 9 in late talking toddlers. *Journal of Speech, Language and Hearing Research, 45*, 360–371.

Schwartz, L., & McKinley, N. (1984). *Daily communication*. Eau Claire, WI: Thinking Publications.

Schworm, R., & Abelseth, J. (1981). Evaluating instructional interactions: Where do we begin teaching? *Learning Disabilities Quarterly, 4*, 101–111.

Simon, C. (1987). Out of the broom closet and into the classroom: The emerging SLP. *Journal of Childhood Communication Disorders, 11*, 41–66.

Wallach, G., & Butler, K. (1994). *Language learning disabilities in school-age children*. Baltimore, MD: Lippincott, Williams and Wilkins.

Chapter 7

AN OVERVIEW OF MULTICULTURAL ISSUES IN COMMUNICATION DISORDERS

Whether employed in a clinical/medical setting or an educational environment, the speech-language pathologist (SLP) comes in daily contact with a very heterogeneous population of clients and families. The people who seek the services of SLPs come from a variety of socioeconomic levels, cultural backgrounds, races, and ages. They speak a wide variety of languages and dialects and have diverse belief systems about disabilities and their remediation. It would be a horrendous mistake to assume that all clients are the same, especially in a field that involves the development of a clinical relationship with a person and his or her family. This chapter introduces you to the importance of multicultural considerations in the work of the communication disorders professional, teachers, and healthcare providers.

POPULATION AND PROFESSIONAL TRENDS

The Bureau of Labor Statistics predicts that by the year 2050, white Americans with European ancestry will no longer be the largest population group in the United States. At present, white Americans make up about 75 percent of the population, but by midcentury their numbers will be reduced to approximately 50 percent. This is because the Hispanic, Asian, and African American populations are growing at a much faster rate as a result of immigration patterns and increased birth rates. Currently, there is an increased emphasis on multiculturalism in business, medicine, education, religion, and other areas as these disciplines struggle to deal with bilingualism and cultural practices that may not reflect the mainstream values of the past century. In the last quarter century, significant increases in sensitivity to other cultures and languages in the United States has occurred. You need only open the directions for a new appliance and see multiple translations of instructions for assembly. Many businesses have multilingual menus on their Web sites or telephone banks. Even in major department stores, clerks have access to translators via telephone that can interpret the needs of customers who speak most of the world's languages. American society is no longer like it was in the 1950s where the predominant assumptions were that everyone speaks English and all people hold the same cultural values.

These trends are also evident in medical and educational settings. Most medical environments are capable of dealing with patients who speak languages other than English. It is easy to see the importance of communication to diagnosing and treating patients with medical problems. Similarly, in school settings, educators are faced with children who represent multiple cultures and ethnicities and who often speak two or more languages. For many of these students, English is not their first language, yet they must enter a school system that is still largely geared for speakers of English. School systems have gradually integrated information from other cultural groups in history courses and social studies classes. Contributions of African American, Hispanic, Asian American, and Native American groups are now included in the curriculum. English as a Second Language (ESL) classes are offered to assist students who are not proficient in speaking English.

Thus, the SLP working in a medical/clinical environment must be aware of possible cultural and linguistic differences in clients and so must other allied health professionals working in such settings. Similarly, the SLP and educational professionals must take into account cultural and linguistic factors when dealing with students from kindergarten through high school. We discuss in later sections some specific ways in which language and culture might affect a client's performance in assessment and treatment of communication disorders.

BILINGUALISM AND DIALECTAL VARIATION

Professionals who work in medical/clinical and educational settings must realize that dialects and bilingualism are both similar and different. First, consider **bilingualism**. If a person originally from Mexico is bilingual, he or she has a first language (e.g., Spanish) and a second language (e.g., English). But turn this example around. For purposes of this illustration, assume that an American student grew up speaking English as a first language and has taken several Spanish courses in high school and college so that she is proficient in speaking Spanish. This student probably has a stronger first language (English) as compared to her second language (Spanish). Of course, the more Spanish courses the student takes and the greater her opportunities to speak Spanish, the stronger the second language becomes. There is a continuum of proficiency with a second language based on training and practice. With lots of training and practice, the student could speak Spanish with native speakers and discuss complex and abstract issues such as philosophy, economics, and politics. With less training and practice, the student might be able only to ask for directions to the train station or order food in a restaurant.

When initially learning a second language, a person is at a considerable disadvantage in communicating, especially if the communication involves complex issues. Picture a Hispanic family who has just immigrated to the United States and has minimal English speaking skills. If a member of this family had a stroke and had to go to an American hospital, it would be difficult for family members to communicate significant medical and case history information to the medical staff with their limited proficiency in English. Similarly, if a student enters the school system with limited English speaking skills, he is at a distinct disadvantage in learning complex concepts taught in English by the educational staff. Thus, when you consider bilingualism, you must take into account the proficiency level a person possesses in speaking the second language and the effect this has on basic communication skill.

Dialect is a complex topic. A dialect is a variation of a national language shared by a particular speech community. Dialects are not totally different languages. A dialect can be regional (Southern, Northeastern, Cajun) or be associated with a particular group of individuals (African American dialect, Hispanic English, Asian English). Thus, when we consider dialect, we are talking about relatively minor changes to a national language. African American speakers speak English, but with an African American dialect. Another way to think of a dialect is as an "accent." Most people can listen to someone on the telephone who is speaking English and know if they "sound" African American, Hispanic, Asian or like they are from New York. This is because the person on the telephone is speaking a dialect of English that is associated with a particular group. To continue the preceding example of the Hispanic family who immigrated to the United States, say the family has been in the country for five years, has taken classes in English as a Second Language (ESL), and has had consistent opportunities to practice speaking, reading, and writing English on a daily basis. A person from this family might be able to communicate quite well in English, even about abstract and complex topics, so basic communication is not impaired. He or she might be able to go to a medical facility and communicate efficiently with the medical staff. In educational settings, this person can participate in classroom activities with minimal difficulty. But in both cases, the person might speak a Hispanic dialect. For example, when she says the word *shoe*, she might produce it as "choo." English speakers can understand her, but they perceive her as having a dialect. Similarly, she might make syntactic changes to sentences such as "I talk to her yesterday" instead of "I talked to her yesterday." Dialect speakers can be bilingual, and they may be farther along toward the more proficient end of the continuum, but they may speak English with a Hispanic dialect. It is always important to realize, however, that such a dialect speaker may have the ability to deal with only basic aspects of communication, and when more complex issues are discussed, she may be unable to understand or produce messages. Dialect speakers who have little difficulty with communication can get their point across, but are perceived by listeners as having "an accent." Bilingual speakers can also communicate well (with a dialect) if they have had training and practice speaking English; however, they can experience major communication problems if they are only beginning to learn English and have had little opportunity to practice. For SLPs, medical staff, and educational professionals it is important to realize that when communication is impaired in a bilingual individual, it is important to have the ability to translate information so that it can be understood.

It is also important to mention here that a person can have a dialect and not be bilingual. Speakers of English use regional dialects of English (e.g., Southern) or the African American English dialect without the direct influence of a first language.

PERCEPTIONS OF DISABILITY

Most people are unaware that different cultures have quite disparate perceptions of disabilities and therefore varying ideas of what should and should not be done with people who have disorders. For example, in some cultures, a disability is viewed as something that is visited upon a person because of sins of ancestors or divine providence. In such cases, the disability is that person's lot in life and not something to be remediated. In the United States, most people believe that a person born with a disability or someone who acquires a disorder later in life should be immediately assessed and treated so that he or she can participate in society to the greatest extent possible. The implication is that most immigrants to the United States carry with them cultural values from their country of origin and it may take time to alter these views or they may never change their perception of disability. Professionals in medical/clinical or educational settings may not be able to convince certain clients of the critical nature of early assessment and intervention for family members with communication or other disorders. Whereas most Americans view intervention and assessment activities as worthwhile and indeed their right, it may not be so for people who have recently immigrated. Thus, it is important that professionals are aware of cultural differences in the perception of disability and can provide counseling and information that might make families aware of their options in clinical assessment and intervention.

CLIENT-CLINICIAN RELATIONSHIPS (INTERVIEWING/COUNSELING)

Client–clinician relationships are often a challenge because the client comes to a professional with a problem. During the clinical interaction, the clinician must obtain from the client information of a personal nature about the onset and development of the communication disorder and how the condition is affecting the person and his family. Sometimes, such disclosures are emotional and the client may be revealing such information and feelings for the first time. As you can imagine, clinicians must handle such interactions carefully and professionally so that the client feels as comfortable as possible in an admittedly sensitive situation.

These types of interactions can be difficult even when the client and clinician are similar in race and cultural backgrounds and they are speaking the same language. It is even more problematic when the client and clinician do not share the same cultural values and may be speaking different languages. Thus, clients who speak English as a second language may be at a disadvantage when asked to explain background information or their feelings about their communication disorder. In some cases, the speech-language pathologist uses an interpreter to make certain that the information provided by the client is transmitted accurately and the client's feelings are understood as fully as possible.

Even when a client and clinician speak the same language, cultural differences can make a clinical relationship more difficult. Earlier, we indicated that different cultures may have differing views of disability and what should be done about a disorder. People of some cultures are resistant to providing personal information until they develop a stronger relationship with the clinician. If the clinician tries to move too swiftly in obtaining personal data, the client may not return. The point here is that clinicians must always be sensitive to linguistic and cultural differences in clients and accommodate these in clinical relationships. As you learn in this textbook, to remediate many communication disorders the SLP must counsel and train clients and family members about the problem. Counseling must always rest on a strong relationship between client and clinician, or it is doomed to failure. Thus, linguistic and cultural issues affect the very basis of providing clinical services because services are provided in the context of an interpersonal relationship.

INCIDENCE/PREVALENCE

Certain communication disorders affect people from different racial groups disproportionately. For example, Asians have a higher incidence of cleft palate compared to Caucasians and African Americans. African Americans and Hispanics are more prone than are Caucasians to neurological disease leading to stroke, hypertension, aphasia, and motor speech disorders. Certain types of vocal disorders (e.g., hoarseness) tend to be higher in Hispanics in certain areas of the country. African Americans have a higher incidence of laryngeal cancer compared to other populations. There are more premature births and less neonatal care in lower-socioeconomic populations that are highly composed of African Americans and Hispanics. Thus, it is not simply the ethnicity of a group, but an interaction of many social and economic variables that account for incidence differences. The point here is that professionals must be prepared for disproportionate numbers of clients with certain communication disorders and take into account multicultural issues when considering the makeup of their caseloads.

ASSESSMENT ISSUES

Especially in the areas of phonology and language, the type of test administered by the SLP is critical. Likewise, the interpretation of test results is crucial to an effective diagnosis. In cases where the client does not speak English or has limited English proficiency, it is difficult for that person to perform well on a test that was designed in English and normed on English-speaking individuals. Such a person could fail the test simply because he or she does not have proficiency in English, not because of an underlying communication disorder. For instance, if a Hispanic person has a stroke and has difficulty communicating, it is important to test that individual in his language of greatest proficiency. Many test developers constructed examinations in several languages, and the clinician must select the test that is most appropriate for the client. Sometimes translators are used in administering screening tests to account for linguistic differences. Decades ago, Hispanic schoolchildren were administered intelligence tests written in English, and based on their results some were diagnosed with cognitive impairments. This was not because of a cognitive problem, but simply because they were being tested in a language with which they were not familiar. Currently, students must be tested in the language in which they have the most proficiency. Even for nonstandardized methods of assessment, instructions/directions must be given to the client so that they are understood before the client can perform tasks accurately.

As stated earlier, an important part of assessment is the diagnostic interview. In this interview, the professional finds out about historical information, the onset of the disorder, and the course the problem has taken since its inception. If the client is not proficient in English, the clinician must obtain the services of a translator so that historical information is elicited in as accurate a fashion as possible.

TREATMENT ISSUES

The treatment of any communication disorder takes place in the context of an interpersonal relationship through interaction. The SLP provides stimuli, cues, and feedback to the client in activities designed to improve whatever aspect of communication is affected. Thus, it should be clear that communicating with clients might have to be done with the services of a translator if the clinician is not bilingual.

DIALECTS

The issue of social dialects is a highly controversial topic. On one hand, several popular sociopolitical movements advocate that all Americans should speak only English and that even the use of dialectal variations should not be encouraged or tolerated in educational and business environments. On the other hand, sociolinguists promote the view that multiculturalism and its associated language differences are not disorders and should be embraced because they are an inherent part of a person's culture. In fact, *everyone* speaks a dialect. This perspective is well supported by federal laws mandating bilingual education for students and guidelines regarding nondiscriminatory testing for non-English-speaking persons.

It is even controversial to talk about the type of language to which professionals compare a dialect. For instance, speech professionals have used the term **Standard American English (SAE)** for years when describing the contrastive features of dialects. Professionals compare the grammatical, phonological, morphological, and pragmatic rules of a dialect with SAE to illustrate language differences. A problem, however, is that SAE does not actually exist in reality. Lippi-Green describes SAE as a "bias toward an abstracted, idealized, homogeneous spoken language which is imposed and maintained by dominant bloc institutions" (Lippi-Green, 1997, p. 64). The institutions she refers to are the mass media/ entertainment industry, the educational system, and corporate America. Typically, the "standard" language is the one used by people with power and money in a society that is best understood by the majority of people. Another commonly cited component of SAE is that it does not carry with it regional or ethnic variations. The most common area of the country identified as speaking SAE is the Midwest. These notions carry with them some significant problems. First, if SAE is the "prestigious" language spoken by those with institutional power and wealth, then other forms of language (e.g., dialects) are automatically devalued, along with the people who speak them. Just the name "Standard English" implies that dialects may be "substandard" versions of English. A second problem is that if SAE is Midwestern, it is really just another regional dialect itself. A recent PBS documentary titled "Do You Speak American?" lamented, "Ask a group of experts to define Standard American English, and you'll find, paradoxically, there's no standard answer." Some suggest the use of the term "mainstream American English (MAE)" or "general American English (GAE)," but in reality, these are not much better than SAE because they have their own set of implications and problems. In this textbook, we continue to use SAE to refer to the mainstream language variety.

To address cultural issues, many school systems have incorporated a more multicultural approach to teaching academic content that includes examples and contributions from a variety of cultures. Although specific data on the issue are difficult to obtain, the present authors believe that most students in this country are being taught using SAE curriculum materials with some degree of sensitivity to cultural variations. We discuss this in more detail in a later section.

Speaking a dialect can carry with it certain disadvantages when the educational "standard" is SAE. In special education, for example, SLPs are aware that students who are bilingual or bidialectal may perform poorly on standardized tests because of linguistic interference or cultural factors (van Keulen, Weddington, & DeBose, 1998; Haynes & Pindzola, 2007). There are unfortunate examples from decades ago when children who spoke another language were tested in SAE. Historically, many more children of color were in special education programs receiving special education services, and in the case of communication disorders, many of these "problems" were language-based (van Keulen et al., 1998). A significant percentage of these children no doubt had normal language skills within their dialect or language group but performed poorly on tests that focused on Standard English and were culturally biased. In the past 20 years, test developers have made a concerted effort to reduce linguistic and cultural bias on tests and to include a variety of cultural groups in normative samples. Today, most school systems have increased their vigilance to ensure that a disproportionate number of "minority" students are not enrolled in special education programs as a result of cultural or linguistic interference factors.

Despite these advances, you might still hear occasional tales of misdiagnosis and insensitivity to multicultural issues.

A major issue implied in the controversy mentioned here is whether a person speaking a dialect of English has a *disorder* of language and whether that person should be enrolled in therapy to change her way of talking. Whereas some people may not see this as a problem, the SLP certainly is faced with the issue on a daily basis. If he is required to work with students on changing their dialect, then he is ultimately faced with an overwhelming caseload of children who are essentially "normal" with regard to their language community. With a caseload of this size, there would be little time to serve those students with legitimate communication disorders in the areas of voice, fluency, language, and phonology. Thus, you will find that most SLPs have a clear "position" on what constitutes a "disorder" and what, if anything, to do with dialect speakers.

One goal of this chapter is to illustrate the significant impact of social dialects on communication and academic performance in educational settings and how bilingualism and dialect affect the role of the SLP in medical environments. It is impossible to cover all regional, ethnic, and racial dialects of English in a single chapter and include all their rules, conventions, and differences from Standard English. Therefore, we elect to illustrate social dialects using **African American English (AAE)** and **Hispanic English (HE)**. Census figures from the year 2000 show that Hispanics and African Americans are the largest minority population groups in the United States. This means that most professionals will encounter African American and Hispanic individuals in educational and medical settings. Although we use AAE and HE as examples of social dialects in the present chapter, you should bear in mind that the points we make could be applied to *any* dialect of English. If you are a teacher in a system that has a large Hispanic population, we hope that you become familiar with information on local Hispanic dialectal variations and cultural mores. Similarly, if you teach Navajo children or Asian/Pacific Islanders, you should familiarize yourself with important cultural mores and dialectal variations.

Most people tend to be **ethnocentric** (Lynch & Hanson, 1992). That is, they view the world from the perspective of their own culture and place value judgments on the practices, mores, and languages of other cultural groups. Ethnocentricity may be a natural tendency, but it is one that can be overcome with exposure to other cultures and systematic study. People are said to have increased their *cultural literacy* when they have learned about and accept the value of the differences among various cultural groups. Cultural literacy is not the province of *any* cultural group. For example, being a member of a minority group does not guarantee a person has a high level of cultural literacy. The only road to cultural literacy is the study of and experience with other cultures and keeping an open mind. Historically, school systems in the United States have been based on a largely white, European, middle-class value system, although this has changed significantly in the last quarter century. Failure to consider other cultures and their contributions is an example of ethnocentricity and results in a relatively narrow view of the world.

Interestingly, if you look at the broader picture, you find that almost 85 percent of the world's population is made up of "people of color." Recent population projections in the United States suggest that by the year 2050, one half of the U.S. population will be nonwhite. In some states at the present time (e.g., California, Texas, New Mexico), whites are in the minority or are approaching this status. This gives a whole new meaning to the notion of *minority group* for many readers. Whether or not someone is considered a minority is largely a matter of context. An African American in Utah may be a minority, but in Washington, DC, he is a majority group member. Many people today reject the term *minority* because it changes with context. Also the term *minority* suggests that the group is less important as compared to a *majority*. There is also ethnocentricity with regard to languages. Most people feel that their own language is the "best." It is interesting that in the United States some feel that citizens should learn and speak only English. Yet, bilingualism, not monolingualism, is the norm throughout the world. There are more than 3,000 different languages/dialects in the world and more than 150 in the United States. Most people in the world speak several languages.

As mentioned previously, school systems and medical settings have made significant changes in recent decades to include more sensitivity to cultural variations. This practice allows medical and educational professionals to move away from an ethnocentric view that white, European, middle-class expectations and practices have value for all clients regardless of cultural group. It also prepares professionals for the inevitable future in which they will see a steady increase of different cultural groups in all work environments. There are many different cultural groups represented in medical and educational settings, and professionals must develop strategies for accommodating all clients regardless of their background.

Most people are aware that there are a number of different ways to speak in the United States. For instance, it is not uncommon to hear reports that African Americans or Hispanics speak differently from whites. People of Italian, Polish, or German descents often speak with an "accent." Further, it is often said that people from lower socioeconomic levels speak differently from middle- or upper-class persons. Regional differences abound in this country, with people in the South speaking differently from those in the Midwest or on the eastern seaboard. Despite these manifold racial, ethnic, social, and regional differences in speech and language, Americans seem to be able to communicate with each other. Although it may take some careful listening for an Anglo to understand a heavy Hispanic dialect, ideas *can* be passed from one person to another. The fact that communication can take place between these diverse groups attests to the fact that (1) they are all basically speaking English, and (2) there are many more similarities than differences among the various versions of English.

A dialect is a "variety of a national language" (Taylor, 1986, p. 386) that is shared by a particular speech community for purposes of frequent interaction. A **speech community** may reflect any of the groups mentioned, such as racial, ethnic, social, or regional. According to Taylor, these variations in language may be the product of any of the following: (1) the languages brought to the country by various cultural groups; that is, speakers of English, Polish, Chinese, Wolof, and such; (2) the indigenous Native American languages spoken in the country; (3) the mix of the various communities and regions where the cultural groups settled; (4) the political and economic power wielded by the various cultures settling in the regions; (5) the migration patterns of the cultural groups within the country; (6) geographic isolation caused by rivers, mountains, and other features, as in the dialects of the Ozark and Appalachian mountains; and (7) self-imposed social isolation or legal segregation (Taylor, 1986, p. 395).

In the sections that follow, we describe and give examples of how a variety of factors affect the way people speak English. None of these versions of English are defective, and thus, none require speech or language therapy.

THE DIFFERENCE-DEFICIT ISSUE

Historically, there was a time when various authorities thought dialectal variations represented a *deficit* in language ability. Dialects, then, were viewed by some as impoverished forms of English, spoken by people who were attempting to use Standard English, but who were falling short of their goal (Rickford, Sweetland, & Rickford, 2004). Some deficit theorists even implicated the intellectual abilities of certain groups. Their reasoning was that because language is used in the service of thought and these speakers practiced imperfect language, they also must have impoverished thinking abilities. Certain groups, especially African Americans, were singled out as examples of the deficit model.

On the other hand, people were quite generous with some dialects in attributing them to the mixing of two different languages. For instance, most people viewed a German or French accent as charming and attributed the language changes in these dialects to the influence of a person's native language. Hispanic English is clearly the result of mixing Spanish and English, resulting in changes in the features of English as influenced by Spanish linguistic conventions. These generous views were not always extended to African American English. Many thought it was neither charming nor legitimate because it had no obvious linguistic roots to another language and because of underlying racism.

As linguists began to investigate African American English, however, they determined that it does, in fact, have its roots in the languages of the western coast of Africa (Dillard, 1972). A well-developed historical path could be traced from African American English back to African languages, and this connection gave African American English the same legitimacy accorded to other dialects. You can find features in African languages similar to those used in African American English. This historical validation shows that African American English is not simply an impoverished version of Standard English, but a dialect that has its roots in African languages. AAE, like other dialects, is rule-governed, which further demonstrates its status as a language system, not a deficiency.

Today, linguists prefer to talk about dialects as being **language differences** as opposed to **language deficits**. This term means that dialects are simply different ways of speaking English, and no implication is made regarding levels of acceptability, capabilities of speakers, or the superiority of one dialect over another.

Many different regional and ethnic dialects are spoken in the United States. However, it is beyond the scope of the present chapter to delineate the critical features of each dialect of American English. Instead, we choose to include some examples of major differences among Standard English, Hispanic English, and African American English. Classroom teachers in larger cities and southern states can attest to the fact that Hispanic and African American students often constitute the largest groups of dialect speakers in their classes. Speech-language pathologists, medical professionals, and teachers in specific areas of the country may teach other groups of minority students (e.g., Native Americans, Hispanics, Asians), and many of the basic principles discussed in this chapter apply to these groups as well. They have specific dialects of English, and professionals should become familiar with the impact of these dialects and their differences from Standard English. A good place to start is to contact the SLP, who should have some information on regional and local dialects and differences from SAE.

ETHNICITY, RACE, AND FIRST LANGUAGE COMMUNITY

Every culture has its customs, social conventions, and linguistic differences. These unique characteristics are interwoven in a very complex manner, and it is difficult to define a culture without delineating its peculiar differences. Language is an integral part of a person's cultural or racial definition that cannot be removed without irreversibly altering the nature of the ethnic or racial group. For instance, a speaker of Yiddish may use unique vocabulary (e.g., *nebbish, schlemiel, putz*) and distinct stress and intonation patterns when talking to members of his ethnic group. Rosten provides an example from Yiddish that illustrates: "*Two* tickets for her concert I should buy?" (Rosten, 1971, p. 72). Littell gives examples of syntax differences in Pennsylvania Dutch, such as "Don't eat yourself so full already—there's cake back yet," and "Sally, you chew your mouth empty before you say" (Littell, 1971, pp. 85–86). African American speakers may also use vocabulary (e.g., *crib* = residence; *kicks* = shoes; *homey* = friend; *tight* = pleasing to the eye) not typically spoken by people who are not members of this culture.

Every racial or ethnic group has its own unique vocabulary items, sentence structures, ways of changing the sounds of English, and different social uses of language. These linguistic changes are part of the complex of behaviors that actually define the culture. When people make fun of the way ethnic or racial minorities talk, they are really disrespecting an important determinant of a person's culture. Further, if a speech-language pathologist or medical or educational professional suggests that a person must change the way he or she talks, this really amounts to altering a significant aspect of a person's culture and should not be done lightly. Essentially, if you say that a person's dialect is unacceptable, you are really saying that the culture is also unacceptable.

In the United States, the two largest racial/ethnic groups are African Americans and Hispanics. These groups have distinct dialects, of which we give examples later in this chapter. Other groups are immigrants or refugees from East Asia, Southeast Asia, and the Pacific Islands. The Asian/Pacific Island people in the United States speak the following major languages: Mandarin, Cantonese, Taiwanese, Hakka, Tagalog, Ilocano, Japanese, Korean,

Vietnamese, Khmer, Lao, Hmong, Mien, Chamorro, Samoan, and Hindi (Cheng, 1989). Most white Americans have not even heard of these languages, but as these speakers are incorporated into the mosaic of U.S. culture, dialects and language differences will emerge.

Most Americans are familiar with the language differences in first-generation immigrants from Europe (e.g., Germany, Poland, Italy, Ireland, France, Czechoslovakia, and Russia). These dialects have been portrayed in many popular films, and in large cities, you can still hear the various ethnic language variations being perpetuated by second- and third-generation Americans. Finally, professionals in some areas of the country will encounter other major dialectal variations when dealing with Native American, Eskimo, and Hawaiian children. Each of these cultural groups has its own variety of English.

REGIONAL VARIATIONS

Most Americans are aware that people in various parts of the country speak a dialect of English that is peculiar to their geographic region. There are many more **regional dialects** in the eastern portion of the United States and regional differences become far less dense in the western states. For example, dialects in Boston, New York City, and Pennsylvania are quite different within a relatively small geographic area; however, it is sometimes difficult to hear differences in dialects in individual states west of the Mississippi River. Some dialects are composed of many variations from the Standard English pattern, and others have only a few features that distinguish them from other regions. Note that each region might have its own unique alterations in speech sounds, syntax, vocabulary, and social language rituals. For instance, carbonated beverages are known in the Midwest as *pop*, on the East Coast as *soda*, and in the South as *co-cola* (even if the person is referring to root beer). People in the Midwest say *hi* or *hello* when greeting someone, while people in the South say *hey*. People in Chicago use a *shopping cart* and Southern shoppers use a *buggy*. As Owens says, "The Italian sandwich changes to submarine, torpedo, hero, wedge and hoagie as it moves about the United States" (Owens, 1988, p. 366). He could also add *grinder*, commonly used in Rhode Island, to the sandwich list. These are just examples of semantic differences around the country.

Various regions also demonstrate differences in use of phonetic elements. Most people are aware that speakers in Massachusetts and Maine pronounce the /r/ sound differently from how speakers in the Midwest do. In Maine, a person might say, "paak youh caa" for "park your car." Actually, this grossly resembles the Southern pronunciation of the same sentence because in Southern dialect the /r/ sound also is affected. Even syntax is influenced by regional dialect variation. In the South, for instance, acceptable sentences may involve two modals such as, "He might could do that." In the Midwest, "might" and "could" would not be placed together in the same utterance. In the South, people are always "fixing to go" somewhere. People on the East Coast, however, do not "fix to go" anywhere; they just go. Thus, there are many regional alterations to language, and professionals must be aware that these variations are part of a particular culture and acceptable to use in that region.

SOCIAL CLASS VARIATIONS

Every culture has a number of social classes. You might recall the classic film *My Fair Lady* in which a speech expert named Henry Higgins stood outside a theater after a performance and was fervently scribbling phonetic transcriptions of speech he overheard from the patrons. When a flower girl named Eliza Doolittle spoke, Higgins knew exactly not only where she was from geographically, but also to which social class she belonged. Similarly, in some lower-socioeconomic areas in New England, people might say things like "youse guys" and "dere" for "there." These are examples of social class variations in language. Many people from lower socioeconomic classes use "ain't."

Studies of the language used by lower social classes reveal that they speak a **vernacular** of English that has a system all its own. The term *vernacular* refers to an informal way of expressing ideas within a speech community. These investigations also show that most versions of a language spoken by lower social classes are more restricted than the elaborated standard language. By restricted, it means that many words are omitted or shortened by the speakers of a vernacular of a language than in the standard language. Thus, "I am not going" is less restricted than is "I ain't goin'."

PEER GROUP IDENTIFICATION

When a teenager or adult becomes a member of a definable peer group, a language variation often occurs. Parents complain that their teenage sons and daughters do not speak English, or that they are sloppy in the way they talk. Although not a dialect per se, peer group variations are unique ways of talking and these linguistic varieties include all areas of language (e.g., syntax, semantics, pragmatics). Instead of a dialectal variation, many consider peer group language as slang, which serves a very important social solidarity function for group members. Not long ago, teenagers showed their respect for someone by saying, "You're the bomb!" This, of course, had nothing to do with explosives. They may also acknowledge a mistake by saying, "my bad." Specific groups such as street gangs, military personnel, musicians, and such have many distinct language variations when compared to Standard English.

COMMUNICATIVE CONTEXT

Throughout the day, every speaker experiences a variety of communicative contexts. *Communicative context* means the situation in which communication takes place. It is not simply the physical place of communication but also includes the identity and characteristics of the listener. For instance, an adult Standard English speaker might speak differently to a group of African American teenagers because of a variety of factors (age, cultural differences, and social class differences) from how that person might address a family member. People change the way they talk depending on the circumstances of communication.

You probably talk quite differently to your roommate than you do to the president of the university. You talk differently to a person with a hearing loss than you do to a person with normal hearing. You talk to a 4-year-old differently from how you talk to a teenager. You talk differently in a neighborhood bar from how you talk at a formal dinner.

The many changes that a person makes in language as a response to communicative context is called style shifting or code switching. **Style shifting** has been studied in the African American culture. It has been reported that many speakers of AAE change their style of communication when addressing members of mainstream culture (Seymour & Seymour, 1979; Hecht, Collier, & Ribeau, 1993). Cazden examined African American children and found that they used a **street register**, which was a relaxed manner of talking to their peers at school and on the street (Cazden, 1970). They also used a **school register** when addressing authority figures in the school environment. Interestingly, examples of the school register used shorter sentences, were less syntactically complex, were more disfluent, and had quite different content as compared to examples of the street register. Like any other dialect, communication style differences in AAE are affected by such variables as age, gender, and socioeconomic status. These examples illustrate the process of a speaker switching the way she talks to fit the communicative context. In reality, most speakers engage in style shifting. For instance, an African American physician might use some features of an African American dialect when talking to patients of his own cultural group and switch to more of a Standard English production when dealing with white patients.

THE DIALECTAL CONTINUUM

When talking about the dialects spoken by various groups in the United States, it would be erroneous to give the impression that every member of a particular culture, region, or peer group speaks the same way. For example, the term *African American English* is somewhat inaccurate because it gives the impression that everyone who is of African American descent speaks this dialect. In reality, there are many African Americans who speak SAE or some regional dialect that has no features of African American English. There are many New Yorkers who are African American and simply sound like they are from New York. We know of some white children in the rural South who attend a predominantly African American school and incorporate many features of AAE in their language. Many people from lower socioeconomic levels speak more of a middle-class version of English. There are teenage girls from the Valley area in southern California who do not sound like Valley girls. Thus, it is productive to think of every dialect and vernacular of English as existing on a continuum.

For example, say that AAE and SAE have about 29 features that are produced differently from one another (Williams & Wolfram, 1977). One African American speaker may incorporate all 29 of the features and thus represent a maximal difference between African American English and SAE. Another African American speaker, however, may incorporate only 10 of the possible 29 features and thus shows more similarity to a SAE speaker. Finally, a third speaker may use only 2 or 3 of the features of AAE and represent a language use that is almost indistinguishable from Standard English. These examples could be from

Hispanic English or regional dialects as well. A person in Maine may or may not have a heavy New England dialect for a variety of reasons (business, long-standing cultural ties, and frequent moves around the country). Speech professionals, therefore, should not stereotype a person in terms of language just because that person represents a particular group or region of the country. There is a **dialectal continuum** upon which each person falls depending on how many or few of the features of a dialect that speaker uses.

Another important notion is that dialects are in a constant state of flux. Whenever two dialects are put in geographic proximity to one another a phenomenon takes place that is known as **dialect importation**. This means that each dialect borrows from the other, and they have a mutual influence on each other. For instance, in south Texas there is a way of speaking called "Tex-Mex," which is a special dialect created because of the influence of the geographic relations of Mexico and Texas. In Europe, many small countries are located right next to each other, and in the border areas distinct dialects have developed as a result of the influences of two languages. Some linguists indicate that Southern English may have been influenced by African American English because historically many Southerners were raised by African Americans who worked on plantations caring for children. Some authorities indicate that the Southern dialect is becoming less pronounced (no pun intended) because of the large influx of "northerners" moving to warmer climates. Thus, dialects influence each other.

It has been said that America is a melting pot in which many cultures become homogenized. This is partly true with dialects because the ways of talking influence each other and dialects gradually change. Others say that a better analogy to characterize America is a salad. In a salad, the ingredients are together in a bowl but to a large degree retain their identities. Although dialects change very gradually over time, they are a reflection of a person's culture, and there is much preservation of dialects as well as a result of the perpetuation of important cultural attributes. There are many reasons why dialects are preserved. For example, forced or voluntary segregation is one factor. Many large cities have areas where concentrations of ethnic/cultural groups live and work. Some cities have areas known by names like "Chinatown" or "little Italy." In some cities where there are large Latino populations, the signs on businesses are written in Spanish. This kind of segregation helps to preserve dialects. Another example of preserving dialects is illustrated by different socioeconomic groups. When people from lower socioeconomic groups live in close proximity, it helps to perpetuate their use of the vernacular of their dialect. Thus, forces exist to both perpetuate and change dialectal forms.

SPECIFIC DIFFERENCES BETWEEN AFRICAN AMERICAN ENGLISH AND STANDARD ENGLISH

In this section, we compare Standard American English (SAE) and African American English (AAE) to illustrate some specific differences between the dialects. It is important to remember that differences between SAE and AAE can be phonological, syntactic, semantic, and even pragmatic. **Table 7–1** and **Table 7–2** outline only some of the more

TABLE 7–1 Selected Phonological Features of African American English

Consonant Cluster Reduction

If a consonant cluster (blend) is located in the final position of a word (e.g., *test, build*), one member of the cluster may be deleted or reduced in African American English. There is a very specific rule that operates here so that only certain cluster types experience deletion. For instance, if both members of the cluster are the same with regard to voicing (both voiced sounds or both voiceless sounds), the final member will be reduced. Some examples of words that end in clusters that are both voiceless are as follows: *test, mask, gasp, gift, wished* (wisht). These words would be pronounced "tes," "mas," "gas," "gif," and "wish." The same rule applies if both members are voiced sounds: *build, hand, warmed.* These words would be pronounced "buil," "han," and "warm." When the two members are different in their voicing (e.g., one voiced and one voiceless), the cluster is typically not reduced. For instance, in the words *jump, count, rent, belt,* and *gulp* the two sounds in the cluster differ in terms of voicing, where one is voiced and the other is voiceless. These words would be said with both members of the cluster present.

Thus, the cluster reduction rule in African American English is lawful in nature. Clusters at the beginning and middle of words are not reduced.

The /th/ Phonemes

The voiced and voiceless /th/ sounds in Standard English are changed in a lawful way in African American English. The specific changes made depend on the position of the TH sound in the word. In the initial position, the voiceless /th/ can be changed to a /t/ sound ("tink" for *think*). The voiced /th/ sound can be changed to a /d/ sound ("dem" for *them*). When the voiceless /th/ sounds are in the medial or final word position the /f/ sound is substituted for them. For example, a child may say "bafroom" for *bathroom*. A similar rule applies for the voiced /th/ sound in the medial position ("bruvah" for *brother*). At the end of a word the same rule applies with the substitution of /f/ and /v/ for the voiceless and voiced /th/ sound ("baf" for *bath*: "bave" for *bathe*).

The /r/ and /l/ Phonemes

A very similar rule applies in African American English and in Southern English regarding /r/ and /l/. In both dialects, the /l/ or /r/ often become /uh/ as in "sistuh" for *sister*. Also, the /r/ and /l/ are sometimes absent in both dialects ("hep" for *help*; "doe" for *door*; "foe" for *four*; "show" for *sure*).

Final /b/, /d/, and /g/ Devoicing

At the end of a syllable, voiced plosives (b, d, g) may be replaced by their voiceless counterparts (p, t, k). Thus, an African American speaker may say "pik" for *pig* or "but" for *bud*.

Final Omission of Nasal Sounds

At the end of words the nasal phonemes (m, n, ng) are often omitted and the preceding vowel is nasalized (e.g., "pa" for *pan*, "ma" for *man*). This is often noted as one of the economical features of African American English because the nasal feature of the word is superimposed on the vowel, thus making the nasal consonant at the end of the word redundant.

str Blends

The str blends in African American English are often changed to skr (*string* and *street* are changed to "skring" and "skreet").

TABLE 7–2   Selected Syntactic Features of African American English

Past Tense -*ed*

In African American English, the bound morpheme -*ed* is omitted because of the consonant cluster reduction rule referred to in Table 7–1. When an SAE speaker puts the -*ed* ending on a word, it is sometimes pronounced as one phoneme, either a T or a D. Thus, making the word *walk* past tense involves adding a *t* to the end of the word as in "walkt." Because both members of this cluster (kt) are voiceless, the consonant cluster reduction rule would eliminate the T sound in pronunciation. So, the following words would be pronounced without the -*ed* ending: *cashed, cracked, named,* or *slammed.*

Third Person Singular Present Tense -*s*

In Standard English, when a third person form is used (*he, she, the boy*) it is required that an -*s* be attached to the verb (he runs, she cooks, the boy eats). In African American English, the -*s* is omitted (he run, she cook, the boy eat).

Absent Forms of the Verb to Be

In Standard English, sentences must either have a verb or a form of the be verb such as *is, am,* or *are.* In African American English, these forms of *be* can be omitted in many sentences. The forms are not totally absent in African American English because certain sentence types do include them such as tag questions (She not going, is she?) or exposed clauses (I know where he is).

Invariant Be

The be verb in Standard English changes its form depending on the type of sentence spoken. For example, *be* changes among *is, am, are, was, were* with the effect of tense, plurality, and person. In African American English, *be* does not change its form and may even be used as *be* (He be workin).

Double Negatives

Like many other dialects and languages, African American English uses double negatives (Couldn't nobody do it?).

Possessives

In African American English, the possessive morpheme -*s* can be omitted (the girl car). Possession is indicated by the order and proximity of words rather than adding the apostrophe *s*.

Plurals

In Standard English, the -s morpheme is placed at the end of words to mark plurality (e.g., *cars, cats, dogs*). African American English speakers omit the plural morpheme largely because of the consonant cluster reduction rule and also because of the nonobligatory nature of the plural morpheme when talking about nouns of measure (money, time, and such). This leads to utterances such as "two dollar," "three year," and "two cat."

obvious phonological and syntactic features of African American English taken from a variety of sources.

Many descriptions of AAE linguistic features consider this topic in great detail (Rickford, 1999; Green, 2002), but these are beyond the scope of the present chapter. Rickford and Rickford provide a readable summary for those without a background in linguistics (Rickford & Rickford, 2000). Clearly, if you consider all of the grammatical rules in SAE and the relatively few differences between AAE and SAE, you can see that there are far more similarities than differences between the dialects. Tables 7–1 and 7–2 illustrate that a small number of linguistic differences can explain many of the variations speech professionals may encounter in the speech and writing of African American students. Rickford, Sweetland, and Rickford report that there is great variation in teacher preparation programs in terms of including information on dialectal features (Rickford et al., 2004). Many of the variations are accounted for by the consonant cluster reduction rule, which affects not only final consonant blends, but also the inclusion of past tense, possessive, and third person -s markers. The other major rule that affects many types of utterances is the use of the verb "to be" and its variants.

From a semantic standpoint, we have already mentioned that a host of words and phrases in African American English is unique to this dialect (Major, 1994; Smitherman, 2000). Many of these terms become popular in the general American culture (e.g., *chillin* = relaxing; *hood* = neighborhood; *the man* = police; *sup* = what's up?), and then are often gradually relinquished by the speakers of African American English (Andrews & Owens, 1976).

The syntactic changes listed in Table 7–2 are certainly not all-inclusive. Some other subtle differences between Standard and African American English are beyond the scope of the present chapter. The differences, however, represent some major points of dialectal variation of syntax in African American English and should allow professionals to recognize some of the ways dialects differ. We could illustrate differences between SAE and Hispanic English or Asian dialects of English in a similar manner. For an introductory course, however, it is enough to make the point using only one dialect.

In terms of language use, it is important to note that speakers of AAE prize the ability to communicate effectively. A speaker's ability to "rap" or use language in social rituals of one-upmanship is valued in African American culture.

THE EFFECTS OF DIALECTAL VARIATION ON THE STUDENT

There are two major implications of speaking a dialect in the school systems. First, most school systems are largely geared to speaking, reading, and writing in SAE. Early surveys of parents of African American children overwhelmingly support the idea of using SAE in the schools (Taylor, 1971). In fact, early attempts at teaching literacy through the use of reading books written in AAE have not had a history of acceptance. Van Keulen, Weddington, and DeBose indicate, "The failure of a pilot series of dialect readers to gain widespread acceptance is often attributed to Black parents' rejection of the concept" (Van Keulen et al., 1998, p. 198). Perhaps the most popular approach to dealing with dialectal variation in schools is **bidialectalism** (Rickford et al., 2004). According to Rickford, Sweetland, and Rickford, bidialectalism refers to

> the perspective that vernacular speakers can and should command the standard variety as well as their native vernacular. It is an additive, rather than an eradicative,

perspective, in that it seeks to expand speakers' linguistic repertoires instead of replacing one linguistic competence with another, more prestigious competence. (Rickford et al., 2004, p. 234)

Thus, AAE speakers are entering a system that uses and reinforces language that is different in some respects from the language that they speak, and this can create some potential problems in learning (Laffey & Shuy, 1973; Harber & Bryen, 1978; Gemake, 1981). Imagine, for instance, that the dialect you speak has phonological and syntactic differences from the language you are being taught to read and write. Some sentences will have extra words in them, as in the case of *is* or *was* for an African American English speaker. Some words will have extra sounds or letters in them, as in the case of plurals, possessives, and consonant clusters for the AAE speaker. Hispanic speakers may have the same difficulties of being faced with a code to learn that differs from the one they typically use. Reading and writing are difficult enough to learn for young SAE speakers, but AAE and Hispanic speakers are at an even greater disadvantage. Thus, one effect of speaking a dialect is that you may have a bit more difficulty learning to read, write, and speak Standard English. This difficulty may result in lower grades, lower self-esteem, and less success in school.

The second implication is that a dialect speaker may be at a disadvantage when taking tests that are designed for Standard English speakers. Fagundes, Haynes, Haak, and Moran discuss some of the types of bias associated with standardized testing:

The typical types of bias on standardized tests that can have a negative effect on culturally diverse children are *situational bias* (examination format is threatening to child), *directions bias* (directions for test can be misinterpreted by child), *value bias* (asking child to give moral/ethical judgments that may differ culturally from the examiners'), *linguistic bias* (presumption that the child is a standard English speaker), *format bias* (test procedures are inconsistent with child's cognitive style), *cultural misinterpretation* (negative interpretation of client behavior when it is culturally appropriate), and *stimulus bias* (test is highly object/picture-oriented when child is socially oriented). (Fagundes, Haynes, Haak, & Moran, 1998, p. 148)

Although standardized language testing has a long history of not considering multicultural variables in test development, more recently developed examinations have been designed to remedy this important problem. For example, most newer tests depict people from a variety of cultures and norms have been developed using standardization samples that include groups/numbers of children consistent with recent census information. In fact, Seymour, Roeper, and deVilliers have developed a criterion-referenced test that is specifically designed to take dialectal variation into account (Seymour, Roeper, & deVilliers, 2003).

Other nonstandardized testing approaches have also made significant contributions to reducing cultural bias in language testing. For example, some researchers have developed a "minimal competency core" that includes types of language that any child, regardless of dialect, should be able to produce because the items are not specific to a particular culture

(Stockman, 1996; Schraeder, Quinn, Stockman, & Miller, 1999). Another approach involves the use of "contrastive analysis" where spontaneous language samples are gathered and analyzed to determine whether any variations produced by the child can be accounted for by a dialect or the variations are not dialectal and possibly evidence of a language disorder (McGregor, Williams, Hearst, & Johnson, 1997; Seymour, Bland-Stewart, & Green, 1998).

Finally, some researchers have found that children with language impairment have difficulty repeating sequences of nonsense words, and because the stimulus items are not part of any culture, these "processing tasks" can be used to discriminate children with disorders from those who are speaking dialects (Bishop, North, & Donlan, 1996; Campbell, Dollaghan, Needleman, & Janosky, 1997; Dollaghan & Campbell, 1998; Ellis-Weismer et al., 2000; Rodekohr & Haynes, 2001).

The SLP must constantly be aware of the possible negative effects of dialectal variation on formal tests and carefully examine errors to see whether they are possibly the result of a student's dialect or culture. Taylor indicates:

> The use of culturally and linguistically discriminatory assessment instruments is specifically prohibited by such federal mandates as The Education for All (Handicapped) Children Act of 1975 (PL 94-142) and its updated version (PL 98-199); The Bilingual Education Act of 1976 (P.L. 95-561); and Title VII of the Elementary and Secondary Education Act of 1965. In addition, several legal decisions have declared illegal the use of culturally and linguistically discriminatory assessment procedures for determining the presence of handicapping conditions. (Taylor, 1986, p. 405)

The two implications of speaking a dialect discussed previously cannot be overemphasized. Classroom teachers must deal with the first problem of learning to read and write. This requires that teachers be more aware of the characteristics of dialects spoken by their students so that they might be more able to effectively teach these children differences between SAE and their dialect. It is especially important for the teacher to be able to understand that a student may be confused about certain reading or writing fundamentals because of interference from his or her dialect (Van Keulen et al., 1998). We discuss this issue in greater detail in a later section. The second problem of test construction currently is being addressed by major test developers in terms of careful selection of norming samples. The American Speech-Language-Hearing Association (ASHA) has instructed SLPs to familiarize themselves with the characteristics of various social dialects and methods of culturally unbiased testing (Battle et al., 1983).

HOW CAN THE CLASSROOM TEACHER DEAL WITH THE DIALECT ISSUE?

Like any controversial issue, dealing with dialectal variations in the school curriculum has been approached from a variety of directions (Rickford et al., 2004). As mentioned earlier, bidialectal approaches emphasize the learning of SAE while still respecting a student's dialect. Some classroom materials have been developed specifically for a bidialectal approach

(Mantell, 1974; Anderson, 1990; Love, 1991; Parker & Crist, 1995). Some of the earlier bidialectal approaches emphasized drill work that was not as engaging for students, but some of the more recent programs incorporate literature, the media, and writing in exercises that are more interesting (Maddahian & Sandamela, 2000; LeMoine, 2001; Rickford, 2002). Some successful programs have even enlisted students in the gathering and analysis of various linguistic samples to emphasize dialectal differences (Wolfram, Adger, & Christian, 1999).

One of the primary aspects of any bidialectal approach is that the teacher communicate respect for all varieties of English during interactions, classroom assignments, and discussions (Alexander, 1985; Birch, 2001). The following suggestions are taken from Alexander and are ways the teacher can work more effectively with students who speak dialects.

1. Develop an understanding of language and how it develops and changes.
2. Become familiar with the dialects of students.
3. Develop a respect for American dialects as language systems that reflect culture.
4. Transmit this respect to all students.
5. Recognize that some dialects are low-prestige dialects and that some students are very aware of this.
6. Demonstrate to students your belief that they are capable of handling two or more dialects.
7. Introduce them to other English dialects, such as those to which students are exposed when they travel in the United States.
8. Help students to understand the role of lingua franca. At one time, French was the international language. Today, English is a language that is spoken all over the world. Advise students that they may have no idea now of what paths they will take when they are older and that it is wise to be prepared and to learn this standard language now.
9. Have the students read literature by African American, Hispanic, and Asian writers, which offers opportunities for performance and discussion. Currently popular rap music also provides many examples of the use of dialect in a musical art form that students can analyze and discuss along with other types of poetry or lyrics.
10. Read aloud or play recorded passages in other English dialects to help students to appreciate the variability of English and the legitimacy of their own dialect.
11. Teach the grammatical constructions of Standard English dialect. Provide time for practice of these grammatical constructions and show how speakers of different dialects might change the SAE sentences to express the same thought.
12. Have the students conduct a television survey or evaluate current motion pictures and note which programs use noticeable dialects. (Alexander, 1985, p. 24)

Many examples are available of effective teaching that takes these issues into account (Foster, 2001; Bohn, 2003; Irvine, 2002). Some of the points mentioned here are overlapping; however, these suggestions basically support the notion that teachers and other education professionals *should* emphasize SAE in the school environment. It is unrealistic for teachers to be expected to instruct students in a variety of dialects or have differing criteria for correctness in grading papers based on dialectal variation. A teacher with several different types of minority students in a class would have difficulty with such an approach.

From reading a broad base of sociolinguistic literature we conclude that the majority of authorities advocate the teaching of SAE in the educational system together with sensitivity to dialectal variation in instructional methods. Further support comes from sources suggesting that more than 90 percent of African American parents surveyed think that their children should be taught in Standard English (Taylor, 1971). The suggestions also strongly support the practice of teaching SAE not as a substitute for an impoverished language system, but as a socially, educationally, and possibly economically advantageous linguistic code in the larger society.

Many children will style-shift between SAE and AAE as appropriate and when dictated by various social contexts. Speech professionals are not in the business of eradicating dialectal variations, only increasing the students' linguistic facility to switch between SAE and AAE when it is appropriate. Students must not be made to feel that their dialect is wrong. Many of these suggestions also emphasize that *all* students should be made aware of the many dialects in the United States, and an attitude of acceptance of these varied ways of talking should be fostered. This practice broadens the views of Standard English–speaking students as well as the other dialect speakers and perhaps increases tolerance among all students and teachers. In using such an orientation, however, it is important that teachers are very clear about their criteria for grading in terms of language use. If departures from Standard English in written work are to be penalized in grading, teachers should clearly state this at the outset. It may not be a realistic expectation for teachers to assume dialect speakers can speak Standard English in oral reports and then penalize students for dialect usage. Although students may attempt to style-shift into their "best" approximation of Standard English, there may always be some features of their dialect that remain. Teachers should be realistic about expectations for oral performance.

DIALECTS, TEACHERS, AND THE SPEECH-LANGUAGE PATHOLOGIST

In the day-to-day interactions of teachers and SLPs, scenes like these often unfold.

VIGNETTE 7–1

Mrs. Steele, the second-grade teacher, has asked the speech-language pathologist to listen to Maurice, an African American child in her class. She says that Maurice leaves certain words out of sentences, omits sounds, and is generally hard for her to understand. When the SLP observes Maurice in the classroom setting, she notes that he omits *is*, plurals, and possessives and reduces consonant blends at the ends of words. The SLP tells Mrs. Steele that Maurice is not exhibiting a communication disorder and is simply speaking African American English. As a result, the SLP recommends that the teacher not initiate a referral for a speech/language evaluation. Mrs. Steele very politely nods her head, glaring at the SLP with her mouth drawn back in a tense red line.

VIGNETTE 7–2

Hernando Sanchez was having a lot of trouble in school. His grades were low and his parents were worried. Mrs. Sanchez talked to his teacher and was told that Hernando was having trouble because he was not learning English well enough to read or speak effectively. The teacher went on to say that Hernando speaking a Hispanic dialect was probably the cause of his academic difficulties. She indicated that she would not refer him for an evaluation to determine whether he needed any special services. The parent wisely requested that the speech-language pathologist and learning disabilities teacher examine Hernando. It was later found that the child had a significant language problem that was unrelated to his Hispanic dialect and also had a learning disability.

It is exactly these kinds of interactions that result in miscommunication among professionals and parents. If the SLP had been performing in-service training with teachers regarding dialectal variations, these situations may never have occurred. The two most common problems that teachers have are (1) referring *all* dialect cases to the SLP because of lack of knowledge about social dialects, and (2) not referring *any* minority students because the teacher assumes that all of their language differences are because of dialectal influence. Make *no* mistake: Children who are dialect speakers can also have coexisting communication disorders such as language problems, articulation problems, fluency disorders, voice disorders, and other difficulties. If the teacher even suspects that a child is experiencing a legitimate communication disorder, it is best to have that child screened by the SLP.

SLPs typically resist working with dialect cases in the absence of a communication disorder for a number of important reasons:

1. *The **ASHA position***: The American Speech-Language-Hearing Association has indicated that the SLP has a primary responsibility to those children with significant communication problems (stuttering, voice problems, language delay, articulation problems, cerebral palsy, cleft palate, hearing impairment, and such) (Battle et al., 1983). If the SLP's caseload were filled with children who were *normal* and speaking dialects, the SLP would not be able to serve children with communication disorders. The ASHA position is clear in that it states the SLP should give preference to individuals with disorders. The ASHA position also indicates that the SLP must become familiar with features of various dialects so that discrimination in testing or enrollment does not occur.

2. *No problem exists:* To enroll a child in therapy implies that the child has a disorder. If a child is enrolled for dialectal variations and is a dialect speaker, by definition, no problem exists. Thus, children and their parents may object to placement in speech therapy. In fact, this issue was taken to court, as explained by Taylor:

   In 1977, a group of parents in Ann Arbor, Michigan, filed suit in Federal Court on behalf of 15 African American preschool and elementary children, charging that teachers in a local school had failed to adequately take into account the children's home dialects in the teaching of the language arts. Among their charges, the parents claimed that the teachers were not sufficiently knowledgeable about these dialects and, as a result, did not fully appreciate their intrinsic worth and usefulness in the educational environment. In several cases, children of the plaintiffs had been inappropriately enrolled in speech programs to "correct" their home dialects. The judge in the case concurred with the parents and ordered the Ann Arbor School Board to develop an educational plan which, among other things, would educate the teachers in the students' dialects and in how knowledge and value of the dialects can be used constructively in the language arts curriculum. (Taylor, 1986, p. 408)

The SLP may be the person in the school system most knowledgeable regarding dialectal variation. Information about social dialects is incorporated into every ASHA-accredited training program, and SLPs are encouraged to provide in-service training to interested teachers about dialects and to communicate their important role in dealing with dialectal variation.

So, how *does* the SLP deal with dialect in the educational setting? First, the SLP can provide in-service training to classroom teachers and assist in providing resources for teachers as they try to incorporate dialectal variations in their instruction. A most important point is for teachers to become familiar with the various dialects in their classroom so that they are aware of how to help individual students in learning Standard English. The SLP is an invaluable resource in this effort. For example, an African American child may want to receive some specific instruction in Standard English because of a particular vocational or higher education target that may be more attainable by learning Standard English. The SLP may act as a consultant in helping the classroom teacher design a cooperative program to increase Standard English proficiency. Koenig and Biel reported an innovative program in an Ohio school system that teaches English as a Second Language (ESL) to bilingual students and English as a Second Dialect (ESD) to students who speak dialects of English (Koenig & Biel, 1989). The ESD program is available for students K–12 and provides instruction to facilitate speaking, reading, and writing skills in Standard English. Students can enter the program through teacher, parent, or self-referral. The goal is to develop effective cross-cultural communication skills that can generalize to academic areas. The program is conducted by language aides working with students individually and in groups several times per week. The aides are under the supervision of the SLP and undergo intensive training sessions prior to working with students. Underlying the whole program is the philosophy that students "are taught with respect for the integrity of the native language, home dialects and cultures" (p. 347). Such a program allows the SLP to offer services to dialect speakers through the judicious use of aides and still not spend significant time away from the caseload of children with clinically significant communication disorders.

Resources are available in some school systems that have high concentrations of bilingual students. Some of these school systems employ ESL teachers to teach Standard English.

Parents and older students also may avail themselves of night classes offered in many communities that teach English. Teachers, however, are a critical influence in helping minority children to learn Standard English, and it is their *attitude* that is a crucial variable.

The issue of how to deal with social dialects in an educational setting is a touchy one. No one yet has the definitive answer as to how to incorporate minority language into a Standard English curriculum without offending someone. All we can say at the present time is that dialects are *not* disorders, dialects *are* important parts of cultures and should *not* be derogated, and that greater understanding of social dialects can benefit all the people involved in this thorny issue. The classroom teacher is at the forefront of this complex situation and is faced daily with minority students. We can only encourage teachers to: (1) provide good models of Standard English, (2) be consistent and up-front about their language expectations for grading purposes; (3) allow each student the courtesy of expressing ideas in his/her own dialect in appropriate situations; (4) try to be sensitive to the possible influence of dialect on errors they find in their students' work and compensate for these in their teaching; (5) attempt to incorporate examples of a variety of social dialects into teaching of language arts, social studies, history, drama, and other relevant topics; and (6) do not regard dialects as pathological and something to be referred to the SLP for correction.

The next few decades, as American society becomes even *more* multicultural, will present exciting opportunities to teach and provide clinical services. The school systems and clinical settings must rise to this challenge.

Terms to Know

Bilingualism	Regional dialects
Dialect	Vernacular
Standard American English (SAE)	Style shifting
African American English (AAE)	Street register
Hispanic English (HE)	School register
Ethnocentric	Dialectal continuum
Speech community	Dialect importation
Language differences	Bidialectalism
Language deficits	ASHA position

Study Questions

1. What potential problems do dialect speakers face in an educational environment that emphasizes and rewards use of SAE? Focus on social, academic, and psychological aspects.

2. What do you feel would be the prevailing attitude of teachers and laypeople in your geographical area toward the notion of dialect in minority speakers? What are the possible reasons for these attitudes being negative or positive?

3. What are five specific ways a teacher could address the dialect issue in language arts classes?
4. Learning SAE can have several potential advantages for dialect speakers. Discuss the advantages of learning SAE.
5. Discuss ways in which parents, teachers, SLPs, and students can cooperate in dealing with the dialect issue in the public school system.

Bibliography

Abrahams, R., & Gay, G. (1975). Talking African American in the classroom. In P. Stoller (Ed.), *African American English.* New York, NY: Delta.

Alexander, C. (1985). African American English dialect and the classroom teacher. In C. Brooks et al. (Eds.), *Tapping potential: English and language arts for the African American learner.* Urbana, IL: National Council of Teachers of English.

Anderson, E. (1990). Teaching users of diverse dialects: Practical approaches. *Teaching English in the Two Year College, 17*(3), 172–177.

Andrews, M., & Owens, P. (1976). *African American language.* Berkeley, CA: Seymour-Smith.

Battle, D., Aldes, M., Grantham, R. Halfond, M., Harris, G., Morgenstern-Lopez, N., Smith, G., Terrell, S., & Cole, L. (1983). Position paper on social dialects. *Journal of the American Speech-Language-Hearing Association, 25,* 23–24.

Birch, B. (2001). Grammar standards: It's all in your attitude. *Language Arts, 78*(6), 535–543.

Bishop, D., North, T., & Donlan, C. (1996). Nonword repetition as a behavioral marker for inherited language impairment: Evidence from a twin study. *Journal of Child Psychology and Psychiatry, 36,* 1–13.

Bohn, A. (2003). Familiar voices: Using Ebonics communication techniques in the primary classroom. *Urban Education, 38*(6), 688–707.

Campbell, T., Dollaghan, C., Needleman, H., & Janosky, J. (1997). Reducing bias in language assessment: Processing dependent measures. *Journal of Speech, Language and Hearing Research, 40,* 519–525.

Cazden, C. (1970). The neglected situation of child language research and education. In F. Williams (Ed.), *Language and poverty: Perspectives on a theme.* Chicago, IL: Rand McNally.

Cheng, L. (1989). Service delivery to Asian/Pacific LEP children: A cross-cultural framework. *Topics in Language Disorders, 9*(3), 1–11.

Covington, A. (1976). African American people and African American English: Attitudes and deeducation in a biased macroculture. In D. Harrison & T. Irabasso (Eds.), *African American English: A seminar.* Hillsdale, NJ: Erlbaum.

Craig, H., & Washington, J. (2002). Oral language expectations for African American preschoolers and kindergartners. *American Journal of Speech-Language Pathology, 11*(1), 59–70.

Craig, H., & Washington, J. (2004). Grade-related changes in the production of African American English. *Journal of Speech, Language and Hearing Research, 47*(2), 450–463.

Dillard, J. (1972). *African American English.* New York, NY: Random House.

Dollaghan, C., & Campbell, T. (1998). Nonword repetition and child language impairment. *Journal of Speech, Language and Hearing Research, 41,* 1136–1146.

Edwards, W. (1985). Inner city English. In C. Brooks et al. (Eds.), *Tapping potential: English and language arts for the African American learner.* Urbana, IL: National Council of Teachers of English.

Ellis-Weismer, S., Tomblin, J., Zhang, X., Buckwalter, P., Chynoweth, J., & Jones, M. (2000). Nonword repetition performance in school age children with and without language impairment. *Journal of Speech, Language and Hearing Research, 43,* 865–878.

Fagundes, D., Haynes, W., Haak, N., & Moran, M. (1998). Task variability effects on the language test performance of southern lower socioeconomic class African American and Caucasian five year olds. *Language, Speech and Hearing Services in Schools, 29*(3), 148–157.

Fasold, R. (1990). *The sociolinguistics of language: Introduction to sociolinguistics* (Vol. II). Oxford, UK: Blackwell.

Foster, M. (2001). Pay Leon, pay Leon, pay Leon paleontologist: Using call and response to facilitate language acquisition among African American students. In S. Lanehart (Ed.), *Sociocultural and historical contexts of African American English* (pp. 281–298). Philadelphia, PA: John Benjamins.

Gemake, J. (1981). Interference of certain dialect elements with reading comprehension for third graders. *Reading Improvement, 18*(2), 183–189.

Green, L. (2002). *African American English: A linguistic introduction.* Cambridge, UK: Cambridge University Press.

Harber, J., & Bryen, D. (1978). Black English and the task of reading. *Review of Educational Research, 46,* 387–405.

Haynes, W., & Pindzola, R. (2007). *Diagnosis and Evaluation in Speech Pathology* (7th ed.). Boston: Allyn & Bacon.

Hecht, M., Collier, M., & Ribeau, S. (1993). *African American communication.* Newbury Park, CA: Sage.

Irvine, J. (2002). *In search of wholeness: African American teachers and their culturally specific classroom practices.* New York, NY: Palgrave.

Koenig, L., & Biel, C. (1989). A delivery system of comprehensive language services to a school district. *Language, Speech and Hearing Services in Schools, 20*(4), 338–365.

Laffey, J., & Shuy, R. (1973). *Language differences: Do they interfere?* Newark, DE: International Reading Association.

LeMoine, N. (2001). Language variation and literacy acquisition in African American students. In J. Harris, A. Kamhi, & K. Pollock (Eds.), *Literacy in African American communities* (pp. 169–194). Mahwah, NJ: Erlbaum.

Lippi-Green, R. (1997). *English with an accent.* New York, NY: Routledge.

Littell, J. (1971). *The language of man* (Vol. 5). Evanston, IL: McDougal, Littell.

Love, T. (1991). *A guide for teaching Standard English to black dialect speakers.* ERIC Document Reproduction Service no. ED340248.

Lynch, E., & Hanson, M. (1992). *Developing cross-cultural competence.* Baltimore, MD: Brookes.

Maddahian, E., & Sandamela, A. (2000). *Linguistic affirmation program evaluation report.* Program Evaluation and Research Branch. Los Angeles: Los Angeles Unified School District.

Major, C. (1994). *Juba to jive: A dictionary of African American slang.* New York, NY: Penguin.

Mantell, A. (1974). Strategies for language expansion in the middle grades. In B. Cullinan (Ed.), *Black dialects and reading* (pp. 55–68). Urbana, IL: NCTE.

McGregor, K., Williams, D., Hearst, S., & Johnson, A. (1997). The use of contrastive analysis in distinguishing difference from disorder: A tutorial. *American Journal of Speech-Language Pathology, 6,* 45–56.

Owens, R. (1988). *Language development: An introduction.* Columbus, OH: Merrill.

Parker, H., & Crist, M. (1995). *Teaching minorities to play the corporate language game.* Columbia, SC: National Resource Center for the Freshman Year Experience and Students in Transition. University of South Carolina.

Rickford, J. (1999). *African American vernacular English: Features, evolution, educational implications.* Oxford, UK: Blackwell.

Rickford, J. (2002). Linguistics, education and the Ebonics firestorm. In J. Alatis, H. Hamilton, & A. Tan (Eds.), *Round table on language and linguistics, 2000: Linguistics, language and the professions* (pp. 25–45). Washington, DC: Georgetown University Press.

Rickford, J., & Rickford, R. (2000). *Spoken soul: The story of black English.* New York, NY: Wiley.

Rickford, J., Sweetland, J., & Rickford, A. (2004). African American English and other vernaculars in education. *Journal of English Linguistics, 32*(3), 230–320.

Rickford, R., & Rickford, A. (1995). Dialect readers revisited. *Linguistics and Education, 7*(2), 107–128.

Rodekohr, R., & Haynes, W. (2001). Differentiating dialect from disorder: A comparison of two processing tasks and a standardized language test. *Journal of Communication Disorders, 34,* 255–272.

Rosten, L. (1971). The joys of Yiddish. In J. Littell (Ed.), *The language of man.* Evanston, IL: McDougal, Littell.

Schrader, T., Quinn, M., Stockman, I., & Miller, J. (1999). Authentic assessment as an approach to preschool speech-language screening. *American Journal of Speech-Language Pathology, 8,* 195–200.

Seymour, H., Bland-Stewart, L., & Green, L. (1998). Differences versus deficit in child African American English. *Language, Speech and Hearing Services in Schools, 29,* 96–108.

Seymour, H., Roeper, T., & deVilliers, J. (2003). *Diagnostic Evaluation of Language Variation (DELV) Criterion-Referenced.* San Antonio, TX: Psychological Corporation.

Seymour, H., & Seymour, C. (1979). The symbolism of Ebonics: I'd rather switch than fight. *Journal of Black Studies, 9,* 397–410.

Smitherman, G. (2000). *Black talk: Words and phrases from the hood to the amen corner.* Boston, MA: Houghton Mifflin.

Stockman, I. (1996). The promises and pitfalls of language sample analysis as an assessment tool for linguistic minority children. *Language Speech and Hearing Services in Schools, 27,* 355–366.

Taylor, O. (1971, Spring). Some sociolinguistic concepts of African American language. *Today's Speech,* 19–26.

Taylor, O. (1986). Language differences. In G. Shames & E. Wiig (Eds.), *Human communication disorders: An introduction.* Columbus, OH: Merrill.

Thompson, C., Craig, H., & Washington, J. (2004). African American and Caucasian preschoolers' use of decontextualized language: Literate language features in oral narratives. *Language, Speech and Hearing Services in Schools, 35*(3), 240–253.

Van Keulen, J., Weddington, G., & DeBose, C. (1998). *Speech, language, learning and the African American child.* Needham Heights, MA: Allyn & Bacon.

Williams, R., & Wolfram, W. (1977). *Social differences vs. disorders.* Washington, DC: American Speech and Hearing Association.

Wolfram, W., Adger, C., & Christian, D. (1999). *Dialects in schools and communities.* Mahwah, NJ: Erlbaum.

<table>
<tr><td>

Chapter

8
</td><td>

FLUENCY DISORDERS
</td></tr>
</table>

The word *fluency* means flowing along (Starkweather, 1981). Speech is **fluent** when words are produced easily, effortlessly, smoothly, quickly, and in a forward flow. Speech is **disfluent** when one word does not flow smoothly and quickly into the next.

Speakers occasionally exhibit disfluencies, such as pausing, interjecting "um," backing up and revising the wording of an utterance, or repeating part of the utterance. These are routine, nonworrisome errors in speech fluency, as judged by society, and everyone commits them from time to time. Some fluency failures are not judged so kindly by society. Persons that utter too many disfluencies or say types that are conspicuously unusual are considered to have a **fluency disorder**. Disorders of fluency include developmental stuttering (often just called stuttering or stammering), cluttering, and acquired stuttering, either neurotic or neurogenic in nature. This chapter discusses each of these fluency disorders, with emphasis on stuttering because it is the fluency disorder teachers most often encounter in the classroom.

Stuttering is a disorder affecting the rhythm of speech. The individual knows precisely what he or she wishes to say, but at the time is unable to say it because of an involuntary repetition, prolongation, or cessation of a sound. Clearly, the loss of fluency conveyed in this definition is involuntary in nature and is the result of a temporary loss of speech production ability rather than a problem with language formulation.

Authorities have struggled for years to agree on the best definition of stuttering. The classic definition provided by Wingate probably best differentiates nonstuttering disfluencies from pathological stuttering:

> The term *stuttering* means . . . disruption in the fluency of verbal expression, which is characterized by involuntary, audible or silent, repetitions or prolongations in the utterance of short speech elements, namely: sounds, syllables, and words of one syllable. These disruptions usually occur frequently and are

usually marked in character and are not readily controllable. Sometimes the disruptions are accompanied by accessory activities involving the speech apparatus, related or unrelated body structures, or stereotyped speech utterances. These activities give the appearance of being speech-related struggle. Also, there are not infrequently indications or reports of the presence of an emotional state, ranging from a general condition of "excitement" or "tension" to more specific emotions of a negative nature such as fear, embarrassment, irritation, or the like. The immediate source of stuttering is some incoordination expressed in the peripheral speech mechanism. (Wingate, 1966, p. 488)

In clinical practice, many speech-language pathologists (SLPs) use simplified operational definitions for identifying and counting stutter moments. Some count syllables stuttered as a function of syllables spoken (Lincoln & Harrison, 1999) while others advocate counting stuttered words per minute of talking (Ryan, 1974; Ryan & Ryan, 1999). Regardless of the frequency method used, it is common practice to assess types of stuttering in terms of whole word repetitions ("My my ball went under the car"), part-word repetitions ("B-but you said I could"), prolongations ("Mmmmmy dog had puppies"), and instances of struggle behavior (e.g., squinting of the eyes while trying to get a word out). Indeed, these are the types of disfluencies that teachers, healthcare workers, and society in general are apt to notice in speakers young or old, and they suggest a true fluency disorder.

Because stuttering typically begins in the preschool years and because preschool children who are not developing stuttering are also disfluent at this same period of time, what is the difference? Parents, pediatricians, educational personnel, and especially speech-language pathologists need to know. The often-cited works by Yairi's research team segmented **stuttering-like disfluencies (SLDs)** from **other disfluencies (ODs)** (Yairi & Lewis, 1984; Ambrose & Yairi, 1994, 1999; Yairi & Ambrose, 1992; Yairi, Ambrose, & Niermann, 1993). The types of disfluencies that characterize SLDs and ODs are shown in **Table 8–1**.

The World Health Organization scheme known as the International Classification of Impairment, Disabilities, and Handicaps (ICIDH-2) focuses attention on the *consequences* of stuttering, not the underlying causes (Yaruss, 1998; Yaruss & Quesal, 2004). Thus, the impairment of stuttering (the interrupted forward flow of speech) is both disabling and

TABLE 8–1 Stuttering-Like Disfluencies Compared to Other Disfluencies

SLDs (stuttering-like disfluencies)	ODs (other disfluencies)
Part-word repetitions	Interjections
Monosyllabic word repetitions	Polysyllabic word repetitions
Sound prolongations	Phrase repetitions
Blocks	Revisions
Broken words	

handicapping: Stuttering and its affective, behavioral, and cognitive reactions limit a child's or adult's ability to communicate with others or to engage in social, academic, or vocational activities.

THE INCIDENCE AND PREVALENCE OF STUTTERING

You may wonder: "How many people stutter?" There are two ways to answer this question. The prevalence of stuttering is somewhat less than 1 percent. The **prevalence** of a disorder indicates how many people are afflicted by it at any given point in time. Hull, Mielke, Willeford, and Timmons (1976) assessed the speech of 38,802 public school students in the 1st through 12th grades and found 0.8 percent of them to stutter. Furthermore, the study confirmed a well-established observation that males who stutter outnumber females who stutter 3 to 1. Young (1975), in reviewing the literature on prevalence of stuttering, suggests that a reasonable figure for both school-age and young adults who stutter is 0.7 percent of the population. With the population of the United States being approximately 281 million (*Encyclopaedia Britannica Almanac 2003*, 2002), these data suggest that more than 1.9 million Americans stutter.

A second way to address the question of how many people stutter is to measure its incidence. The **incidence** of a disorder can be measured over time to include those who presently stutter, as well as those who used to stutter but do so no longer. The incidence of stuttering among the general population is approximately 4–5 percent (Bloodstein, 1995; Conture, 2001), suggesting that, indeed, many recover from stuttering. Estimates are that some 50–85 percent of the children who stutter undergo **spontaneous recovery** (Andrews & Harris, 1964; Martin & Lindamood, 1986; Yairi & Ambrose, 1992; Yairi et al., 1993). Most children outgrow their highly disfluent speech by age 9 years; others still manage to recover by puberty. Recovery ranges, however, are so great that it makes clinical use of the information difficult. Yet this is an important aspect of stuttering that merits further study. No doubt, teachers, pediatricians, and SLPs are asked many questions about recovery.

Parents want to know the probability of *their* child outgrowing stuttering. There is no easy answer, but the speech-language pathologist may be the person most equipped with knowledge of the disorder, and knowledge of the child, to formulate the best response. Research shows that a child's chances of outgrowing stuttering worsen with age, the **severity** of characteristics exhibited, and the length of time stuttering has existed. A generalization is that a child who has stuttered for more than one or two years and/or who is past age 9 years probably will not recover without help. Parents, pediatricians, and teachers may wonder, then, whether it might be best to postpone fluency treatment in hopes the child will outgrow stuttering. The prevailing clinical opinion, however, is not to wait. Early intervention is important. Stuttering is a simpler problem to treat in a young child. With Public Law 99-457, schools are responsible for handicapped children ages 3 through 5 years, facilitating such early intervention. Prevention and early intervention of stuttering are extremely important. It should be emphasized, though, that treatment is appropriate at any age. Successful outcomes are reported for a variety of approaches for children, adolescents, and adults.

There are many other interesting aspects of stuttering. Following is a list of some of these facts.

- Stuttering is universal. The disorder has existed throughout recorded history and is found among all peoples of the world.
- Stuttering almost always begins in childhood, usually before age 6 years. Ages 2 to 4 years are particularly common periods for the onset of stuttering.
- Stuttering occurs more often among males than females. Reports of sex ratio vary from 3:1 to as high as 6:1.
- Stuttering tends to run in families. Family studies have shown that the risk of stuttering in relatives of a person who stutters is increased over that for the general population. Furthermore, the pattern of transmission in families is consistent with predictions derived from genetic models (Cox, 1988), yet genetic components of stuttering have not been proved.
- The amount of stuttering varies widely with situations. Persons who stutter often report excessive speech difficulties when they are excited or feel under pressure. Saying their name, talking on the telephone, ordering in a restaurant, talking to a person in authority (e.g., a teacher), and talking in front of a group (as in a classroom) also are situations that elicit much stuttering. Additionally, speakers have good days and bad days, meaning that the frequency and severity of their stuttering fluctuate.
- Stuttering is reduced or eliminated in a variety of conditions as well. Most affected people report being able to sing, whisper, and talk to themselves or their pets fluently. By talking in a prolonged, slow fashion, most become stutter free. Choral or unison speaking and talking to a rhythmical beat also improve fluency.
- For those who do not outgrow it, stuttering tends to change—and worsen—as the person matures. What began as a speech problem evolves into a personal-social-psychological problem.
- Stuttering need not hold a person back from achieving full potential. Many famous, brilliant, and talented people stuttered, such as Winston Churchill, Moses, Marilyn Monroe, Sommerset Maugham, Isaac Newton, Mel Tillis, Bob Newhart, and James Earl Jones.

This list of interesting facts points to aspects of stuttering of which you, as an educator or healthcare professional, need to be aware. Many items on this list also have obvious implications for treatment.

CAUSATION AND DEVELOPMENT OF STUTTERING

Stuttering remains a mystery. The ultimate cause of this perplexing speech disorder is unknown, yet theories abound. Parts of the stuttering problem seem to be learned behaviors; still other evidence suggests that there are neurophysiological reasons for the loss of speech coordination. Psychological theories, once popular, seem to have suffered from a lack of verifiable causal evidence. It is beyond the scope of this chapter to critically examine all of the theories of etiology. However, years of research reveal that no intellectual or emotional behaviors distinguish children who stutter from those who do not (Zebrowski & Schum, 1993; Bloodstein, 1995).

No matter what the cause or causes of stuttering, the child begins trying too hard to speak and starts having more and more trouble. Although the onset of stuttering is usually gradual, worrisome behaviors emerge and, over time, the symptoms change and worsen. It is a vicious cycle unless caught in time. It is incumbent upon classroom teachers and pediatricians to refer children who show any signs of stuttering to the speech-language pathologist in an effort to prevent a more severe situation in the future. Furthermore, although parents most certainly do not cause their child to stutter, one can speculate that there are some behaviors in the home environment that might contribute to its exacerbation and continued development. Clearly, then, certain environmental conditions need to be addressed through intervention.

EARLY SIGNS OF CONCERN

Parents and teachers of young children often worry that a particular child might be beginning to stutter. Speech-language pathologists are trained to recognize early signs of concern and to differentiate them from other, non-stuttering-like disfluency. It is important for parents, teachers, and pediatricians to know that all children periodically demonstrate disfluencies; however, these instances are of particular types and do not occur too often. The following are some examples of these so-called other disfluencies (ODs) where speech errors in children need not be of concern.

1. Whole-word and phrase repetitions: "My, my ball went under the car." "I want, I want some ice cream."
2. Sentence revisions: "It went—My ball went under the car."
3. Pauses filled with *um, ah, uh*: "I want some . . . um . . . ice cream."
4. Unfilled pauses or relaxed hesitations: "Daddy, I want (pause) some ice cream."
5. Infrequent, easy, single part-word repetitions: "B-but you said I could."

Certain early signs of concern should alert parents, teachers, pediatricians, and speech-language pathologists that stuttering may be developing. Symptoms of stuttering-like disfluencies (SLDs) include the following.

1. Frequent part-word repetitions, especially when part-word repetitions occur more often than whole-word or phrase repetitions: "B-but" more likely than "But-but"
2. Part of a word repeated more than two or three times: "Ba-ba-ba-ba-ball"
3. Repetitions having an irregular rhythm: "B-ba-buh-b-ball"
4. A sound held conspicuously long (perhaps prolonged 1 second or more): "Mmmmmmmmmmmy ball"

Other early signs of concern may be present in addition to the disfluencies themselves. As stuttering develops, children might exhibit tension and fear. Excessive tension in the speech musculature may cause explosive enunciations of speech sounds, voice tremors, or rises in pitch when speaking. Muscles in the neck and face may distend as children struggle to talk. Children may even show fear when anticipating a difficult word and may, in fact, learn to substitute easier words. Avoidance behaviors become habituated shortly after the child becomes adept at anticipating difficulties. By this time, stuttering is beyond its beginning stages.

These early signs of concern appear gradually in a child's speech. Stuttering rarely occurs overnight! This dissolution of fluent speech often follows a predictable pattern of development.

DEVELOPMENTAL PHASES

Developmental stuttering is so called because it begins in early childhood, especially between ages 2 and 4 years, and its characteristics and symptoms worsen with time. No assumption is made about the original cause of the stuttering. The majority of stuttering cases begin and develop with a regular, predictable pattern. Bloodstein (1960), after a cross-sectional investigation of more than 400 persons who stutter, describes four phases through which stuttering typically develops. These now classic results are shown in **Table 8–2**.

In another classic work, Van Riper (1982) also describes the onset and developmental course of stuttering, which, he says, can proceed in any of four different directions. These developmental scenarios are termed Tracks (Track I, II, III, IV). The onset and developmental course of the most typical form of stuttering constitutes Track I. Track I encompassed all of Bloodstein's (1960) phases with cardinal characteristics including onset in the preschool years; normal speech and language development; previously fluent; easy and rhythmic repetitions predominate; episodic fluctuations in fluency; unawareness of speaking difficulties; and absence of avoidance behaviors. It is no wonder that these early characteristics were termed **primary stuttering**. However, the assumption that young children lack awareness is not supported because 3-year-old children are aware of their speech differences and 5-year-olds even more so (Ezrati-Vinacour, Platzky, & Yairi, 2001). In primary stuttering, with the passage of time, the symptoms worsen to include tension in the speech musculature, appearance of irregular part-word repetitions followed by prolongations and struggle behaviors, the awareness and predictability of speaking difficulties, and the development of a stylized system of avoidance behaviors to reduce or conceal stuttering. The person, by this time in the development of the disorder, truly has the self-concept of being a person who stutters. Although the development of this **secondary stuttering** form requires conditioning through experience and the passage of time, it can occur at any age. Young children can have confirmed stuttering.

The Track I developmental scenario accounted for 54 percent of the more than 300 cases Van Riper (1982) studied, including 44 clients followed longitudinally. An additional 14 percent

TABLE 8–2   The Classic Four Phases in the Development of Stuttering

Phase One

1. The difficulty has a distinct tendency to be episodic, that is, to come and go in cycles.
2. The child stutters most when excited or upset, when seeming to have a great deal to say, or under other conditions of communicative pressure.
3. The dominant symptom is repetition.
4. There is a marked tendency for stutterings to occur at the beginning of the sentence, clause, or phrase.
5. In contrast to more advanced stuttering, the interruptions occur not only on content words, but also on the function words of speech (pronouns, conjunctions, articles, and prepositions).
6. Most of the time children in the first phase of stuttering show little evidence of concern about the interruptions in their speech.

Phase Two

7. The disorder is essentially chronic.
8. The child has a self-concept as a stutterer.
9. The stutterings occur chiefly on the major parts of speech (nouns, verbs, adjectives, and adverbs).
10. Despite a self-concept as a stutterer, the child usually evinces little or no concern about the speech difficulty.
11. The stuttering is said to increase chiefly under conditions of excitement or when the child is speaking rapidly.

Phase Three

12. The stuttering comes and goes largely in response to specific situations.
13. Certain words or sounds are regarded as more difficult than others.
14. In varying degrees, use is made of word substitutions and circumlocutions.
15. There is essentially no avoidance of speech situations and little or no evidence of fear or embarrassment.

Phase Four

16. Vivid, fearful anticipations of stuttering.
17. Feared words, sounds, and situations.
18. Very frequent word substitutions and circumlocutions.
19. Avoidance of speech situations, and other evidence of fear and embarrassment.

Source: Bloodstein, 1960.

of the cases fit a different pattern of onset and development, what he called Track II. (Tracks III and IV occur rarely.)

Data reported by Daly (1981) agree well with the commonness of these so-called typical Track I persons. He reports that 54 percent of 138 persons who stutter (treated at the Shady Trails Summer Speech Camp) indeed fit the Track I description. Accounting for

24 percent of the 138 disfluent campers, Track II persons were found to be more common than as reported by Van Riper.

In Track II, fluency problems are evident from the time the child begins to talk. Not only is there no history of good fluency, these children often are also delayed in the onset of talking, have articulation problems, and possess poor language skills. The syllabic repetitions seem hurried and irregular; more silent gaps and hesitations are evident at an earlier stage than in the Track I scenario. Yet, like Track I, Track II persons show little awareness or frustration in the early stage of stuttering development. Fears, especially of speaking situations, develop later.

These children certainly are candidates for team intervention. The presence of weak language skills may affect all academic areas, particularly reading and spelling. The speech-language pathologist also is likely to design a combination of treatment strategies to simultaneously address the fluency, phonology, and/or language disorders of the individual. Data and a research summary reported by Louko, Edwards, and Conture (1999) suggest that, indeed, 33 percent of persons who stutter have coexisting articulation or phonological problems. Less often, they say, persons who stutter exhibit other concomitant disorders.

ASSESSMENT ISSUES

Although typical and atypical forms of stuttering exist, for those who do not outgrow it, evidence suggests that the problem becomes more complex with the passage of time. What starts as overt disfluency evolves into a complicated disorder that affects the person's thoughts, emotions, words, deeds, and lifestyle. Early identification and early intervention are considered critical by many specialists in the area of stuttering (Onslow & Packman, 1999). By knowing the difference between nonstuttering forms of disfluency and beginning stuttering, a classroom teacher can recognize the student exhibiting early signs of concern and make an appropriate referral to the speech-language pathologist. An educator's intuition about and observation of a child's speech, along with parental concerns expressed to teachers, are principal avenues for identifying students in need of fluency management.

The educator refers the student to the speech-language pathologist, who attempts to answer two key questions in a diagnostic evaluation. First, is the person stuttering or not? Fluency may be viewed, quite simply, on a continuum, as shown in **Figure 8–1**. Some speakers are silver-tongued, yet others are highly disfluent. The bulk of the population has average fluency, containing speech errors including pauses, interjections, revisions, and the like (recall Table 8–1). Other speakers are viewed by society as highly disfluent. Where does society draw the line to separate acceptable disfluency from abnormal disfluency? There is no magic number that defines such a border, yet speech-language pathologists collect information and data to do just that. A trained, experienced speech-language pathologist gathers the necessary information to determine whether the person is stuttering or not; this is termed making a **differential diagnosis**. Often the diagnosis is more straightforward in the evaluation of an adult or adolescent than in a young child.

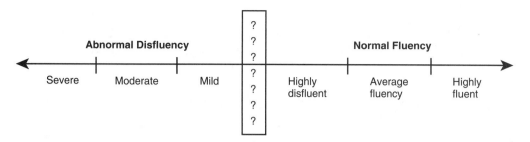

FIGURE 8–1 Fluency depicted on a continuum illustrating the process of differential diagnosis and severity determination.

A second diagnostic question follows the first. If the person is stuttering, how involved is it? Here, the SLP addresses the issue of severity; it, too, can be placed on the continuum, as shown in Figure 8–1. Information and data collected in the diagnostic evaluation help categorize the severity of the stuttering along the dimensions of mild, moderate, or severe.

Many assessment scales exist for the evaluation of a stuttering disorder and a thorough discussion may be obtained in the book by Haynes and Pindzola (2008). An educator also may encounter assessment information through a cooperative, working relationship with the speech-language pathologist. Certainly, information of this kind is contained in the student's speech-language file, is summarized on the student's Individualized Education Program (IEP), and is discussed during the IEP meeting with the classroom teacher present. Two scales typical of stuttering assessment are described—one useful in differential diagnosis and the other a well-known severity scale. Knowledge of their content is a good foundation for understanding the disorder itself.

DIFFERENTIAL DIAGNOSIS

Explicit identification procedures that can distinguish between persons who stutter and those who do not stutter are needed to make a differential diagnosis. Gordon and Luper (1992) reviewed six often-used protocols for identifying beginning stuttering, including *A Protocol for Differentiating the Incipient Stutterer* (Pindzola & White, 1986; Pindzola, 1988, 1999). This is an appraisal tool that synthesizes existing knowledge into a format that guides the speech-language pathologist through clinical observations, data collection, and interpretation. The protocol quantifies eight auditory behaviors perceived by the listener, assesses visual evidence of speaking difficulties, and examines subjective feelings as well as historical and psychological indicators of chronic stuttering.

The speech-language pathologist administers the protocol by obtaining a sample of natural speech. Often this is done by the SLP in a clinical interview. Listening to the student on the playground, in the cafeteria, or in the classroom also may provide the SLP with a natural sample of speech for analysis. The protocol uses a numerical scale for rating behaviors.

The auditory and visual sections of the protocol yield a total score of between 14 and 42. Preliminary standardization studies (Pindzola, 1988) suggest that a total score of 14–21 is within normal limits, but a score greater than 21 may be indicative of incipient or confirmed stuttering. Some important information about stuttering from the protocol is highlighted in the following sections.

The predominant type of disfluency that a speaker typically uses and the size of the speech unit affected by the disfluency influence the listener's judgments of speech normalcy. For example, repetitions of whole phrases are quite normal; whole-word repetitions are disfluencies typical of both stutterers and nonstutterers. Yet the predominance of part-word repetitions distinguishes stuttering from nonstuttering preschoolers (Yairi & Lewis, 1984). Hesitations or pauses before phrases or before words may, likewise, be less innocuous than such gaps within words (e.g., preceding syllables or sounds). The rule of thumb that Perkins (1971) suggests is that the smaller the speech unit affected, the more abnormal the disfluency. Recall again the types of speech errors listed in Table 8–1.

The frequency with which disfluent behaviors occur has long been recognized as important in the diagnosis of stuttering. There are various ways the SLP can determine frequency, and there are various data for interpreting normalcy. Suffice it to say that frequencies in excess of 2 percent, 5 percent, or 10 percent suggest a stuttering disorder, depending on the strictness of the criterion used by the SLP.

The duration of the disfluency may be expressed in two ways, either as number of times for repetitions or as length of time for prolongations. For example, in the sentence "My my my cat had kittens," the whole word *my* is produced twice before being uttered meaningfully. Likewise, silent or audible prolongations may be measured with a stopwatch or simply estimated. If the typical duration of prolongations exceeds 1 second, or if repetitions involve numerous reiterations, the SLP may interpret these behaviors as signs of stuttering.

Audible signs of effort while speaking generally are not noted among nonstuttering speakers and, therefore, are indicative of abnormality. A complete listing of these audible behaviors is not realistic, but typical behaviors include disrupted airflow, hard contacts (explosive, crisp articulation), and effort or tension heard in the voice.

Van Riper (1982) provides clinical reports that disfluencies within normal limits and perhaps very early stutterings are characterized by repetitions that preserve the rhythm and rate of speech. Not until the tempo of the reiterations speeds up or their rhythm becomes irregular and choppy is there substantial reason for concern. The speech-language pathologist is asked to judge subjectively the student's rhythm, tempo, and the speed of disfluencies in using the protocol.

Behaviors that may be audible and learned are thought to develop as a means of minimizing stuttering. The person who stutters may use concealment devices, such as word substitutions ("big fries" substituted for "large fries" to avoid the troublesome /l/ sound) or circumlocutions (talking around *blue* by describing the color of the sky), to avoid feared words. Postponement devices may consist of maneuvers (e.g., interjections) to delay attempts on a feared word, and the individual may use starting tricks (e.g., humming prefixed to the feared word) to assist in initiating feared words. These and other mannerisms may help the SLP discriminate between stuttering and nonstuttering.

The second part of the protocol assesses visual evidence of a stuttering disorder. Visual signs of effort suggest to the listener that the act of speaking is unduly difficult. Such signs may reflect that a student is aware of the speaking difficulties, that he or she is trying to do something about the moments of difficulty, and that the disfluency has developed into a more severe disorder. The SLP records the specific behaviors displayed by the student in the facial, head, and body regions. Frequently observed contortions are blinking, wrinkling of the forehead, distortions of the mouth, and overt tension in the jaw. Rhythmical head movements, head jerks, and the more subtle head turnings to divert eye contact also are observable in some persons who stutter.

The third section of the protocol assesses historical and psychological indicators of stuttering. The subjective evaluations made by a speaker while experiencing speech disfluencies, and in reaction to them, are diagnostically important. These covert reactions have been studied through the introspection of older persons who stutter but also may be present to some degree in younger children who stutter. Whenever possible, the speech-language pathologist should explore the student's perception of the problem; additional information collected from parental reports and teachers is useful also. It is not uncommon for even young children to be aware and concerned about their disfluent speech as evidenced by parental reports of their child's being upset at peer teasing or crying over not being able to talk. Clearly, this early concern is testimony to the reality of a disfluency problem. Evidence exists that even preschool children are aware of stuttering (Ambrose & Yairi, 1994) and their degree of awareness may relate back to the developmental progression discussed earlier in the chapter (see Table 8–2).

The SLP can explore these and other historical and psychological factors by using Pindzola's *Protocol for Differentiating the Incipient Stutterer.* Clearly, SLPs should collect much information on a student and use it to shape clinical opinion. Only after weighing the evidence can a speech-language pathologist make an accurate diagnosis regarding stuttering.

JUDGING SEVERITY

The Individualized Education Program adopted by most school districts requires a statement regarding the severity of the handicapping condition. The speech-language pathologist attempts to categorize the severity of the student's stuttering along the continuum of very mild to very severe. Many aspects of the stuttering condition contribute to such a severity determination, yet three parameters seem to be the most important: The SLP should quantify the frequency, duration, and physical concomitants of the stuttering. The *Stuttering Severity Instrument* (Riley, 2009), a severity scale in wide use, assesses these three parameters. The classroom teacher should be versed in the process of determining severity to appreciate what the modifiers *mild*, *moderate*, and *severe* represent and to contribute meaningfully to the discussions of a particular student during the IEP meeting.

The *Stuttering Severity Instrument* (Riley, 2009) is useful with both children and adults and has provisions for testing those who can and cannot read. The speech-language pathologist computes the number of syllables stuttered and the number of total syllables spoken as the student reads or is engaged in conversation. The SLP then computes frequency, expressed as percentage of stuttering (number of stuttered syllables divided by total syllables spoken multiplied by 100 equals the percentage), and converts it to a corresponding task score. The SLP also monitors the amount of time a student is stuck during stuttered blocks and averages the three longest. This measure is converted into a task score. Last, the speech-language pathologist watches and carefully listens to the student during reading and conversation samples and rates the presence and conspicuousness of physical behaviors accompanying the speech attempts. The SLP makes a separate rating (on a 0 to 5 scale) for each anatomic area (facial, head, and extremity) and for distracting sounds; their sum constitutes the task score. The SLP then combines frequency, duration, and physical concomitant task scores for a total score. The severity of the student's stuttering can be ascertained by comparing the total score to the normative data provided by Riley. In this manner, the SLP can describe stuttering severity as very mild, mild, moderate, severe, or very severe.

COMMON AVOIDANCE AND CONCEALMENT TECHNIQUES

Sometimes a stuttering problem is not so obvious to a classroom teacher. Persons who stutter may become very adept at using **avoidance behaviors**, even at an early age. Avoidances are tricks and crutches. They are a complex series of behaviors that children and adults can use to cope with and perhaps hide stuttering. They are learned tactics. Persons who stutter begin to disguise behaviors by having someone talk for them, by refusing to talk at all, or by giving up and saying "I don't know." Fear grows and spreads; the student worries and may develop a low self-concept.

VIGNETTE 8–1

Mario is moving through the school's cafeteria line. One of the day's selections is his favorite, spicy chicken tortilla soup. He wants to ask for some but has a feeling he will block on the word *soup*. He says to the cafeteria worker, "I'd like some chicken, urn, so to speak, uh some chicken s-s-s-s—." The cafeteria worker hastily interrupts and says, "You want what?" Mario responds saying, "A cup of—you know—that stuff with chicken, onions, celery. . . ." "You mean chicken salad?" snaps the cafeteria worker while trying to hand it to Mario and continuing, "You have to keep the line moving." Mario, in frustration, ekes out, "Well, just give me some fingers!" Mario continues down the line thinking to himself how sick he is of eating chicken fingers! In this scenario Mario is using a variety of avoidance tactics to postpone (**postponement devices**) and/or start (**starter devices**) saying the feared word *soup*. By describing the ingredients, Mario is using the technique of **circumlocution** to talk around the feared word. Finally, in disgust, he gives up and **substitutes** an easier word, ordering fingers.

The presence of repetitions, prolongations, and struggle behaviors often is obvious. A teacher who hears and sees these behaviors in a child should refer the student to the speech-language pathologist. Avoidance behaviors, by their very nature, obscure recognition of a person who stutters. The covert tricks disguise speech difficulties; teachers may find it harder to recognize this type of stuttering in the classroom. The following is a list of commonly used avoidance techniques. Teachers should familiarize themselves with these techniques to be able to spot such cases.

- Remaining silent; giving the impression of being a quiet or shy person
- Avoiding situations that demand speech (e.g., not using the telephone, not participating in show-and-tell, not contributing to group discussions, refusing to give an oral report)
- Seldom interacting with the teacher and other persons in authority
- Agreeing easily; avoiding speaking by concurring with others rather than explaining reasons for disagreement
- Rehearsing speech and using preparatory techniques
- Using fillers excessively, such as *like, well, um,* and so on
- Avoiding certain words by substituting others
- Looking away while speaking; maintaining poor eye contact with a listener
- Pretending to think during pauses while really blocking
- Feigning a cough or yawn or shielding the mouth during a block
- Talking while moving a body part (e.g., foot tapping, arm swinging) or talking to a rhythm
- Altering breathing patterns during speech or before speech

INFORMATION THE TEACHER CAN PROVIDE

An open, working relationship between the classroom teacher and the speech-language pathologist is important. Teachers serve as a prime referral source of persons who stutter to the intervention program and can provide valuable information about the student's behaviors. The following list of teacher observations, compiled by Pindzola, may be useful to the speech-language pathologist:

1. Describe as completely as possible what the child is doing that makes you suspect a stuttering problem exists.
2. Describe how often or with what frequency the stuttering occurs in your class.
3. How does the student react to the stuttering?
4. What struggle behaviors and facial contortions, if any, have you observed?
5. Are there particular situations or activities in school that seem to worsen the stuttering (e.g., during show-and-tell, oral book reports, on the playground)?
6. Are there situations or activities that the student tries to avoid because stuttering might occur?

7. Describe the student's peer relationships (e.g., well liked, shy, teased).
8. What is known about the home situation (e.g., pace of living, organization, discipline, sibling rivalry, divorce, emotional tension)? (Pindzola, 1988)

In concert with a determination of fluency characteristics and disfluency severity, a thorough communication assessment is necessary, including appraisal of language and phonology skills. The SLP tries to determine the extent of the student's handicapping condition and this is discussed in the IEP meeting. Teachers and parents can be extremely valuable in helping the SLP make an accurate determination of the degree to which the student is handicapped by the stuttering problem (i.e., educationally, psychologically, and economically).

THERAPEUTIC PRINCIPLES

The speech-language pathologist should discuss a particular student's treatment approach with the classroom teacher and, whenever possible, enlist the teacher's aid and support. Although it is beyond the scope of this chapter to discuss the myriad of treatment programs available, an overview of therapeutic principles is warranted. Before proceeding, we wish to alert teachers that children who display additional speech and language difficulties, or cognitive/intellectual deficits concomitant with stuttering, generally present a poorer prognosis in fluency treatment than those with "pure" stuttering (Louko, Edwards, & Conture, 1990).

TREATMENT OPTIONS FOR THE YOUNG STUDENT

Different philosophies exist regarding the treatment of young persons between the ages of 3 and 9 years who stutter. Treatment options are shown schematically in **Figure 8–2**.

In the first option, environmental treatment, the speech-language pathologist determines that the most prudent course of action is to work through the significant others in the child's life—parents and teachers—to modify the daily environment. The goal is to structure the child's environment to make it more conducive to fluency. The child is not seen for treatment; typically, parents and teachers meet regularly with the SLP to discuss environmental modifications and results. Opting for only environmental treatment is commonly done for the child at risk for developing stuttering or for the child beginning to stutter who displays early symptoms. Modifying parental and teacher reactions to disfluencies, altering the pace and organization of home and classroom, and generally educating significant others about fluency, disfluency, and the modeling of good speech habits are beneficial. Reduction in communicative pressures that the child is vulnerable to is a necessary and important aspect of treatment. **Table 8–3** describes some common forms of communicative stress. Because these situations can occur at home and in school, it is vitally important that both the parents and teachers work with the SLP to reduce and, whenever possible, eliminate them. The payoff of environmental treatment for young children beginning to stutter or those at risk for this disorder generally is improved fluency in the child and the likelihood of recovery.

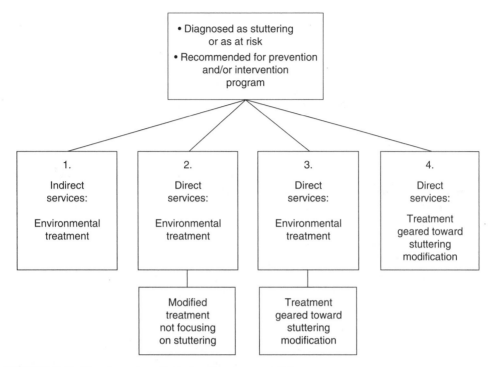

FIGURE 8–2 Treatment options for the young child.

TABLE 8–3 Some Forms of Communicative Stress

1. Listener loss
2. Interruptions
3. Competition for the conversational floor (i.e., an uninterrupted turn to talk)
4. Cross-examination kind of questioning
5. Demands for display speech (e.g., "recite your poem for Grandma")
6. Demands for confession
7. Having to talk under conditions of strong emotion (e.g., guilt, fear, anger), or when fatigued or distracted

Source: Van Riper, 1982.

A second treatment option (see Figure 8–2) is to combine the environmental treatment with direct but modified therapy for the child. Sessions may be individual but are often in groups. The treatment is considered modified because it does not focus on specific symptoms of stuttering. Rather, treatment may emphasize the concept of rhythm by having children sing, speak to a rhythm, practice rhymes, use choral speaking, and just generally experience much success in easy, fluent speech. Modified treatment often involves the strategies of language learning and discourse manipulation (Weiss, 2004a). The language skills of a young child who stutters may be somewhat delayed. The length and complexity of utterances affect the likelihood of even normal speakers having a disfluency. By shoring up weak language skills, and by systematically controlling the linguistic output of young clients (regarding sentence length and syntactic complexity), speech-language pathologists are able to reduce or eliminate stuttering (Weiss & Zebrowski, 1992; Weiss, 2004b). Additionally, some speech-language pathologists may include in the modified program mention of "smooth" and "bumpy" speech and train the children to identify samples of each. Altering the "bumpy" speech, however, is not done in this form of treatment.

A third option of treatment for the young person who stutters (see Figure 8–2) is to combine the environmental approach with direct intervention. The child attends individual or group treatment sessions (depending upon the severity of the problem) with the purpose of modifying specific stuttering symptoms. A variety of therapeutic emphases is possible. The student may be taught a new, fluent way of talking by learning patterns such as slow speech; breathy speech; stretchy speech; an easy speaking voice; slow, easy speech; and other similar strategies for fluency. Discussions of feelings and attitudes may be a component of the treatment program for children ready to address personal issues surrounding their speech difficulties.

The fourth option of direct stuttering modification alone (see Figure 8–2) expands the details involved in mastering strategies, techniques, or targets for fluency. The absence of simultaneously occurring environmental treatment may be a function of: (1) the setting in which services are provided (parents may not be available to participate fully in the intervention program); or (2) the possible progression of the student's stuttering symptoms beyond the level where environmental manipulations would be expected to have much effect. In such cases, efforts need to be focused on direct treatments using greater specificity.

Regardless of the option pursued, stuttering intervention with young children is both effective and efficient in clinical settings. An excellent overview of the leading approaches to childhood stuttering is in the book by Onslow and Packman (1999). Gregory (1990), however, cautions that for treatment to be effective, it should be fairly intensive in the early stages. He recommends at least three individual sessions of 30–50 minutes a week. Gregory goes on to say that one of the problems of effective stuttering treatment in the school setting has been the infrequency and short duration of the sessions. Innovative models of service delivery, such as the consultative/collaborative approaches discussed in this book, should be of great benefit to students who stutter.

TREATMENT FOR THE OLDER STUDENT

The treatment of stuttering among older children, adolescents, and adults of all ages is of the direct type. Obviously, programs differ in complexities and emphases for these disparate age groups. Because negative feelings and attitudes develop late in the evolution of stuttering, treatment for the older student may involve explorations into these psychological topics. The emotional crisis of stuttering escalates during the teenage years when social interactions become so critical. Physiological modifications of speech are often components in adolescent and adult fluency programs. Physiological targets may include breathing, voice onset, and rate, as well as a host of others. Computerized instrumentation may help in the training of these speech targets. Much practice is necessary to habituate new speaking patterns, and support from family, friends, and school personnel can be critical to success. Some children who stutter, particularly older school-aged children and teenagers, do not want to participate in treatment. This desire to refrain from treatment may be related to such feelings or beliefs as fear of peer group judgments, fear of change, fear of failure to change, fear of disappointing oneself and one's family if progress in treatment is not made, lack of concern about stuttering, lack of sufficient motivation to work toward making changes in speech fluency, and the like.

Gregory (1987) describes why participating in class activities, interacting with fellow students and teachers, and receiving treatment as a school activity are topics that teenagers who stutter think about a great deal. Examples of school situations follow; it is useful for teachers to consider what they might do to alleviate these anxious times.

- Almost all who stutter have experienced the frustration of saying, "I don't know," when they did know, rather than take the chance of stuttering as they answered a question in class.
- Students who stutter refer to the anticipation of what they call "reading up and down the rows." They scan ahead in a reading passage to see if there are words on which they may stutter in the passage anticipated for their turn. Not only does the student fear being blocked, but also being laughed at.
- Giving reports is another commonly feared situation. (Some find that practicing a report many times alone makes it easier when giving the report in class.) Also, it is hard for the student to participate in class discussions when stuttering is anticipated. Avoiding these situations only increases tension and eventual stuttering.

WAYS TEACHERS CAN ASSIST IN THE INTERVENTION PROGRAM

Once the speech-language pathologist establishes a treatment program, significant others in the student's environment can—and should—contribute. The roles of the parents and teachers cannot be overemphasized. The student who stutters needs help and much practice to carry over, or generalize, the newly learned speaking patterns that may be part of the intervention program. Classroom teachers can assist both the student and the speech-language pathologist in this practice. The following list of suggestions may be useful.

1. Encourage the student to talk about the speech management sessions and to explain the fluency strategies that he or she is learning.
   Rationale:
   Explaining something newly learned helps cement the student's understanding of it. Talking openly about problems also is very therapeutic. It is healthy to admit a

problem, and treating or overcoming it can be a source of pride. Furthermore, this discussion informs the classroom teacher of the fluency strategies being used (if any) so that the teacher may model them as well. By knowing the strategies, the teacher can monitor their application and reinforce their use or provide subtle reminders when they are needed.

2. Provide help with speech assignments. Work closely with the speech-language pathologist in adapting classroom activities to practice time, where fluency strategies may be applied in real situations. The speech-language pathologist will want to observe the student in real communication in the classroom, particularly in the later stages of treatment.

Rationale:

Newly acquired behaviors need much practice to become habituated. Also, mastery of a skill in the therapy room is meaningless until the skill can be applied in the real world.

3. Provide frequent verbal and social reinforcement for the student's use of fluency strategies. It is particularly important to reinforce fluent speaking in situations that have been difficult in the past.

Rationale:

Reinforcement increases the likelihood that the behavior will recur. Reinforcement of fluency and the use of strategies is done by the speech-language pathologist in the treatment session, but it is more important that such reinforcement be given outside in the real world.

4. Be a good speech model for the student to imitate. The following specific suggestions apply when speaking directly to the child who stutters; some, however, may be used routinely in addressing the entire class:

   a. Use short sentences.

   b. Use vocabulary appropriate for the child's age; do not pressure the child to be more advanced in language usage than other children of the same age.

   c. Speak slowly. An unhurried rate of talking is a good model for fluency.

   d. Pause before responding to a student's utterance. This models the concept of taking one's time and ignoring the pressures to speak quickly.

   e. Avoid interrupting the conversational speech of others. Through such modeling, students learn the importance of turn-taking, which is not only polite but is a pragmatic feature of language. Interrupting and being interrupted both tend to generate disfluent speech.

   f. Blend words together smoothly; speech should not sound choppy. Keeping the voice and air flowing between words in a sentence is a good fluency model.

   g. Model speaking in a soft manner. A voice that is not loud and has less muscular effort driving it is less likely to tense or block (and result in stuttering). A concise motto for teachers to remember in modeling good speech is simply to talk in a manner that is "soft, smooth, and slow." (Pindzola, 1988)

When there is a student who stutters in the classroom, the teacher may find it helpful for all students to discuss openly and in a nonjudgmental manner the nature of stuttering. To promote adjustment and understanding, the teacher may wish to infuse literature that deals with stuttering into the language arts curriculum. Bushey and Martin (1988) critiqued 20 works of children's fiction in which a character stutters. A sampling of this literature is shown in **Table 8–4** and is listed according to reading age level.

TABLE 8–4   Stuttering in Children's Literature

- *Emily Umily*, by Kathy Corrigan. Toronto: Annick Press, 1984. Reading level: ages 4–7 years. Emily begins kindergarten reluctantly. She tries to participate like all the other children, but is quite disfluent. The children laugh at her as she says "umm" every few words—hence the nickname Umily. Emily's emotional reactions worsen in the story until she experiences positive attitude changes.

- *Don't Worry Dear*, by Joan Frassler. New York: Behavioral Publications, 1971. Reading level: ages 4–8 years. This book is useful as a tool for counseling parents. The character, Jenny, sucks her thumb, wets her bed, and stutters on some words. Surrounded by warmth and acceptance, she is given an opportunity to overcome these habits.

- *The Legend of the Veery Bird*, by Kathleen Hague. San Diego, CA: Harcourt Brace Jovanovich, 1985. Reading level: ages 4–10 years. This modern fairy tale is of a boy named Veery who stutters and lives at the edge of a forest. As a misunderstood child, he shuns the human world and embraces the world of the forest. The magical forest keeper helps him deal with his sorrows and grants him a lovely singing voice. The beautiful story is also emotionally satisfying and deals as well with the death of parents.

- *Glue Fingers*, by Matt Christopher. Boston: Little, Brown, and Company, 1975. Reading level: ages 5–9 years. In this sports story, Billy Joe is afraid of rejection, so he decides not to play football until he stops stuttering. Reluctantly, he joins the team late in the season and becomes the star. His teammates are impressed with his athletic prowess and accept his stuttering.

- *Seal Secret*, by Aidan Chambers. New York: Harper and Row, 1980. Reading level: ages 9–12 years. This is a wonderfully written adventure story in which stuttering is only a minor theme. Two very different boys are forced to become playmates at their vacation seaside home. One plans to keep a baby seal trapped in a cave to raise for meat and skins. The other boy is outraged and plans to rescue the seal. He is successful but injures himself and nearly loses his life in the process.

- *The Skating Rink*, by Mildred Lee. New York: Seabury Press, 1969. Reading level: ages 13–18 years. Tuck is looking forward to his 16th birthday when he can drop out of school. He walks 2 miles to school every day to avoid his classmates' ridicule about his stuttering. Then, he meets a husband and wife skating team who are building a rink. Tuck befriends them both only to discover his own hidden skating talents. The story is rich in details of stuttering experiences and explores many theories and superstitions about stuttering.

Source: Bushey & Martin, 1988.

TEACHER TIPS FOR CLASSROOM MANAGEMENT

A classroom teacher has an opportunity to participate in the prevention and treatment of stuttering by properly structuring class activities. A teacher can structure the classroom environment to *facilitate* fluency or to *inhibit* it. Naturally, a good teacher will want to provide experiences that encourage fluency, but what is said, what is done, and how things are done make a difference. The disfluent student needs flexibility, not sympathy from the teacher. Good judgment is important. The following guidelines may help in the development of flexible classroom management skills (Pindzola, 1988).

- The student must not develop the attitude that normal responsibilities can be avoided because of stuttering. Classroom duties and responsibilities should be assigned as they are for other children. Perhaps modification or substitution of some activities is appropriate from time to time.
- Call on the person who stutters to answer questions in class but take care in phrasing the questions so that the answers may be very short. (Short sentences elicit less stuttering than do long ones.) Call on the student who stutters only when you are confident he or she knows the answer. Avoid calling on the student on days when his or her speaking is unusually difficult.
- Oral recitation and reading aloud activities need not be abandoned just because a student who stutters is in the class. Excluding a person who stutters denies the chance for improvement and forces the acceptance of this defect. A chance to participate verbally helps establish self-confidence. Consider different methods of doing recitative and reading activities. Choral reading is especially good; rather than individual performances, have the students read or recite simultaneously with a partner.
- Reading aloud in a slow, easy manner with light articulation is a good method; this is an ideal time to practice fluency strategies learned in therapy. For severe cases, the student may practice reading for the teacher before reading to the class. It is characteristic of stuttering to adapt or become more fluent with successive readings of the same passage.
- It is best to call on students randomly. Activities such as alphabetical roll call or answering questions down rows of desks can create anticipatory anxiety. Anxiety interferes with the ability to coordinate speech muscles; stuttering often results. Make no great issue of speech and be patient. Give the student *time to speak* without pressure. Eye contact is important; show by your expression that you are interested in *what* the student has to say, not *how* it is said.
- Be a good listener; listen in a calm, relaxed manner. Allow the student to complete the sentence without being interrupted and without having the words supplied.
- Insist on conversational manners in the classroom. A person speaking should not be interrupted. No one should monopolize a conversation. Let the student who stutters have a chance to talk.
- Create an atmosphere of ease and relaxation in the classroom. Avoid an atmosphere of tension and pressure.

- Conduct the school day in a routine manner. Stick with a schedule so that the student does not need to be hurried. Surprise and unexpected events seem to trigger more stuttering.
- Insist on discipline. Teachers and parents of children who stutter need to know that structure reduces anxiety. When children are not sure what is expected of them and/or what will happen next, uncertainty breeds anxiety and worry. Anxiety is an exacerbating component in children's stuttering problems (Zebrowski & Schum, 1993). In this context, then, both parents and teachers should be encouraged that positive discipline (i.e., setting firm and realistic limits in a positive manner) can reduce anxiety.
- Avoid competition among the students. Do not favor one student over the others. In particular, do not overprotect, pamper, or be extremely anxious about the student who stutters.
- Do not allow ridicule or sarcasm from class members. Discipline the guilty participant as you would under other circumstances. Educate the class to be tolerant of the differences among people. Just as some students have trouble with math or reading, others have trouble with talking.
- Think of the child who stutters as a normal student who presently has difficulty talking. The student is not learning disabled, retarded, or emotionally disturbed. Do not let the stuttering bias your educational expectations.
- If the student mentions frustration about the inability to talk fluently, reassurance that everyone finds it difficult to talk at times may help. Remind the student that the new way of talking (as learned in management sessions) would be appropriate and helpful in getting over the difficult moments.
- Talk openly about stuttering. It can be most helpful if parents and teachers engage children in objective, nonjudgmental discussions of stuttering. Indeed, when a child is experiencing a lengthy or struggled block, much support can be intimated by saying, "I can tell you're having a hard time," or by physical contact (touching the arm, shoulder, or back without verbalizing) (Zebrowski & Schum, 1993).
- Be frank with the student. If the student is called a stutterer or is teased and becomes embarrassed by the speech difference, it is wise to state that you recognize the hesitations and repetitions, but if he or she uses the new techniques learned in speech treatment it will be easier to talk.
- In the classroom, model *delayed responding* by taking a second before answering. The student who stutters should adopt this habit of taking some thinking time before responding and your assistance and understanding can be crucial.
- In the classroom, provide a model of smooth, unhurried talking. Speaking in a softer voice is also a good model for all students to emulate.

Table 8–5 provides additional information on booklets, videos, and Web sites that may be of interest to both students who stutter and their teachers.

TABLE 8–5 Selected Booklets, Videos, and Web Sites on Stuttering Useful for Classroom Teachers and Their Students Who Stutter

- A homepage on stuttering is maintained by a faculty member at Minnesota State University–Mankato at www.mnsu.edu/comdis/kuster. This excellent site also includes special pages, "Just for Kids" and "Just for Teens," as well as covering frequently asked questions and special topics, such as how to handle teasing or tips on making a presentation. A "kid-to-kid" chat room also exists at this Web site as does information on cluttering.

- The American Speech-Language-Hearing Association maintains basic information on fluency disorders, risk factors, and communication tips for the general public at www.asha.org/public/speech/disorders/stuttering.

- The National Stuttering Association is a self-help and support organization for people who stutter. The Web site www.nsastutter.org also provides information on local support groups, adult workshops, youth days, and the like.

- *Stuttering: Straight Talk for Teachers* is a video and booklet set designed for every classroom teacher with a child who stutters; also useful for SLPs working with teachers individually or leading inservices. Covers teachers' frequently asked questions and has classroom suggestions. Available for $5 from The Stuttering Foundation at www.stutteringhelp.org.

- *Notes to the Teacher: The Child Who Stutters at School* is a brochure with useful tips for teachers and parents, and is also available in Spanish. Available for 10 cents from The Stuttering Foundation at www.stutteringhelp.org.

- *Stuttering: For Kids by Kids* is a videotape (or DVD) that uses cartoon characters and real kids to talk about what stuttering is, what to do when teased about stuttering, what bugs a child who stutters, and what helps. Available for $10 from The Stuttering Foundation at www.stutteringhelp.org.

- *Sometimes I Just Stutter* is written for children who stutter. This 40-page booklet with activity pages provides helpful information on stuttering, why stuttering fluctuates, why teasing occurs, and what teachers and family members should know about stuttering. Available in English and in Spanish for $2 from The Stuttering Foundation at www.stutteringhelp.org.

- *The School-Age Child Who Stutters: Working Effectively with Attitudes and Emotions* is a 192-page workbook for speech-language pathologists. It works with feelings and beliefs of school-age children and includes reproducible handouts and tasks to gather information from children, parents, and teachers. Available for $15 from The Stuttering Foundation at www.stutteringhelp.org.

ADULT ASSESSMENT AND TREATMENT ISSUES

At the beginning of this chapter, we introduced fluency disorders and stuttering and the notion that its prevalence (less than 1 percent) is less than its incidence (about 4–5 percent). People can recover from stuttering spontaneously, through development, or with intervention. Yet other people have mild to severe persistent fluency issues in adulthood. In addition, there are cases of acquired stuttering, though less rare and usually associated with brain injury such as stroke. Adults with untreated developmental stuttering or adults with persisting stuttering may seek the services of a speech-language pathologist. Adults who stutter may seek intervention at different periods of their life and self-refer to a private community clinic or medical outreach facility. Hospital healthcare workers are more likely to encounter adults with acquired fluency disorders. Either way, the speech-language pathologist applies similar assessment and treatment principles.

The SLP begins an adult assessment by collecting a case history, with particular interest in date of stuttering onset, history of any treatment, and motivation for currently seeking help. The SLP assesses overt features of the disfluency, in particular frequency, duration of the moment of disfluency, and presence of any concomitant behaviors (e.g., facial contortions). A commonly used tool for assessing severity of stuttering in adults is the *Stuttering Severity Instrument* (Riley, 2009). The SLP also assesses covert features of stuttering that include tricks to hide or conceal the stuttering, such as avoidance behaviors. The degree of psychological and social consequences of stuttering in adults certainly can affect the person's quality of life. This topic is explored further in Chapter 14.

In treating adults who stutter, the speech-language pathologist has an array of options. In "stutter more fluently" approaches, the adult is taught ways to modify the moment of disfluency such as regaining control of articulation and smoothly pulling out of the block so that speech can continue forward. There are a myriad of strategies within this type of intervention. Another set of approaches has been termed "speak more fluently" treatment. In this collection, fluency-enhancing strategies such as soft, smooth, slow, or even syllable-timed speech and prolonged speech are used with the result of slightly altered rate and naturalness but with nonstuttered speech. Still other therapies focus more on the covert side of stuttering and work to improve the person's fears, avoidances, and other emotional aspects of stuttering. In principle, the goal here is to help the person who stutters be well adjusted in daily activities. Finally, aids can assist a person who has not shown improved fluency through traditional therapies. Voice-activated auditory feedback placed directly into the speaker's ear has been shown to help persons with persistent stuttering. The SpeechEasy is an example of such a device (Janus Development Group, 2009).

OTHER FLUENCY DISORDERS

A rare acquired fluency disorder is that of neurotic or hysterical stuttering, called Tracks III and IV by Van Riper (1982). **Neurotic stuttering** is characterized by a sudden onset of rather severe stuttering. The onset may occur at any age, including adulthood, yet usually happens in an older child. Some psychological trauma, emotional upheaval, or stress seems to precipitate the occurrence of stuttering (Deal, 1982; Van Riper, 1982; Mahr & Leith, 1992). The psychogenic stuttering pattern is severe from the beginning, with unvoiced prolongations, laryngeal blocks, tension, and/or lengthy repetitions typical. Although highly aware of these sudden and severe disfluencies, the person may or may not be frustrated by them. The level of concern and motivation to change are important elements for the speech-language pathologist to assess in determining a therapeutic outcome.

Stuttering also may be acquired following specific nervous system damage, such as from stroke, head trauma, infection, or tumor. Although similarities exist, there are enough characteristic differences to insist that such a fluency disorder is not true (developmental) stuttering. The term **neurogenic stuttering**, then, establishes this as an acquired fluency disorder that results from neurological damage. Neurogenic stuttering may occur in conjunction with bilateral or unilateral brain damage, with focal or diffuse lesions, or with cortical or subcortical damage to the central nervous system (Van Borsel, Van Lierde, Van Cauwenberge, Guldemont, & Van Orshoven, 1998).

There are numerous reports of neurogenic stuttering in patients with aphasia, apraxia, cerebral palsy, neurological diseases (e.g., Parkinsonism), dementias (including dialysis dementia), and substance abuse issues. Although nervous system damage can occur at any age (even prenatally), most instances of neurogenic stuttering occur in adults.

Cluttering is a fluency disorder, but not *just* a fluency disorder. Cluttering has varied symptomatology and occurs simultaneously with other speech, language, and behavioral disorders. According to Weiss (1964, 1968), cluttering symptoms may be categorized into obligatory, facultative, and associated types. The five obligatory symptoms of cluttering include part- and whole-word repetitions, lack of awareness of the disorder, short attention span, perceptual weakness, and poorly organized thinking. Among facultative symptoms are excessive speech rate (tachylalia), interjections, articulatory and motor disabilities, and grammatical difficulties. Some associated symptoms include reading and writing disorders, lack of rhythm and musical ability, and restlessness and hyperactivity.

Similarly, Daly views cluttering as a fluency disorder syndrome. The many facets of the condition are noted in his definition:

> Cluttering is a disorder of both speech and language processing that frequently results in rapid, dysrhythmic, sporadic, unorganized, and often unintelligible speech. Accelerated speech (tachylalia) is not always present, but impairments in formulating language almost always are. . . . Those who clutter confuse their listeners with incomplete and awkward sentences, false starts, sound sequencing errors, and word-retrieval problems. Their garbled speech is confounded by a lack of clarity of inner language formulation. Equally frustrating for clinicians are the absence of self-awareness and the unconcerned attitude of many clients who clutter. Their self-monitoring skills for speech and social situations are deficient. (Daly, 1993, p. 7)

In contrast, St. Louis and colleagues (St. Louis, 1992; St. Louis, Raphael, Myers, & Bakker, 2003; St. Louis, Myers, Faragasso, Townsend, & Gallaher, 2004) regard that rate problems are somehow central to cluttering, stating that persons who clutter talk too fast and fail to maintain normally expected sound, syllable, phrase, and pausing patterns. St. Louis and his colleagues do not include language difficulties in their definition of cluttering, noting that there are a few persons who clutter who do not evince language problems. Still, they cite other symptoms that are optional, if not frequent, in persons who clutter: lack of awareness of the problem; family history of fluency disorders; poor handwriting; confusing, disorganized language or conversational skills; temporary improvement when asked to slow down or pay attention to speech; misarticulations; poor intelligibility; social or vocational problems; distractibility; hyperactivity; auditory perceptual difficulties; learning disabilities; and apraxia.

With such a host of possible symptoms affecting all channels of communication and behavior in general, the teacher may have little difficulty in recognizing such an unusual child in the classroom, yet may not realize that speech-language problems are at the core. Referral to a speech-language pathologist is appropriate. As espoused by Preus (1996), cluttering is not only related to stuttering, but also to other disorders, notably psycholinguistic disorders, minimal brain dysfunction (MBD), language learning disorders (LLDs), attention deficit disorders (ADDs), and central auditory processing disorders (CAPDs). The relationship between cluttering and a series of learning and related disorders necessitates interdisciplinary cooperation. After differential diagnosis of cluttering and all its components along the lines suggested by St. Louis et al. (2003), the speech-language pathologist can devise a treatment plan. Therapeutic efforts may be directed toward rate of speech, heightened monitoring, clear articulation, language formulation and organization, speech naturalness, attention and concentration skills, and remedial reading. A team of special education professionals should be involved in the total intervention program, with the classroom teacher as the central figure.

VIGNETTE 8–2

The fourth-grade teacher referred Adam to the school SLP, concerned that he might be stuttering because of his repeating and unclear speech. In the assessment, Adam displayed a rapid rate of speech (as measured by overall syllables per minute but especially during articulatory rate when only fluent segments were measured). His speech sample was sprinkled with many syllable and word repetitions as well as numerous incomplete sentences. When answering specific questions it was necessary for the speech clinician to ask him to repeat many answers because it was difficult to understand what he had said. Intelligibility for spoken words and short phrases was excellent. No struggle behaviors were noted and Adam, upon questioning, was oblivious to any speech differences he might have. In follow-up with the classroom teacher, the SLP learned that Adam was a poor reader and that his handwriting was hard to read because it was both sloppy and contained many misspelled words. The school reading specialist was called in for assessment of possible dyslexia. At the IEP meeting, the father, who was a physics professor at the nearby university, was observed to speak rapidly. The father also noted that growing up he "had stuttered" but not as badly as an uncle who was plagued with it his whole life. The intervention decided upon was a team approach with classroom teacher, reading specialist, and speech-language pathologist working closely together. Among the initial strategies for speech were to increase Adam's awareness of his output and to train a slower, syllable-timed speech pattern.

Terms to Know

Fluent	Secondary stuttering
Disfluent	Differential diagnosis
Fluency disorders	Avoidance behaviors
Stuttering (developmental stuttering)	Postponement devices
Stuttering-like disfluencies (SLDs)	Starter devices
Other disfluencies (ODs)	Circumlocution
Prevalence	Substitutions
Incidence	Neurotic stuttering
Spontaneous recovery	Neurogenic stuttering
Severity	Cluttering
Primary stuttering	

Study Questions

1. How can you distinguish between a child who is beginning to stutter from a child who is normally disfluent? Cite some of the danger signs for which you might look.
2. Describe, as if talking to a parent, the typical developmental sequence of stuttering.
3. Describe and give examples of stuttering behaviors, including repetitions, prolongations, and struggle behaviors.
4. Communicative stress is known to disrupt fluency. Cite common classroom examples of the stresses listed in Table 8–3. Be able to discuss these fluency disruptors without relying on the table.
5. Discuss as many techniques as you can think of that a teacher should use when a child who stutters is in the class.
6. List as many examples as you can think of that a teacher should not do when a child who stutters is in the class.
7. What are some of the factors a speech-language pathologist might assess during an evaluation of a person suspected of stuttering? Include in your discussion factors pertinent to making a differential diagnosis and in determining severity.
8. What are avoidance behaviors? Identify as many behaviors as you can that might suggest a person who stutters is in your class even though you have never heard him or her repeat or prolong sounds.
9. Differentiate between developmental and acquired types of fluency disorders.

Bibliography

Ambrose, N., & Yairi, E. (1994). The development of awareness of stuttering in preschool children. *Journal of Fluency Disorders, 19*(4), 229–246.

Ambrose, N., & Yairi, E. (1999). Normal disfluency data for early childhood stuttering. *Journal of Speech, Language, and Hearing Research, 42,* 895–909.

Andrews, G., & Harris, M. (1964). *The syndrome of stuttering*. London, England: Heinemann Medteal Books.

Bloodstein, O. (1960). The development of stuttering: II. Developmental phases. *Journal of Speech and Hearing Disorders, 25*, 366–376.

Bloodstein, O. (1995). *A handbook on stuttering* (5th ed.). San Diego, CA: Singular.

Bushey, T., & Martin, R. (1988). Stuttering in children's literature. *Language, Speech, and Hearing Services in Schools, 19*(3), 235–250.

Conture, E. G. (2001). *Stuttering: Its nature, diagnosis, and treatment*. Needham Heights, MA: Allyn & Bacon.

Cox, N. J. (1988). Molecular genetics: The key to the puzzle of stuttering? *ASHA, 30*, 36–40.

Daly, D. A. (1981). Differentiation of stuttering subgroups with Van Riper's developmental tracks: A preliminary study. *Journal of NSSLHA, 9*(1), 89–101.

Daly, D. A. (1993). Cluttering: The orphan of speech-language pathology. *American Journal of Speech-Language Pathology, 4*(2), 6–8.

Deal, J. (1982). Sudden onset of stuttering: A case report. *Journal of Speech and Hearing Disorders, 47*, 301–304.

Encyclopaedia Britannica Almanac 2003. (2002). Chicago: Encyclopaedia Britannica.

Ezrati-Vinacour, R., Platzky, R., & Yairi, E. (2001). The young child's awareness of stuttering-like disfluencies. *Journal of Speech, Language, and Hearing Research, 44*(2), 368–380.

Gordon, P., & Luper, H. (1992). The early identification of beginning stuttering, I: Protocols. *American Journal of Speech-Language Pathology, 1*, 43–53.

Gregory, H. (1987). Coping with school. In J. Fraser & W. H. Perkins (Eds.), *Do you stutter?: A guide for teens*. Memphis, TN: Speech Foundation of America.

Gregory, H. (1990). Integration: Present status and prospects for the future. In J. Fraser (Ed.), *Stuttering therapy: Prevention and intervention with children*. Memphis, TN: Speech Foundation of America.

Haynes, W. O., & Pindzola, R. H. (2008). *Diagnosis and evaluation in speech pathology* (7th ed.). Boston, MA: Pearson Education.

Hull, F. M., Mielke, P. W., Willeford, J. A., & Timmons, R. J. (1976). *National Speech and Hearing Survey* (Final Report, Project 50978). Washington, DC: Health, Education, and Welfare, Office of Education, Bureau of Education for the Handicapped.

Janus Development Group. (2009). SpeechEasy Web site. Retrieved June 3, 2010, from http://www.SpeechEasy.com.

Lincoln, M., & Harrison, E. (1999). The Lidcombe program. In M. Onslow & A. Packman (Eds.), *The handbook of early stuttering intervention*. San Diego, CA: Singular.

Louko, L. J., Edwards, M. L., & Conture, E. G. (1990). Phonological characteristics of young stutterers and their normally fluent peers: Preliminary observations. *Journal of Fluency Disorders, 15*, 191–210.

Louko, L. J., Edwards, M. L., & Conture, E. G. (1999). Treating children who exhibit co-occurring stuttering and disordered phonology. In R. Curlee (Ed.), *Stuttering and related disorders of fluency* (2nd ed.). New York, NY: Thieme Medical.

Mahr, G., & Leith, W. (1992). Psychogenic stuttering of adult onset. *Journal of Speech and Hearing Research, 35*, 283–286.

Martin, R. R., & Lindamood, L. P. (1986). Stuttering and spontaneous recovery: Implications for the speech-language pathologist. *Language, Speech, and Hearing Services in Schools, 17*, 207–218.

Onslow, M., & Packman, A. (1999). *The handbook of early stuttering intervention*. San Diego, CA: Singular.

Perkins, W. H. (1971). *Speech pathology: An applied behavioral science*. Saint Louis, MO: Mosby.

Pindzola, R. H. (1988). *Stuttering intervention program: Age 3 to grade 3*. Austin, TX: Pro-Ed.

Pindzola, R. H. (1999). The stuttering intervention program. In M. Oslow & A. Packman (Eds.), *The handbook of early stuttering intervention*. San Diego, CA: Singular.

Pindzola, R. H., & White, D. T. (1986). A protocol for differentiating the incipient stutterer. *Language, Speech, and Hearing Services in Schools, 17*, 2–15.

Preus, A. (1996). Cluttering upgraded. *Journal of Fluency Disorders, 21*(3–4), 348–358.

Riley, G. D. (2009). *Stuttering severity instrument for children and adults* (3rd ed.). Austin, TX: Pro-Ed.

Ryan, B., & Ryan, B. (1999). The Monterey fluency program. In M. Oslow & A. Packman (Eds.), *The handbook of early stuttering intervention*. San Diego, CA: Singular.

Ryan, B. P. (1974). *Programmed therapy for stuttering in children and adults*. Springfield, IL: Charles C. Thomas.

St. Louis, K. O. (1992). On defining cluttering. In F. L. Myers & K. O. St. Louis (Eds.), *Cluttering: A clinical perspective* (pp. 37–53). San Diego, CA: Singular.

St. Louis, K. O., Myers, F. L., Faragasso, K., Townsend, P., & Gallaher, A. J. (2004). Perceptual aspects of cluttered speech. *Journal of Fluency Disorders, 29*(3), 213–235.

St. Louis, K. O., Raphael, L. J., Myers, F. L., & Bakker, K. (2003). Cluttering updated. *ASHA Leader, 8*(21), 4–5, 20–22.

Starkweather, C. W. (1981). Speech fluency and its development in normal children. In N. Lass (Ed.), *Speech and language: Advances in basic research and practice* (Vol. 4). New York, NY: Academy Press.

Van Borsel, J., Van Lierde, K., Van Cauwenberge, P., Guldemont, I., & Van Orshoven, M. (1998). Severe acquired stuttering following injury of the left supplementary motor region: A case report. *Journal of Fluency Disorders, 23*(1), 49–58.

Van Riper, C. (1982). *The nature of stuttering* (3rd ed.). Englewood Cliffs, NJ: Prentice Hall.

Weiss, A., & Zebrowski, P. (1992). Disfluencies in the conversations of young children who stutter: Some answers about questions. *Journal of Speech and Hearing Research, 35*, 1230–1238.

Weiss, A. L. (2004a). What child language research may contribute to the understanding and treatment of stuttering. *Language, Speech, and Hearing Services in Schools, 35*(1), 30–33.

Weiss, A. L. (2004b). Why we should consider pragmatics when planning treatment for children who stutter. *Language, Speech, and Hearing Services in Schools, 35*(1), 34–45.

Weiss, D. A. (1964). *Cluttering.* Englewood Cliffs, NJ: Prentice Hall.

Weiss, D. A. (1968). Cluttering: Central language imbalance. *Pediatric Clinics of North America, 15,* 705–720.

Wingate, M. E. (1966). A standard definition of stuttering. *Journal of Speech and Hearing Disorders, 29,* 484–489.

Yairi, E., & Ambrose, N. (1992). A longitudinal study of stuttering in children: A preliminary report. *Journal of Speech and Hearing Research, 35,* 755–760.

Yairi, E., Ambrose, N., & Niermann, B. (1993). The early months of stuttering: A developmental study. *Journal of Speech and Hearing Research, 36,* 521–528.

Yairi, E., & Lewis, B. (1984). Disfluencies at the onset of stuttering. *Journal of Speech and Hearing Research, 27,* 154–159.

Yaruss, J. S. (1998). Describing the consequences of disorders: Stuttering and the International Classification of Impairment, Disabilities, and Handicaps. *Journal of Speech, Language, and Hearing Research, 41*(2), 249–257.

Yaruss, J. S., & Quesal, R. W. (2004). Stuttering and the International Classification of Functioning, Disability, and Health (ICF): An update. *Journal of Communication Disorders, 37,* 35–52.

Young, M. A. (1975). Onset, prevalence, and recovery from stuttering. *Journal of Speech and Hearing Disorders, 40*(1), 49–58.

Zebrowski, P. M., & Schum, R. L. (1993). Counseling parents of children who stutter. *American Journal of Speech-Language Pathology, 2*(2), 65–73.

Chapter 9

VOICE DISORDERS AND ALTERED METHODS OF BREATHING

The voice carries a great deal of information about an individual. It is common to be able to identify a friend calling on the telephone when all the friend says is "Hi, how are you doing?" You know in an instant that the caller is Sarah, not Melissa, Kathy, or any of your other friends. It is also common to be able to identify from a voice sample a stranger's sex and approximate age without being able to see who is talking. The voice mirrors people's emotions; you can tell from the tone of a friend's voice if anger, nervousness, or excitement is present. The voice also reflects a person's physical health, as in the statement, "You sound like you're coming down with a cold." Yes, the voice carries a great deal of information and has the responsibility of projecting an individual to the world.

A voice that is perceived as abnormal—too effeminate, too hoarse, too sing-songy, too soft, or too much of anything—may affect an individual's social acceptance, educational expectations, eventual type of employment, or cause that person's personality to be inaccurately labeled (Morton & Watson, 2001; Jotz, Cervantes, Abrahao, Settanni, & Carrar de Angelis, 2002).

This chapter reviews the anatomy and physiology of the larynx as was described more fully in Chapter 2, with an emphasis on normal versus abnormal vocal parameters. Vocal pathologies typically seen in the school-aged population as well as adults are discussed, and the roles of the classroom teacher, allied health professionals, and speech-language pathologists (SLPs) in the management of voice disorders are then delineated. Later, this chapter describes people who, for some medical reason, do not breathe through their larynx and who produce voice in an unusual way. Among other concerns, the environment of the classroom and that of the residential environment area necessitates monitoring for these special students. Similarly, this chapter also discusses adult voice disorders encountered in medical settings, including laryngeal cancer.

It may be wise to state at the outset that voice disorders are typically divided into two types. **Phonatory disorders** are true disorders of the voice because they stem from problems in the laryngeal mechanism. For example, the vocal folds may be inflamed, there may be a growth on or near the folds, or the folds may be paralyzed and unable to move. Voice disorders of this type are the emphasis of this chapter. A second category is **disorders of resonance**. Structural or functional deviations in the vocal tract may affect the tone or resonance of the voice as it passes through the tract. The person may be judged as having a voice disorder because the quality of the voice sounds unusual. Examples include nasal obstruction causing hyponasality (which sounds like speaking with a head cold), velopharyngeal incompetence leading to hypernasality (which may be caused by neuromuscular disorders, clefts of the palate, or tissue deficiencies), or the unusual haunting quality of cul-de-sac resonance, as often heard in the speech of persons with a severe hearing impairment. Disorders of resonance are discussed only briefly in this chapter because they are mentioned again in Chapters 10 and 11. The present chapter concludes with an overview of persons with altered methods of breathing, which surely affects vocalizing.

THE NATURE OF VOICE PRODUCTION AND VOICE DISORDERS

When a person wishes to talk, the respiratory musculature delivers exhaled lung air up through the bronchial passages and into the trachea. This air passes freely through the larynx when the vocal folds are opened, or **abducted**, merely to be compressed at some point in the upper vocal tract, perhaps by the tongue, teeth, and/or lips, into sound. What is articulated, then, is a voiceless speech sound (such as the sounds associated with the letters *p, t, s, f,* and so on). Conversely, the air released from the lungs may be momentarily blocked at the level of the larynx by vocal folds that are closed, or **adducted**. This blocked air accumulates and increases in pressure until it is strong enough to literally blow open the closed folds. The pressure beneath the vocal folds is termed **subglottic pressure**; not only does it blow the folds apart, but the rapid pressure changes and air velocities associated with this subglottic pressure explosion suck the folds together again. With continued air being supplied from the lungs, the folds are once again blown apart. This process of opening-closing-opening-closing continues at an incredibly rapid rate—more than 100 times per second in an average adult male and about 200 times per second in an average adult female. Each opening-closing cycle of the vocal folds is termed a cycle of **vibration**, and the number of cycles per second is the **fundamental frequency** of vocal fold vibration. This vibratory pattern causes rapid, regular fluctuations of air pressure in the vocal tract and hence a crude sound is phonated. Simply put, voice is produced at the larynx, yet this sound wave must travel up the vocal tract to be shaped and articulated into recognizable (voiced) speech sounds (such as b, d, z, v, and all vowels).

It should be obvious from the foregoing discussion of voice production that problems may arise at many different levels. Voice disorders may be related to problems with the respiratory system and the generation of insufficient subglottic air pressures to drive the laryngeal mechanism; there may be laryngeal muscle weakness or paralysis affecting abduction and adduction abilities; or there may be growths, swellings, or sores on the glottal edges of the vocal folds that interfere with the regular and smooth vibrations so typical of healthy folds. These and myriad other problems may cause voice disorders.

To summarize, then, the normal voice is supported by a healthy respiratory system, strong and coordinated laryngeal muscles, and even and smooth glottal edges that can vibrate regularly with changes in air pressures. Normal laryngeal conditions lead to normal parameters of the voice, meaning those attributes that compose listeners' overall impression of a voice.

Voice disorders are prevalent in about 6 percent of the school-aged population (as reviewed by Wilson, 1987); this suggests an average of 2 students per class of 33 pupils has a voice disorder. However, it should be pointed out that the frequency of vocal deviations fluctuates as a function of age—higher in young children, and lower after adolescence. Of children with voice disorders, some 45–80 percent of cases are the result of vocal abuse, a type of **phonotrauma** (Herrington-Hall, Lee, Stemple, Niemi, & McHone, 1988). The vocal activities of children, especially boys, include frequent loud talking, yelling, and strained phonation.

Students in middle school through high school, although they may have a lower prevalence of voice disorders, nevertheless are at risk for developing problems. Students in these grades are likely to engage in extracurricular activities, such as cheerleading and competitive sports, in which vocal abuse frequently and insidiously becomes part of the activity. Adults have some of the same vocal issues as do students but also a host of other medically based vocal problems.

CAUSATIONS OF COMMON VOCAL DISORDERS

Table 9–1 lists common etiologies or conditions that bring about voice problems, as typically seen in schools. The table also lists the most frequently occurring laryngeal conditions seen by **laryngologists**, or throat doctors, in a pediatric population ranging in age from 3 days to 18 years (Dobres, Lee, Stemple, Kummer, & Kretschmer, 1989). The implication is that, by the school years, some of the more serious medically related voice problems have been treated. Phonatory disorders, those caused by laryngeal mass or movement problems, are much more commonly encountered than are resonance problems of the vocal tract. Of this list, the conditions called nodules and edema are the most frequent causes of a voice disorder in the school years. The principal feature of both is hoarseness. Some of the conditions listed in the table are discussed separately.

TABLE 9–1   Common Voice Disorders in Children and Youth

Phonatory Disorders Commonly Seen in Schools

1. *Nodules:* Calloused growths on the vocal folds; see text.
2. *Edema:* Swelling of the vocal folds; see text.
3. *Papilloma:* Clusters of wartlike growths; see text.
4. *Paralysis:* One or both vocal folds are unable to move; if unable to open, the ability to breathe may be impaired; if unable to close, voice may be weak and breathy. Paralysis may be caused by trauma (such as nerve damage in an automobile crash) or by a virus (with a good chance for spontaneous recovery).
5. *Polyps:* Fluid-filled growths on or around the vocal folds; often likened to "blisters" on the folds; usually caused by vocal abuse/misuse and linked to smoking as well. Vocal symptoms are similar to nodules, particularly hoarseness and low pitch.
6. *Idiopathic:* No visible pathology is present, yet the voice is judged to be abnormal sounding.

Pediatric Laryngeal Pathologies Commonly Seen by Laryngologists (and Frequency of Occurrence)

1. *Subglottic stenosis* (31.2 percent): A narrowing of the trachea; usually detected in infancy.
2. *Nodules* (17.5 percent): See above.
3. *Laryngomalacia* (11.9 percent): Usually seen in the newborn and often outgrown by age 2 years; a flabbiness of some laryngeal structures causing them to be indrawn during inhalation. Stridor (noisy inhalation) and dyspnea (shortness of breath) usually result.
4. *Idiopathic* (7.7 percent): See above.
5. *Paralysis* (6.2 percent): See above.
6. *Papilloma* (3.8 percent): See above.

Resonance Imbalances Commonly Seen in Schools

1. *Congenital palatal incompetence:* Inability to close off the oral and nasal cavities; may be caused by a variety of velar or pharyngeal problems.
2. *Structural deviations:* Including palatal clefts, submucous clefts, nasal polyps, deviated septa, and such.
3. *Neuromuscular disorders:* Including velar paralysis, dysarthrias, cerebral palsies, and such.
4. *Functional:* No structural cause of the resonance imbalance exists.

And, although hundreds of Web pages that deal with voice disorders exist, **Table 9–2** lists a few that might be of interest, especially those showing photographs of laryngeal conditions. Adults have some of the same types of disorders as do children (notably nodules and edema) as well as a host of other issues.

NODULES

Hoarseness is often caused by the presence of **vocal nodules**. Nodules (or nodes) are calloused growths of tissue on the edge of one or both vocal folds. Whether unilateral or bilateral, nodules appear in the characteristic location shown in **Figure 9–1**, which is the place of greatest impact when the vocal folds adduct. Obviously, if adduction is done in a strained, forceful manner, the tissue here becomes irritated and, over time, thickened. The young, still-forming nodule may be relatively small, soft, and compressible during vocal fold adduction, but with continued irritation, the nodule

TABLE 9–2   Select Web Sites for Information on Voice Disorders

- www.entusa.com/larynx_videos.htm. This is an excellent site for seeing and hearing voice disorders. It is provided by an otolaryngologist, Kevin Kavanagh, MD. Color pictures of healthy and diseased vocal folds—including nodules, polyps, laryngitis, cancers, and paralyses—are shown along with audio samples of disordered voices and video clips.
- www.bcm.edu/oto/othersa5.html. This is the Baylor College of Medicine's guide to otolaryngology resources on the Internet. A large number of links exist for accessing information on laryngeal anatomy, vocal diseases, and a sundry of medical treatments.
- www.asha.org/public/speech/disorders/voice.htm. The American Speech-Language-Hearing Association provides this site for the public. General information on the voice and its disorders is presented along with how to find treatment.
- www.voiceproblem.org/disorders/index.asp. The voice problem Web site provides useful information on the various disorders of voice and is most helpful once a medical diagnosis underlying the vocal disturbance is known.

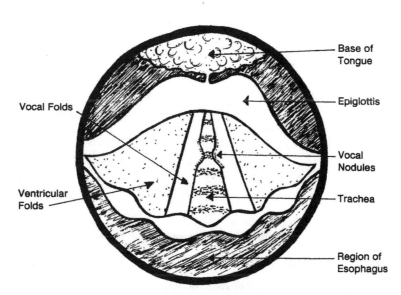

FIGURE 9–1   Schematic drawing of the larynx showing typical location of vocal nodules.

tends to enlarge, harden, and become less compressible. The size and callousness of the nodules may, therefore, interfere with complete closure, leaving instead gaps (or chinks) where air can escape during adduction. The result is a breathy quality to the voice and loss of overall vocal loudness. The nodular growth itself weighs down the small vocal fold and causes the rate of vibration to slow. Consequently, the person's voice sounds lower pitched than it did when it was healthy. The mass also may interfere with the smoothness of these vocal fold vibrations, further adding a rough or harsh quality to the voice. In an attempt to produce a stronger, clearer voice with less breathiness and loss of loudness, the person may use extra tension or effort to close the vocal folds. This, however, begins a vicious cycle in that such strain merely increases the force of impact during adduction and aggravates the irritated nodule even more. **Figure 9–2** schematizes these auditory symptoms of nodules.

As mentioned, nodules may be caused by chronic irritation and the force of impact when the vocal folds are slammed together. What causes some people to drive their laryngeal

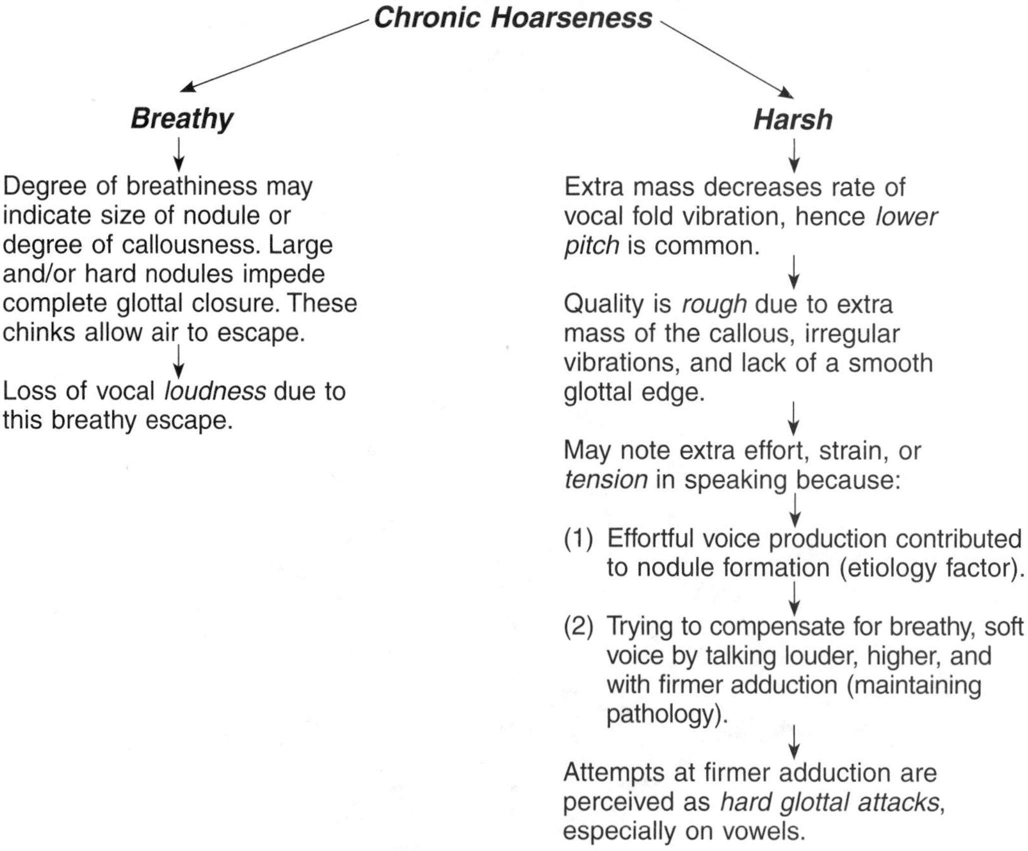

Chronic Hoarseness

Breathy

Degree of breathiness may indicate size of nodule or degree of callousness. Large and/or hard nodules impede complete glottal closure. These chinks allow air to escape.

Loss of vocal *loudness* due to this breathy escape.

Harsh

Extra mass decreases rate of vocal fold vibration, hence *lower pitch* is common.

Quality is *rough* due to extra mass of the callous, irregular vibrations, and lack of a smooth glottal edge.

May note extra effort, strain, or *tension* in speaking because:

(1) Effortful voice production contributed to nodule formation (etiology factor).

(2) Trying to compensate for breathy, soft voice by talking louder, higher, and with firmer adduction (maintaining pathology).

Attempts at firmer adduction are perceived as *hard glottal attacks*, especially on vowels.

FIGURE 9–2   The auditory symptoms of vocal nodules.

mechanism so forcefully? The answer is not exactly clear; frequent situational misuses, even abuses, though not intentional, can cause phonotrauma. In such cases, the implication for treatment is straightforward: identify the types of trauma and any triggering situations and help the person modify or eliminate them. The nodule would, it is hoped, heal and disappear. Although the process really may not be this simple and surgery may prove necessary, the identification of behaviors leading to phonotrauma is a necessary assessment step by the speech-language pathologist and laryngologist. Some common situations leading to phonotrauma are outlined in **Table 9–3**.

Middle- and high school cheerleaders are vulnerable to frequent bouts of vocal stress, laryngitis, and the eventual development of nodules. Also children, particularly physically active boys with outgoing, aggressive, distractible, boisterous, talkative personalities, are predisposed to having nodules.

Nodules and the pattern of vocal trauma that contributes to their formation tend to occur in certain types of people, regardless of age. Teachers, singers, and preachers are engaged in strenuous vocal activity as a function of their occupation. **Table 9–4** provides a word of warning for classroom teachers.

Referral to the school speech-language pathologist is in order when a teacher notices a student with chronic vocal hoarseness. Consultation with a laryngologist may lead to one of three routes of intervention: medical, indirect behavioral (vocal hygiene), or direct behavioral **voice treatment**.

TABLE 9–3 Common Vocal Misuses and Abuses in Students

I. Nonverbal (nonspeech) abuses:
  1. Excessive crying
  2. Frequent throat clearing
  3. Frequent coughing
  4. Smoking (including tobacco and marijuana)
  5. Making strange noises (as in machine gun, growling, siren noises during play, or grunting during football or karate practice)

II. Verbal abuses:
  1. Excessive yelling, screaming, cheering
  2. Talking over noise (TV, radio/stereo, groups of friends, machine environments)
  3. Singing (especially out of natural range or in a forced manner)
  4. Excessive talking (especially if in a strained manner)

III. Misuses:
  1. Speaking at an inappropriate pitch level
  2. Using hard glottal attacks
  3. Speaking with tension
  4. Using excessively loud voice

TABLE 9–4   Information Classroom Teachers Should Heed About Their Own Voice

- Vocal nodules tend to occur in certain occupations, including the teaching profession.
- More than 11 percent of teachers, as compared to 6 percent of nonteachers, experience multiple voice symptoms.
- Vocal problems of teachers, especially elementary school teachers, include the following:
  - Hoarseness
  - Voice/throat discomfort
  - Increased vocal effort
  - Tiring of the voice
  - Voice quality change after short use
  - Difficulty projecting the voice
  - Trouble speaking or singing softly
  - Loss of the singing range
- Teachers report that because of their vocal dysfunction, they tend to reduce classroom activities and interactions with students, which affects the learning environment.
- Teachers feel they would benefit from an SLP's voice hygiene inservice directed at their personal vocal care as well as vocal strategies for handling classroom situations.

Source: Yiu, 2002; Roy et al., 2004.

Based on the student's age and the maturity of the nodule, surgical removal may be recommended. Nodules often are removed by microsurgical stripping techniques or by laser surgery. Medical clearance for behavioral intervention also may be granted. In fact, Moran and Pentz (1987) found that 59 percent of laryngologists polled recommend behavioral intervention as the treatment of choice in children. Only 10 percent of these doctors opted for surgery as the treatment of choice. Once given medical clearance, the speech-language pathologist has the choice of providing voice treatment or a **vocal hygiene approach**, as discussed later in the chapter.

EDEMA

Vocal **edema** refers to an inflamed swelling of the tissues on and around the vocal folds. To be sure, phonotrauma may lead to edema in the formative stages before the nodule appears. Edematous swelling also is commonly associated with respiratory tract infection (e.g., colds, flu) and allergies. Postnasal drip and sinus drainage, whether infected with bacteria or not, can irritate the mucous membrane linings of the larynx and cause fluid retention and edema. This fluid-like puffiness makes the vocal folds heavier. Consequently, they vibrate more slowly and perhaps unevenly. The auditory symptoms of hoarseness and lowering of the pitch are the result.

The teacher and speech-language pathologist need to gather information to help determine whether a student has vocal hoarseness because of edema associated with respiratory infection or allergy or because of some other more serious reason (such as nodules, tumors, cancers, and the like). Student and parent interviews can yield information regarding the student's health, whether the student claims to be experiencing a cold or allergy attack, whether the vocal hoarseness is worse in the mornings (indicating drainage while lying in bed is contributory), and whether the hoarseness is temporary. A student with hoarseness should be watched; colds and upper respiratory infections usually subside within 10 to 14 days. If the hoarseness persists longer than this period of time, a referral to the SLP, then physician, is in order.

Most schools have in place regulations that stipulate that the student must be seen by a laryngologist for differential diagnosis. Certainly, if the hoarseness is not caused by edema but by a more serious, even life-threatening laryngeal condition, this should be discovered as soon as possible. If the hoarseness is attributable to edema, the student may benefit from decongestant or antihistamine medicines to relieve drainage. Care of the voice is important during these times of inflammation and vocal fold edema. The teacher or speech-language pathologist can teach care of the voice through vocal hygiene lessons, as discussed later in this chapter. Voice treatment by the SLP is generally not indicated for such cases.

PAPILLOMA

A serious laryngeal condition is that of **papilloma**, or, more accurately, juvenile laryngeal papillomatosis. Papilloma usually affects children, makes frequent recurrences throughout childhood, and gradually tapers off, becoming rare after puberty. Classroom teachers and special education personnel need to be cognizant of papilloma because of its life-threatening conditions.

Papilloma appears as clusters of wartlike growths and is thought to be viral related. These warty tumors often spread rapidly and interfere with the airway. Getting adequate air is more important than the hoarseness and breathiness that may co-occur with phonation. Students who are hoarse for more than 10–14 days should be referred to the SLP, who will in turn refer them to the laryngologist. Students with hoarseness also should be watched for daily changes in their ease of breathing. Once papilloma is diagnosed, it becomes a medical or surgical problem, especially if any obstruction of the airway is present.

Voice treatment per se by the speech-language pathologist generally is not indicated because it will not resolve the papilloma; yet, vocal hygiene is important to impress on the student during the tumor flareups. Because papilloma tends to grow back quickly, repeated surgeries may be needed. Repeated surgeries scar the vocal mechanism and result in chronically abnormal vocal parameters, usually severe hoarseness, inadequate loudness, intermittent voice stoppages, and a lowered pitch. The SLP can offer voice treatment after surgery to help the student learn to use the scarred mechanism to its maximum potential.

SELECT ADULT VOICE DISORDERS

Much of the preceding information about phonotrauma and vocal fold changes of edema and nodules certainly applies to adults. But there also is a vast array of serious, potentially life-threatening vocal pathologies in adults. The following four categories simplify and cluster the myriad of disorder types common among adults:

1. **Functional voice disorders** are those that show structural changes to the vocal folds but in the absence of any underlying neurological, viral, or cancer types of issues. Functional voice disorders include vocal fold edema, nodules, polyps, cysts, contact ulcers, laryngeal stenosis, and the like. Many but not all functional disorders are the consequence of phonotrauma. Problems plaguing the professional voice user (e.g., singer, actor) also fall into this category.

2. **Psychogenic voice disorders** include some forms of aphonia, elective mutism, mutational falsetto or puberphonia, and transsexual/transgender voice issues.

3. **Neurogenic voice disorders**, as the name implies, are phonatory changes or limitations as a result of neurological damage or disease. One or both folds, for example, may not move or move only weakly, or may exhibit uncontrollable fluctuations in tone. Vocal problems in this category include vocal fold paralysis, paresis, and vocal fold tremors. The dysarthrias are covered in the motor speech section of Chapter 13, but suffice it to say that terms such as *flaccid* and *spastic* may be applied to voice disorders of the neurogenic kind.

4. **Neoplastic voice disorders** is the category of laryngeal pathology involving growths of new tissue; the new mass is termed a *neoplasm*. Whereas neoplasms can be benign growths, most neoplasms carry a heightened sense of concern. Papillomas, discussed previously, are benign neoplasms but with real dangers to breathing, tissue scarring, and voice production. Precancer growths on the vocal folds may morph into a future malignancy; leukoplakia is such an example (white tissue patches are linked to heavy smoking). Cancer anywhere in the larynx is life threatening, and cancer confined to one or both vocal folds is no different. Vocal hoarseness and pitch changes may be symptoms and warning signs of cancer.

VOICE ASSESSMENT AND VOCAL PARAMETERS

Issues in the diagnosis and evaluation of vocal disorders are provided elsewhere, including the overview text by Haynes and Pindzola (2004). Regardless of age, student or adult, an overall judgment of a person's voice is insufficient for an evaluation; each parameter of the voice is best judged separately. The *Voice Assessment Protocol* (Pindzola, 1987) is a useful tool for appraising vocal characteristics. The speech-language pathologist may use this or a similar instrument as a guide in the decision-making process regarding normal versus abnormal voice-related features. The *Voice Assessment Protocol* appraises five parameters of the voice: pitch, loudness, quality, breath features, and rate/rhythm. The first three are by far the most salient of the vocal characteristics. As a teacher or healthcare professional, your knowledge of these parameters can help in the classroom or medical clinic identification of persons with voice disorders and thus may expedite their receiving assessment and intervention services from the SLP.

PITCH

Pitch level during typical conversational speech is determined. This so-called **habitual pitch level** is the speaking fundamental frequency of vibration, and it is merely an overall average of the opening-closing cycles of the vocal folds. It is important for the SLP to determine by using normative data whether pitch level is appropriate for the student's or adult's age, sex, and body stature. Measurements can be of the type to determine voice musical equivalence (such as A3 on the scale for comparison to adult female norms) or more sophisticated instrumentation to determine fundamental frequency of vibration (with a yield such as 150 Hz to compare to norms for a 16-year-old boy).

The normal voice is characterized by variability in pitch known as intonation or inflection. The voice is abnormal when there is a lack of pitch variability, termed **monotone**, or when pitch fluctuations are excessive and sing-songy. Other pitch abnormalities that the SLP should listen for are diplophonia and pitch breaks. **Diplophonia** refers to the presence of two or more simultaneous pitches in the voice. These multiple tones are produced by separate or unequal vibratory sources and may indicate a serious problem with the vocal folds or simply be an innocuous and temporary globule of saliva. **Pitch breaks** are intermittent and sudden changes in the pitch of the voice. The voice may jump upward, even into a squeak, or it may break downward. Frequent pitch breaks are associated with neurological problems and with growths on or around the vocal folds (and therefore may be serious) but also may be associated with normal puberty changes. School teachers who interact with students at the age of puberty should be aware that rapid laryngeal growth during this developmental period, especially in males, causes random fluctuations of vocal fold muscle length and tension. Although upward and downward pitch breaks may be socially embarrassing to the student, they are of no consequence and generally subside within 6 months or so.

LOUDNESS

Of interest during the assessment is whether **loudness** is appropriate for the speaking situation. If a voice is judged too loud or too soft, the speech-language pathologist should investigate possible reasons. The SLP should note whether the student can maintain the typical loudness level comfortably, without tension or strain. Loudness also should be maintained throughout the utterance and not trail off toward the end of the sentence. Furthermore, there should be no breaks or momentary skips of loudness.

It is of great importance for the speech-language pathologist to determine whether loudness abuse occurs. The teacher's daily observations and knowledge of the student's activities may prove extremely helpful here. Adult clients can report their own vocal activities. Loudness excesses are often situation oriented rather than constant throughout the day, but employment in a noisy factory or living with an untreated older relative with hearing impairment who keeps the television on full blast may be notable daylong exceptions. Adults and students may use loud talking, strained phonation, or screaming only in certain situations, such as on the playground, in the cafeteria, during karate class, at sporting events, when singing, or during nightlife activities. A few abusive situations may be perpetuating a vocal disorder and, therefore, must become the focus of an intervention program, as discussed later in this chapter.

QUALITY

The descriptive terminology used with disorders of vocal **quality** reflects the perceptual nature of the judgments. Words like *breathy, harsh, hoarse, strident, rough, denasal, hypernasal,* and *husky* are used commonly. Hoarseness, in fact, is the most common symptom of many vocal disorders.

Because hoarseness is a common symptom of a voice disorder—and possibly of a serious underlying medical situation—it is important that healthcare professionals and classroom teachers be able to recognize a patient or student with a hoarse voice for assessment or monitoring. In its simplest form, hoarseness is a combination of breathiness and harshness. Further attention to a speaker's breath features is warranted.

BREATH FEATURES

Breathing variables affect voice production and, as a result, should be assessed by the speech-language pathologist. The SLP is interested in the adequacy of breath support, how many words (or syllables) are typically spoken per breath, how long the speaker can sustain a voiceless sound (such as s̲) and a voiced sound (such as z̲), and whether there are any distracting breathing noises, particularly during inhalation.

RATE/RHYTHM

The rate at which a person talks can affect other variables of speech and voice. In particular, rate may be related to poor breathing features and improper phrase grouping. The speech-language pathologist can best judge the impact of rate of speech; the healthcare professional or the teacher may lend an overall impression of a speaker's talking rate. The rhythm, smoothness, and coordination of speech reflect an individual's neurological integrity and, so, are assessed by the SLP as well.

INSTRUMENTATION

Instrumental measures of vocal function have become increasingly available in clinical healthcare settings. Less-equipped clinics and school settings can benefit from free online acoustic assessments such as Praat (www.fon.hum.uva.nl/praat). Computer instrumentation holds much promise for enhancing the diagnostic process, treatment planning, and documentation of clinical effect (Behrman & Orlikoff, 1997). A discussion of sophisticated instrumental measures of speech and vocal functions is beyond the scope of this book.

VOICE TREATMENT OPTIONS

Whereas physicians diagnose any medical condition related to the vocal mechanism, the functional vocal assessment performed by the SLP can be invaluable to the physician (laryngologist or ears, nose, and throat [ENT] doctor) in guiding treatment decisions. Depending on the situation, the physician may deem that surgery is necessary, that radiotherapy (radiation) is the best course of action, that medications can improve the situation, that no intervention is warranted, or that the SLP should provide behavioral treatment. Often a combination of these treatment options is pursued; for example, the SLP may work with a patient before and/or after surgery. The SLP also has the option of providing direct versus indirect intervention in some types of situations. This section discusses those options.

Within the educational system, and from the earlier discussion, it should be obvious that the identification of students with voice disorders depends, to a large measure, on the ability of classroom teachers to recognize aberrant voices and make referrals. Classroom teachers tend not to be able to identify voice disorders without training. Recognition of voice disorders improves dramatically when teachers are trained. DeGregorio and Polow (1985) present a model for inservice workshops and planned interactions between teachers and speech-language pathologists. Classroom teachers can be effective listeners and facilitators of good speech and voice practice when taught the importance of their contribution.

Throughout, this chapter alludes to two avenues of voice intervention: The speech-language pathologist may enroll the adult patient or school student in a voice hygiene approach, or in voice treatment. These two avenues differ in their underlying philosophy and goals.

VOCAL HYGIENE PROGRAMS

Voice hygiene programs are designed to be informational and are preventative; they can be offered to anyone and, as such, are the ultimate form of indirect intervention. Students with vocal disorders and even entire classrooms of students with normal voices can benefit from knowledge on the use and care of the human voice. Hygiene programs can be offered by the speech-language pathologist or by the classroom teacher, or the two professionals can work together in designing teaching units. Because no direct manipulation of vocal parameters is attempted, vocal hygiene programs do not require medical clearance, parent permission, or placement in the speech pathology program (hence no Individualized Education Program [IEP] is written).

Vocal hygiene programs share common goals. First, the individual student or the entire class is educated in voice production. This typically entails a description of the normal larynx and how it functions, followed by discussions of what can go wrong. Nodules often are the principal example. This educational unit may be highlighted with pictures, movies, laryngeal models, and taped samples of healthy versus disordered voices. The Web pages cited in Table 9–2 may prove useful. A second goal is to identify any traumas such as abusive voice behaviors that can contribute to a voice disorder. Discussions may proceed from general abuses that anyone might do, to particular abuses that an individual student does. Depending on the maturity level of the student, this goal may be accomplished by brainstorming lists of traumatic behaviors, cutting out magazine pictures of people engaged in such (e.g., screaming at a football game), coloring predrawn pictures symbolic of trauma (e.g., loud voice analogues to heavy walking boots and a soft voice like ballet slippers), and making scrapbooks or bulletin boards from these materials. A third goal of vocal hygiene programs, especially for students with disordered voices, is to help students reduce or eliminate their traumatic behaviors. This may entail suggesting alternative behaviors where such alternatives exist, as in **Table 9–5**. Otherwise, overall reduction or complete elimination of traumatic voice behaviors is necessary, particularly during situations with a high probability for occurrences. **Table 9–6** lists situations that may be troublesome for school-aged students.

The appendix to this chapter summarizes sample hygiene programs for young children such as from Terrell and Morgan (1980) and Scott (1998) for preschool children, Nilson and Schneiderman (1983) for second and third graders, and from Cook, Palaski, and Hanson (1979) for third- through sixth-grade children. These synopses may provide ideas for use in classroom hygiene programs. Such units can be incorporated easily into health or science curricula. Additionally, commercial vocal hygiene programs are available (Moran & Zylla-Jones, 1998; Flynn, Andrews, & Cabot, 2004).

With regard to adolescents, and by way of example, the vocal activities of cheerleading include prolonged and strenuous use of the voice in the presence of tension and with inadequate breath support. It should not be surprising that cheerleading predisposes one to vocal troubles. Aaron and Madison (1991) designed a vocal hygiene program for high school cheerleaders and for their advisors that explained voice production, identification of abusive vocal behaviors, and ways to self-monitor such abuses.

TABLE 9–5   List of Suggested Alternatives to Abusive Behaviors

Abuse	Alternative
Yelling to a friend	Walking closer to the person to talk
	Waving or whistling to get his or her attention
Cheering	Clapping hands
	Shaking a pom-pom at a sporting event
Singing	Mouthing the words to allow voice rest
Coughing	Blow coughing (strong but silent exhalation of air)
	Sipping some water
Clearing throat	Using "sniff and swallow" technique
	Swallowing
	Sipping some water
Yelling for pet	Whistling
	Clicking the tongue

TABLE 9–6   Situations of High Probability for Vocal Abuse

1. Before school (at home in the morning)
2. On the way to school (especially noisy school bus environment)
3. At recess
4. During lunch period
5. In physical education
6. In music class
7. On the way home from school
8. After school (playtime)
9. In the evening
10. During sports (football practice, cheerleading, pep rallies, competitive games or activities)

VOICE TREATMENT

Direct voice treatment is administered only to students and adults who demonstrate a voice disorder and who have a reasonable prognosis for improvement. The National Center for Voice and Speech (1994) indicates that SLPs commonly use about seven genres of voice treatment. Pannbacker (1998) provides an excellent compendium of these voice treatment approaches and a critical review of their effectiveness. The type of voice treatment undertaken depends on the diagnosis, client characteristics, and the speech-language pathologist's preference.

Voice treatment programs for disorders stemming from phonotrauma are strikingly similar to each other and, in the beginning, to vocal hygiene programs as well. Yet voice treatment goes further than vocal hygiene programs and seeks to actually alter vocal parameters. For this reason, voice treatment is always preceded by the SLP's comprehensive assessment, a laryngologist's consultation, and, in the schools, an IEP meeting in which the student's problem and the intervention plan are clearly explained to the parents and teachers. It is important that all of the teachers understand the need for specific recommendations (e.g., no singing for 3 months, return to laryngologist in 6 months, no loud talking or shouting, and the like). The involvement of teachers is therefore critical.

Not unlike vocal hygiene programs, voice treatment for disorders related to phonotrauma usually begins with the same three goals. Goals 4 and 5 are unique to treatment programs and are at the heart of intervention:

1. Education in voice production
2. Identification of behaviors that lead to phonotrauma
3. Reduction and/or elimination of these behaviors
4. Identification of techniques that improve parameters of the voice
5. Modification and habituation of the improved voice

Treatment seeks to achieve a clear vocal tone and may use facilitating techniques to alter the pitch and loudness level; manner of vocal fold adduction; state of muscular tension in the larynx, throat, and mouth areas; depth and manner of respiration; and numerous other subgoals. Suffice it to say that the speech-language pathologist has the responsibility of designing and executing the treatment program to facilitate the best possible voice. Teachers and allied health professionals who actively support voice treatment programs provide immeasurable support to the student trying to master new vocal habits.

SUGGESTIONS FOR TEACHERS

We agree with Kahane and Mayo, who state:

> A major component of the education process should be helping teachers recognize when to refer a dysphonic child to the speech-language pathologist. We need to educate teachers about what we do, the processes involved in remediation, and to encourage their participation in the treatment of the vocally abusive child. The classroom teacher serves as a model of good vocal usage and can facilitate therapy goals by monitoring and reinforcing appropriate targeted behaviors. His or her role in voice therapy should not be underestimated. (Kahane & Mayo, 1989, p. 105)

We hope that this book serves some of these noble purposes, incorporating some of the following suggestions.

1. Participate in teacher inservice programs offered by speech-language pathologists. Your ability to identify and refer students with pitch, loudness, and quality aberrations may depend greatly on your training to listen with a critical ear. Degregorio and Polow (1985) and Deal, McClain, and Sudderth (1976) offer valuable procedures for the design of such inservices.
2. Liberally refer suspected voice cases to the speech-language pathologist. Voice abnormalities may indicate a medically serious problem, or not. It is always best to check them.
3. Volunteer to teach a voice hygiene unit in your class or work closely with the speech-language pathologist's hygiene program. Remember that everyone can benefit from knowledge of the care and use of the human voice.
4. Attend the IEP meeting and discuss a student's voice disorder with the speech-language pathologist. The more you know, the better you will be able to help.
5. Assist the SLP in identifying daily abuses and misuses, and work with the SLP to develop elective methods of reducing abuse in the classroom.
6. Volunteer to assist in the treatment program. Make your classroom a situation of vocal practice and reinforce the work of the speech-language pathologist and the student.
7. Control the noise level in your classroom such that no one needs to speak loudly and forcefully. A quiet, controlled class is not only good for the student with a voice disorder,

but it is also preventative protection of the teacher's voice. A disciplined, quiet-speaking class also is conducive to student learning. To the extent possible, control excessive ambient noise from heaters and air conditioners. Also curtail everyone's talking when the loud grass mower is outside the window!

8. Model a soft speaking voice for your students. Not only is this excellent when a student with a voice disorder is in the class, it is good hygiene for everyone, including the teacher.

9. Avoid modeling whispered speech in the class. Whispered speech that is audible enough to be heard is taxing to the laryngeal mechanism.

10. Allow a student with a voice disorder to drink water in the classroom. Frequent hydration can ease vocal distress and promote healing.

11. Allow a student with a voice disorder to suck on throat lozenges in class, if this is soothing and deemed appropriate by the SLP.

12. Follow and support any SLP recommendations for a particular student. This may involve, for example, altering assignments to involve less speaking, allowing a few days of voice rest, curtailing singing, or other temporary strategies.

FURTHER COMMENTS REGARDING ADULTS IN MEDICAL SETTINGS

Most states have at least one large and well-equipped medical center containing a voice clinic with state-of-the-art equipment including laryngeal videostroboscopy (to view the condition of the vocal folds in motion), assorted computerized acoustic analyses, as well as aerodynamic and other physiological events. As stated earlier in the chapter, much information can be gained by the perceptual analysis of the clinician as the patient sustains a vowel, sings the scale, demonstrates loudness variation, and engages in conversational speech. Instrumental analysis of the voice adds a degree of precision and objectivity to the vocal assessment.

After medical referral and after the SLP has completed the assessment, the treatment of voice, whether done in the medical voice center, community clinic, or other work setting, is tailored to the needs of the patient. Treatment is designed by taking many variables into account: (1) What is the medical diagnosis and prognosis for vocal improvement? Treating vocal nodules in an otherwise healthy school teacher is vastly different from treating an adult with a paralyzed vocal fold secondary to heart disease and laryngeal nerve compression. A progressive disorder such as Parkinson's disease may benefit from short-term training of strategies for enhanced vocal loudness and intelligibility even though the course of the disease is inevitable. (2) What did the assessment reveal as targets for vocal change and, through probing, which techniques were shown to be effective starting points in treatment? By way of example, perhaps the SLP saw poor breath support and plans to begin therapy with respiratory goals. Or perhaps probing during the experimental phase of the diagnostic session revealed improved vocal quality by raising the patient's pitch level. Quality and vocal loudness may need to be adjusted by changing to a soft or hard glottal attack. **Table 9–7** lists commonly used nonstandardized probe and

TABLE 9–7   Some Facilitating Techniques Useful in Probing Improved Vocalization

Change of loudness

Chant talk

Digital manipulation: SLP presses on throat (larynx) in different ways to change voice attributes.

Focus: Redirect focus of resonance to forward, backward, higher, or lower in vocal tract.

Head position: Tilt left or right to improve vocal fold closure.

Inflection methods: Client says "urn hum" using a rising inflection.

Open mouth approach: Client speaks with open, exaggerated articulation.

Pitch range methods: Client intones *do-re-mi* or *ah-ah-ah* or *one-two-three* from lowest to highest. Listen for improved voice on certain note(s).

Pushing or pulling techniques: Client phonates *ah* while pushing down or pulling up on his or her chair.

Relaxation: Client uses techniques such as laryngeal massage and head rolls.

Resonance-swell method: As client hums up the scale, listen for where voice becomes louder or swells.

Vegetative techniques: At what pitch is client's laughter, cough, throat clearing, or grunt? Grunts after pushing or pulling may help elicit a natural tone.

Yawn–sigh: Client yawns with a relaxed, audible sigh.

facilitative techniques. (3) Did the SLP determine that contributing factors warrant thera-peutic attention? It is not unusual for the behavioral triad of smoking, drinking, and frequent loud talking in noisy environments to dictate that phonotrauma therapy is the best course of action. This can be true even in medical cases such as cancer. Treatment akin to the vocal hygiene programs presented earlier for students can be retooled for an adult patient. (4) Have the patient's needs been considered in designing treatment? The age, general health, employment status (vocal demands of the job versus retired), and degree of daily social interactions (use of the voice) are just a few of the many issues that shape the therapeutic process.

In addition to individualized, clinician-designed interventions, published voice treat-ment programs have been available over the years. The Lee Silverman Voice Therapy, known as LSVT, is an effective approach widely used with adults and even the pediatric population. In particular, exercises to improve vocal loudness, intelligibility, and respiratory support for speech have been investigated in neurologically based disorders such as Par-kinson's disease (Baumgartner, Sapir, & Ramig, 2001; Huber, Stathopoulos, Ramig, & Lancaster, 2003; Spielman, Ramig, Will, Halpern, & Petska, 2007).

Whichever approach to treatment the SLP uses, progress or lack of it should be tracked. Improvements may be documented through frequent reassessments.

VIGNETTE 9–1

Mrs. Sanchez was a 28-year-old third-grade teacher. She noticed voice fatigue and increased bouts of her "voice cutting out" over the last 5 months. She reports smoking 3 packs of cigarettes a week and she enjoys her single lifestyle of "going clubbing" in the local nightlife scene. Her voice evaluation revealed a hoarse voice that was lower in pitch than typical for her sex, age, and petite body stature. Her pitch range was restricted, with aphonia noted in the higher notes. Vocal loudness was strong but appeared to be pushed. Conversational speech became fast when excited and her breathing pattern appeared shallow and with shoulder elevation. Resonance was judged to be within normal limits. Fundamental frequency, jitter, shimmer, average intensity, airflow rates, and time of sustained phonation of a vowel were all measured in the voice lab for comparison to norms and for baseline measures should intervention be prescribed. The otolaryngologist diagnosed a right unilateral, soft vocal nodule and opted for the SLP to intervene with treatment rather than phonosurgery to remove the nodule.

Questions for thought based on Mrs. Sanchez's scenario: (1) Why do you think this plan of action was chosen? (2) What behavioral changes might be necessary in the vocal management of Mrs. Sanchez?

TIPS FOR ALLIED HEALTH PROFESSIONALS CONCERNING ADULT PATIENTS WITH VOICE DISORDERS

1. Be aware of any voice or speaking restrictions the patient may have. This is particularly true in the hours and days following phonosurgery.
2. Avoid excess stimulation, excitement, or laughter of patients who had phonosurgery.
3. Be aware that following surgery the patient may have temporary diet restrictions and difficulty swallowing.

BACKGROUND INFORMATION ON ALTERED METHODS OF BREATHING

Not-so-subtle vocal changes or a complete absence of voice may occur in students and adults who have undergone a rerouting of the airway. Following surgery for the management of certain medical conditions, students may be reintegrated into the schools or adults may return to work with altered methods of breathing. Teachers, coworkers, and friends might, at first, feel ill at ease at having a "neck breather" in their midst. Understanding of the condition is a necessary and important first step for structuring the optimal home, classroom, or work environment.

TRACHEOSTOMIZED PERSONS

For various medical reasons, some temporary and some permanent (including neuromuscular disease, head trauma, chronic obstructive pulmonary disease, upper airway obstruction, bilateral vocal fold paralysis, and sleep apnea), physicians may decide that to ensure reliable respiration, a person needs to have a **tracheostomy**. The tracheostomy is an opening made into the trachea just under the larynx. A tracheostomy tube, more simply called a **trach tube**, is inserted to maintain the opening. During inhalation and exhalation, air passes through the tracheostomy tube in the neck rather than through the usual route through the larynx, throat, mouth, and/or nose.

Although the tracheostomy may help solve respiratory problems, it causes the loss of speech. Recall that exhaled lung air must pass through the larynx and blow the vocal folds into vibration to produce voice. With exhaled air routed out the hole in the neck, called a **stoma**, no vocal fold vibration occurs. There can be a simple solution. Most tracheostomized people (using a specific type of trach tube) simply put their thumb over the stoma to divert air back through the larynx when they wish to speak. As a classroom teacher or allied health professional, you should understand this method of speech and recognize the importance of the student or adult maintaining clean hands. Always having to talk with one hand is not convenient, and it limits activities that can be accomplished simultaneously while speaking. Also some people, such as those with quadriplegia cannot raise their hands to occlude the stoma and so are mute. Again, medical technology provides a solution. Specially designed trach tubes cam be used or a speaking valve can be connected to the trach tube at the stoma opening to allow for speech. The one-way valve opens during inhalation and remains open during easy exhalation, allowing for neck breathing to occur. With a more forceful exhalation, the valve closes the stoma opening and directs the air through the trachea, vocal folds, and up the rest of the vocal tract for articulation of speech. The valve, therefore, simply eliminates the need to talk with thumb occlusion. It is appropriate for use with infants, youths, and adults despite whether the tracheostoma is temporary or permanent. Classroom teachers and allied health professionals should understand the basic operation of these valves to be tolerant of the appearance of the apparatus worn at the person's neck. Helpful Web sites are presented in **Table 9–8**.

TABLE 9–8 Web Sites with Further Information on Altered Methods of Breathing and Speaking Valves

- www.asha.org/slp/clinical/Tracheostomy.htm. The American Speech-Language-Hearing Association provides a basic overview of speech issues found in patients with tracheostomies or ventilators. This is an excellent resource for the general public on this subject.
- www.passy-muir.com. This commercial Web site describes tracheostomy and ventilator speaking valves used with children and adults. It contains excellent information and color pictures to aid understanding.
- www.orl.nl/Voice_Rehabilitation/Blom-Singer/blom-singer.html. This site describes an indwelling low-pressure voice prosthesis typically used in a laryngectomy. Also, the site's "image atlas" has interesting pictures.

VIGNETTE 9–2

Tony Dement has the inherited disease of Duchenne muscular dystrophy. As a result of his progressive weakness, Tony became quadriplegic over time and eventually was confined to a wheelchair but continued attending public school. His ability to breathe deteriorated in high school and his doctors decided it would be easier for Tony to breathe with a tracheostomy. Eventually, he was fitted with a speaking valve and operates his computer by voice control.

LARYNGECTOMIZED PERSONS

Laryngectomy is surgical removal of the larynx. Often, this is done when cancer has invaded the larynx, but occasionally removal is necessary in cases of burns (from acids, lyes), gunshot wounds, and other traumatic accidents. Laryngectomy, then, is often a procedure done on adults (especially those older than 60 years with a history of smoking). Though rare, children and infants with laryngeal tumors have been laryngectomized. Because cancer—and the attempt to save a person's life—is the main reason for doing a laryngectomy, it follows that if caught early, the cancer can be treated by radiotherapy (radiation) or by a less extensive surgery. With reconstruction of partially excised area and some potential function, the speech-language pathologist can help the person regain a usable voice. Traditional voice treatment approaches directed at effort, reduced breathiness, and increased loudness may apply. With advanced cancer, the surgeon removes the total larynx and some of the surrounding area. With such total laryngectomy, the person cannot talk and may have trouble swallowing safely. Without a larynx—and no vocal folds—the medical team, especially the surgeon and the SLP, can often devise ways for the person to speak again. The speech-language pathologist trains the person to talk in an alternative fashion, and several options are available.

Artificial larynx speech involves the person holding a battery-powered device to the neck and mouthing the word. The electronic buzz emitted from the device is shaped by the articulators into audible speech. It is good speech yet mechanical sounding. In treatment, the SLP refines efficiency of neck placement to talk, curtails extraneous noise, optimizes articulator excursion and rate, and modulates frequency, amplitude, and pausing.

A second treatment option is **esophageal speech**. You probably have burped and this is stomach gas traveling up the vocal tract and vibrating air along the way to make sound. Try using your articulators (especially the tongue, jaw, and lips) to mouth a few words next time you are burping, and you are doing something akin to esophageal speech. Recall that the person with a laryngectomy lacks vocal folds to vibrate lung air for sound, but also recall that the lung air moves in and out the neck stoma rather than the upper vocal track. By learning techniques to gulp a ball of air in the mouth and then swallow or inject that ball of air into the top of the esophagus (just below where the larynx used to be), the person can then "burp" the air back out and articulate audible speech. Esophageal speech can be difficult to learn and it takes much practice to become proficient. Even good esophageal speakers can say only a few syllables at a time before needing to recharge the air supply. Not being able to speak on lung air is a distinct disadvantage and the speech is quite segmented and of slow rate. In lieu of vibrating vocal folds to create sound, the walls at the top of the esophagus are vibrating to cause sound; hence the name esophageal speech. The esophageal tissue is thick and so vibrates at a low frequency, meaning that the speaker has a low-pitched and hoarse-quality voice. This tends to concern female esophageal speakers more than it does males.

A third type of alaryngeal rehabilitation follows a simple surgical procedure known as tracheoesophageal puncture, or TEP for short. Following total laryngectomy, the surgeon may create a hole in the tissue wall that separates the trachea from the esophagus. This puncture site is roughly below the area when the larynx was removed (and inside the stoma). Importantly, the hole provides an opening for exhaled lung air to pass through into the top of the esophagus. A specially designed tiny prosthesis is fitted through the stoma and into the puncture site to prevent saliva from entering the lungs yet still allow for air to pass through. The person covers the stoma site with their thumb and exhaled lung air travels not out the stoma when occluded but through the prosthesis and into the top of the esophagus. The air vibrates the esophageal wall, making sound that then passes up through the vocal tract so that it can be articulated in the normal fashion for speech. **TE speech**, then, is a hybrid of techniques. Like esophageal speech, the walls of the esophagus are set into vibration to produce sound as a substitute for the missing vocal folds. But, unlike esophageal speech, TE speech has the advantage of using lung air just as normal speakers do. The result is that TE speech rate and word segmentation are nearly normal, yet pitch remains low and quality hoarse. And, unlike esophageal speech, TE speech is easily and swiftly acquired. Rather than using thumb occlusion, the SLP fits a small prosthetic speaking valve device onto the first prosthesis. When not talking, the person breathes air into and out of the lungs through the stoma opening. When ready to speak, a slight increase in exhalation pressure causes the valve to close and divert exhaled air through the prosthetic valve and into the top of the esophagus for vibration and speech production.

TIPS FOR WORKING WITH PERSONS WHO HAVE ALTERED METHODS OF BREATHING

People, especially young children, with tracheostomy tubes (with or without valves) represent a small yet challenging population. They have complex medical treatment needs, and their families often experience high amounts of stress. In medical centers or in large school districts, the SLP may wish to organize a support group for parents of these tracheostomized children, as done by Woodfin (1988).

Teachers and allied health professionals should realize that tracheostomized students are at high risk for many infections. Tracheitis, bronchitis, and pneumonia are frequent and may require ongoing antibiotics or occasional hospital stays. Teachers should assist in limiting exposure of other sick students (those with colds and respiratory infections) to the neck-breathing student. Teachers also should be understanding and helpful as the student works with a homebound teacher to make up missed schoolwork caused by frequent absenteeism.

Teachers, health professionals, and home caregivers should try to maintain a clean environment. Dusty rooms are not good for neck-breathing persons. Also, the temperature and humidity of the room air (or the outdoor seasonal air) are important. Breathing cold air or hot air that is dry can be quite painful to the mucous linings of the trachea, bronchi, and lungs. The person may benefit from operating a humidifier to help adjust the temperature and humidity of the air.

The school nurse needs to be aware that a student who breathes via the neck is in a particular class. It is prudent for the school nurse to review resuscitation techniques with a classroom teacher in case of an emergency. It should be obvious that mouth-to-mouth resuscitation is ineffective for anyone with a stoma; mouth-to-stoma techniques are needed.

Last, the teacher should assist the student in developing a sense of self-worth and of belonging to the class. Social relationships with classroom peers are not easy for the student who is different.

Terms to Know

Phonatory disorders	Neurogenic voice disorders
Disorders of resonance	Neoplastic voice disorders
Abducted	Habitual pitch level
Adducted	Monotone
Subglottic pressure	Diplophonia
Vibration	Pitch breaks
Fundamental frequency	Loudness
Phonotrauma	Quality
Laryngologist	Tracheostomy
Vocal nodules	Trach tube
Voice treatment	Stoma
Vocal hygiene approach	Laryngectomy
Edema	Artificial larynx
Papilloma	Esophageal speech
Functional voice disorder	TE speech
Psychogenic voice disorders	

Study Questions

1. List several behaviors that are considered abusive to the vocal mechanism.
2. Differentiate between disorders of phonation and resonance.
3. What are vocal nodules? Be able to discuss potential causal factors and general principles of intervention.
4. Discuss the major goals to be accomplished in a vocal hygiene program.

5. What are some things a teacher should do when a student with an altered method of breathing is in the class?
6. What substitutes as the vibrating vocal folds to generate sound in artificial larynx speech? In esophageal speech? In TE speech?

Bibliography

Aaron, V. L., & Madison, C. L. (1991). A vocal hygiene program for high-school cheerleaders. *Language, Speech, and Hearing Services in Schools. 22*(1), 287–290.

Baumgartner, C., Sapir, S., & Ramig, L. (2001). Voice quality changes following phonatory-respiratory effort treatment (LSVT®) versus respiratory effort treatment for individuals with Parkinson disease. *Journal of Voice, 15*(1), 105–114.

Behrman, A., & Orlikoff, R. F. (1997). Instrumentation in voice assessment and treatment: What's the use? *American Journal of Speech-Language Pathology, 6*(4), 9–16.

Cook, J. V., Palaski, D. J., & Hanson, W. R. (1979). A vocal hygiene program for school-age children. *Language, Speech, and Hearing Services in Schools, 10*, 21–26.

Deal, R. E., McClain, B., & Sudderth, J. F. (1976). Identification, evaluation, therapy, and follow-up for children with vocal nodules in a public school setting. *Journal of Speech and Hearing Disorders, 41*, 390–397.

DeGregorio, N., & Polow, N. G. (1985). Effect of teacher training sessions on the perception of voice disorders. *Language, Speech, and Hearing Services in Schools, 16*(1), 25–28.

Dobres, R., Lee, L., Stemple, T. C., Kummer, A. W., & Kretschmer, L. W. (1989). *Description of laryngeal pathologies in children evaluated by otolaryngologists.* Paper presented at the Annual Convention of the American Speech-Language-Hearing Association, St. Louis, MO.

Flynn, P., Andrews, M., & Cabot, B. (2004). *Using your voice wisely and well* (2nd ed.). Austin, TX: Pro-Ed.

Haynes, W. O., & Pindzola, R. H. (2004). *Diagnosis and evaluation in speech pathology* (6th ed.). Boston, MA: Pearson Education.

Herrington-Hall, B. L., Lee, L., Stemple, J. C., Niemi, K. R., & McHone, M. M. (1988). Description of laryngeal pathologies by age, sex, and occupation in a treatment-seeking population. *Journal of Speech and Hearing Disorders, 53*, 57–64.

Huber, J., Stathopoulos, E., Ramig, L., & Lancaster, S. (2003). Respiratory function and variability in individuals with Parkinson disease: Pre and post Lee Silverman Voice Treatment (LSVT). *Journal of Medical Speech-Language Pathology, 11*(4), 185–201.

Jotz, G. P., Cervantes, O., Abrahao, M., Settanni, F. A., & Carrar de Angelis, E. (2002). Noise-to-harmonic ratio as an acoustic measure of voice disorders in boys. *Journal of Voice, 16*(1), 28–31.

Kahane, J. C., & Mayo, R. (1989). The need for aggressive pursuit of healthy childhood voices. *Language, Speech, and Hearing Services in Schools, 20*(1), 102–107.

Moran, M. J., & Pentz, A. L. (1987). Otolaryngologists' opinions of voice therapy for vocal nodules in children. *Language, Speech, and Hearing Services in Schools, 18*, 172–178.

Moran, M. J., & Zylla-Jones, E. (1998). *Learning about voice: Vocal hygiene activities for children, a resource manual.* San Diego, CA: Singular.

Morton, V., & Watson, D. R. (2001). The impact of impaired vocal quality on children's ability to process spoken language. *Logopedics, Phoniatrics, and Vocology, 26,* 17–25.

National Center for Voice and Speech. (1994). *Voice therapy and training.* Iowa City, IA: University of Iowa.

Nilson, H., & Schneiderman, C. R. (1983). Classroom program for the prevention of vocal abuse and hoarseness in elementary school children. *Language, Speech, and Hearing Services in Schools, 14,* 121–127.

Pannbacker, M. (1998). Voice treatment techniques: A review and recommendations for outcome studies. *American Journal of Speech-Language Pathology, 7*(3), 49–64.

Pindzola, R. H. (1987). *A voice assessment protocol for children and adults.* Austin, TX: Pro-Ed.

Roy, N., Merrill, R., Thibeault, S., Gray, S., & Smith, E. (2004). Voice disorders in teachers and the general population: Effects on work performance, attendance, and future career choices. *Journal of Speech, Language, and Hearing Research, 47*(3), 542–551.

Scott, A. (1998, July 13). Vocal hygiene for preschoolers. *Advance for Speech-Language Pathologists & Audiologists,* 14.

Spielman, J., Ramig, L., Will, L., Halpern, A., & Petska, J. (2007). Effects of LSVT Extended (LSVT-X) on voice and speech in Parkinson disease. *American Journal of Speech-Language Pathology, 16,* 95–107.

Terrell, S. L., & Morgan, P. A. (1980). *The adventures of Mr. Gruff: A voice therapy program for preschool children.* Paper presented at the Annual Convention of the American Speech-Language-Hearing Association, Detroit, MI.

Wilson, K. D. (1987). *Voice problems of children* (3rd ed.). Baltimore, MD: Williams & Wilkins.

Woodfin, S. T. (1988). A support group for parents of tracheostomized children. *Texas Journal of Audiology and Speech Pathology, 14*(1), 7–9.

Yiu, E. M. (2002). Impact and prevention of voice problems in the teaching profession: Embracing the consumer's view. *Journal of Voice, 16,* 215–228.

SELECTED VOCAL HYGIENE PROGRAMS

HYGIENE PROGRAM BY TERRELL AND MORGAN (1980)

This program for reducing abusive vocal behaviors was designed for preschool children. It consists of an audiocassette recording of a conversation between two animal characters: a hoarse bear named Mr. Gruff, and a normal-voiced kitten named Mr. Gentle. The taped program is only 20 minutes in length but is segmented for use over a number of sessions. Additionally, time is spent each session reviewing portions of the tape through questions, further explanations, and demonstrations to ensure learning. Demonstrations include the use of a flannel board with pictures of Mr. Gruff and Mr. Gentle in various story-like situations.

In the pleasant conversation between the two characters, Mr. Gentle explains to Mr. Gruff the manner in which Mr. Gruff is abusing his voice and alterations that he can make to improve his voice quality. Mr. Gentle also offers a clear, precise explanation of the larynx, the normal vocal folds, vocal folds with nodules, and the ways that various types of vocal abuse can contribute to vocal nodules. Pictures for the flannel board accompany this explanation. At the end of the taped story, Mr. Gruff undergoes a dramatic change from a hoarse voice to a normal voice, much to the approval of Mr. Gentle.

In summary of Terrell and Morgan's program for preschool children, flannel board stories were used to demonstrate:

1. Types of vocal abuse
2. Situations of vocal abuse
3. Explanations of the larynx, including both normal folds and vocal folds with nodules
4. Alternatives for abusive vocal behaviors

HYGIENE PROGRAM BY SCOTT (1998)

A classroom of preschoolers was presented a hygiene program focusing on basic anatomy, using models, activities, and vocal habits, through coloring book activities. Coloring book pictures showed cartoon characters engaging in good and bad vocal behaviors. For example, a picture depicted a cartoon duck singing so loudly that his friend covered her ears. Kazoos were used to explain proper voice quality. By humming into the kazoo, the children focused on vocal quality rather than on meaning or articulation. The children felt their larynx while humming to also understand the source of their voice. Three 1-hour sessions were conducted with the children. One month later in a follow-up evaluation, the children "had retained much of the information about basic anatomy and identifying bad vocal habits in pictures."

HYGIENE PROGRAM BY NILSON AND SCHNEIDERMAN (1983)

Second- and third-grade children were enrolled in a preventative program for vocal hygiene. They did not need to demonstrate vocal abuse or hoarseness to enter the program; the program was administered to entire classrooms with the teacher participating as well. Pretests were given to assess baseline knowledge. Each class received two half-hour sessions per week for 2 weeks. These four lessons are summarized.

Lesson 1: Basic laryngeal anatomy was explained. Quality terms (e.g., rough/smooth, hoarse) were discussed in general, and specific voices of the children were described in particular. Tape recordings of the children were made also.

Lesson 2: Adequate and inadequate voice qualities were discussed as were behaviors that were abusive to the voice. The children discussed alternatives to abusive behavior.

Lesson 3: Vocal qualities, vocal abuses, and abusive situations were discussed further. Lists were generated of abuses and high-probability situations for abuses. The students were read short stories containing characters that abuse and correctly use the voice. The children were encouraged to identify the vocal behaviors.

Lesson 4: All previous lessons were reviewed. Notebooks containing pictures of voice caricatures, the list of abusive and nonabusive voice behaviors, and an award for completing the program were presented to each child. A posttest was then given.

Five months later, the children were again given the posttest to see whether the hygiene information had been retained. It had indeed.

HYGIENE PROGRAM BY COOK, PALASKI, AND HANSON (1979)

Third-, fourth-, fifth-, and sixth-grade children with hoarseness participated in a 6-lesson vocal hygiene program. The program consisted of two half-hour classes per week for 3 weeks.

Instructional materials included tape-recorded voice samples, handouts, and cartoon illustrations (such as Victor Voicebox).

The first lesson began with a 20-item pretest and was followed by an introduction to voice production. Each child's voice was recorded at this session. The second lesson taught concepts of vocal quality; taped examples (such as hoarseness) were played and discussed. Lesson 3 discussed anatomy and voice production in more detail. Lesson 4 discussed abusive vocal behaviors, using cartoon characters as illustrative material. Lesson 5 gave the children an opportunity to determine their own vocal habits and identify possible sources of vocal abuse. A contractual agreement was made with each child to eliminate one form of vocal abuse. Each child received a booklet with pictures that summarized the program. Lesson 6 was a summary of the program with emphasis on personal goals for eliminating vocal abuse. A posttest was given and an analysis of the results indicated that the children learned the vocal hygiene concepts. Through such educational awareness, the children should be able to prevent abuse and its damaging effects on the larynx.

HEARING LOSS

BACKGROUND INFORMATION

NATURE OF THE PROBLEM

A hearing loss can range in severity from mild, similar to having "blocked" ears as the result of a head cold, to profound, where hearing is essentially unusable for any purpose. Obviously, the communication challenges facing individuals with profound hearing losses are different from those faced by people with milder losses. Traditionally, an effort has been made to distinguish individuals with the most severe hearing losses from those with lesser degrees of loss by using the terms **deaf** and **hard-of-hearing**. Deaf describes those whose hearing loss is so great as to preclude the understanding of speech through the ear alone. Hard-of-hearing refers to those whose hearing loss makes difficult, but does not preclude, the understanding of speech through the ear alone (Moores, 1987). The dividing line between deaf and hard-of-hearing is not universally agreed upon, and these terms have been used with much imprecision. Even if the terms were more precisely defined, the hard-of-hearing category is still too broad to be helpful in planning habilitative or rehabilitative intervention.

A more discriminating classification of hearing loss is one based on a measurement of **hearing threshold**. **Threshold** is the lowest intensity at which a person can hear a sound. The higher the threshold, the louder the sound must be to be heard. Recall from Chapter 2 that intensity (which listeners perceive as loudness) is measured in decibels (dB). For children, an average threshold of 0 to 15 dB among the speech frequencies (500 to 2000 hertz) is considered normal hearing. Thresholds above 15 dB indicate a hearing loss that can be categorized according to the following levels: **slight** (15–25 dB), **mild** (26–40 dB), **mild-to-moderate** (41–55 dB), **moderate** (56–70 dB), **severe** (71–90 dB), and **profound** (above 90 dB). **Table 10–1** describes the effect of these categories of hearing loss on communication. These thresholds represent hearing level in the better ear. A person with a hearing loss in only one ear does not face the same challenges as the student whose loss is in both ears. Note that some hearing losses are progressive. Progressive losses become worse over time.

Whereas the preceding categories are more precise than simply using the terms *deaf* and *hard-of-hearing*, the degree of hearing loss is not the only factor to be considered in determining how a hearing loss affects communication ability. Some people with severe or profound hearing losses have excellent speech and language skills and can function quite

TABLE 10–1 Effects of Various Degrees of Hearing Loss on Communication

Hearing Threshold	Effect on Communication
0–15 dB Normal hearing	N/A
16–25 dB Slight hearing impairment	Difficulty hearing faint or distant speech in noise. Possible difficulty with tense and plural markers at the ends of words.
26–40 dB Mild hearing impairment	Difficulty hearing faint or distant speech even in quiet setting. Consonants affected most. May miss up to 50 percent of class discussion. May be fatigued resulting from effort required to try to hear conversation.
41–55 dB Mild-to-moderate hearing impairment	Hears normal speech completely only at close range. Without hearing aid, may miss more than half of the spoken message. Possible limited vocabulary and delayed or defective syntax and speech.
56–70 dB Moderate hearing impairment	Hears only loud conversational speech. Without a hearing aid may miss most of the spoken message. Difficulty in group situations. May miss most or all of classroom discussion. Possible severe language delay, problems with speech intelligibility and intonation patterns.
71–90 dB Severe hearing impairment	Cannot hear conversational speech. Without a hearing aid may not recognize any speech by hearing alone. Spoken language may not develop without early intervention. Possible language delay and intelligibility problems.
>90 dB Profound hearing impairment	May hear or feel loud sounds. Hearing is not a primary communication channel. Possible language delay and intelligibility problems.

Source: Data from Flexer, 1994; Stach, 1998; Tye-Murray, 1998; Anderson & Matkin, 2007.

well in classroom and work settings. Other people with less severe hearing losses may have unintelligible speech, poor language skills, and may experience more difficulty in adjusting to a regular classroom or some work settings. Additional factors that affect communication skills include the frequencies affected by the hearing loss and whether the loss was sudden or gradual (Stach, 1998). However, perhaps the most critical factor to be considered, in addition to the extent of hearing loss is the age at which the hearing loss occurred.

Hearing loss can be **congenital**, that is, present at birth, or it can be acquired at any time during a person's life. With regard to communication skills, a critical distinction is whether the hearing loss occurred before or after the development of speech and language. Hearing loss occurring prior to speech and language development is referred to as **prelingual**, and that occurring after speech and language develop is **postlingual**. Because children typically learn language skills through the auditory channel, prelingual hearing impairment can have a devastating effect on speech and language development.

CAUSES OF HEARING LOSS

Hearing losses are typically categorized as one of three types: **conductive**, **sensorineural**, or **mixed**. The type of hearing loss is determined by the portion of the hearing mechanism that fails to function properly.

A conductive hearing loss results from disorders of the outer or middle ear. Recall from Chapter 2 that the outer ear consists of the pinna and the external canal. The outer ear has little function other than to direct the sound toward the eardrum. Therefore, hearing problems that originate in the outer ear most often result from blockage of the canal. Congenital malformations of the outer ear, known as **microtia** or **atresia**, narrow or occlude the ear canal and can result in a conductive loss. A buildup of excessive ear wax, or **cerumen**, also can impede the transmission of sound through the canal. Blockage of the external canal can also result from the tendency of children to place objects where they do not belong. This apparently powerful drive results in the placement of beans, peanuts, erasers, gum, and a variety of other objects in the ear canal. Fortunately, such obstructions can usually be removed quite easily by a physician. Perforations of the eardrum, or tympanic membrane, which separates the outer ear from the middle ear, also may cause a conductive hearing loss. Perforations of the tympanic membrane may be the result of a middle ear infection (discussed later) or the result of direct trauma. Sticking objects in the outer ear or a severe blow to the side of the head in the area of the pinna may result in a perforation of the tympanic membrane.

Conductive hearing losses more often result from middle ear rather than outer ear disorders. Remember that the middle ear includes the eardrum, or tympanic membrane, and the three bones, or ossicles, known as the malleus, incus, and stapes. The most common middle ear disorder in children is **otitis media**. Otitis media is an inflammation of the middle ear. In most cases, this condition involves the presence of fluid in the middle ear cavity behind the eardrum. When fluid is present, the condition is known as otitis media with effusion (OME). The fluid interferes with the movement of both the eardrum and the ossicles, thereby reducing hearing sensitivity. In some cases the fluid is infectious and, left untreated, may perforate the eardrum, destroy the ossicles, and spread to other parts of the body. If there is no infection present, the existence of the fluid, and therefore the reduction in hearing acuity, may go unnoticed by the parents. Otitis media is extremely common among young children. Klein states, "Otitis media is the most frequent diagnosis for illness when children visit medical facilities" (Klein, 1991, p. 140). Patrick (1987) indicates that in an average kindergarten class of 30 students, there could be between 5 and 11 cases of otitis media at any one time. Many children seem to be "otitis prone." According to Klein (1991), about one third of all children experience recurrent instances of otitis media. Harrison and Belhorn (1991) identify situations and conditions that contribute to making a child otitis prone. These include the following.

- The presence of certain congenital anomalies such as cleft palate and Down syndrome
- A history of upper respiratory infections
- Early onset and frequent occurrences of otitis media
- Secondary or passive smoking (i.e., being around people who smoke)

There is significant disagreement as to whether the mild hearing loss associated with otitis media can delay speech-language development when the condition continues to recur. Several researchers report that speech and/or language may be delayed by the presence of otitis media during the period when a child is developing language (Northern & Downs, 1984; Friel-Patti & Finitzo, 1990; Teele, Klein, Chase, Menyuk, & Rosner, 1990; Robb, Psak, & Pang-Ching, 1993). However, other studies have failed to find a relationship between the presence of otitis media and later language delays (Grievink, Peters, vanBon, & Schilder, 1993; Paul, Lynn, & Lohr-Flansers, 1993; Roberts, Rosenfeld, & Zeisel, 2004).

Otitis media is usually treated by the use of antibiotics over a period of about 2 weeks. However, in recent years a dramatic increase in antibiotic resistance has created great concern about the overuse of antibiotics for the treatment of otitis media. This has caused physicians to be more stringent in diagnosing the various types of otitis media and, in some cases, withholding antibiotics. When otitis media persists over a longer period, the condition may be treated by the surgical insertion of **ventilating tubes** (pressure equalization, or p.e. tubes). These tiny tubes are inserted under general anesthesia through a tiny incision in the eardrum. The tubes ventilate the middle ear cavity, allowing the fluid to dissipate. The tubes typically work their way out on their own after several months.

Another condition that results in a conductive hearing loss, especially in adults, is **otosclerosis**. In this condition, a bony growth occurs around the stapes and the point where it pushes against the cochlea (the oval window). This causes the stapes to become unable to move against the oval window. Otosclerosis seems to run in families and is sometimes associated with hormonal changes during pregnancy. According to the American Academy of Otolaryngology–Head and Neck Surgery (2009), otosclerosis is most common among middle-aged Caucasian women and typically begins in the early 20s.

The second type of hearing loss, sensorineural, occurs as a result of damage to the inner ear or the auditory nerve. There are many possible causes of sensorineural hearing loss. Among the most common are the folllowing.

- *Genetic factors:* Approximately 50 percent of all congenital sensorineural losses are genetic. In some cases of genetic hearing loss, one or both of the parents have a hearing loss and they may have been aware of the chances of having a child with hearing impairment. In other cases, parents with normal hearing may not have realized that they carried a recessive gene and their child's hearing loss may come as a shock. Sometimes a genetic hearing loss is one of several conditions that occur together and constitute a syndrome. There are several hundred syndromes associated with hearing loss (Robin, 2008) including Usher syndrome, Stikler syndrome, and Treacher-Collins syndrome, just to name a few.
- *Maternal infection:* There are several infections that, when they occur in a pregnant woman, may affect her unborn fetus, resulting in a number of congenital disabilities including hearing loss. These infections include a group sometimes known as the **TORCH infections**. TORCH stands for *t*oxoplasmosis, *o*ther diseases such as syphilis and hepatitis, *r*ubella, *c*ytomegalovirus, and *h*erpes simplex viruses (Epps, Pittelkow, & Su, 1995; Klein, Baker, Remington, & Wilson, 2006).
- *Postnatal infection:* Infectious diseases such as bacterial meningitis and encephalitis may be acquired at any age. These diseases tend to attack and destroy portions of the nervous system including those associated with hearing.
- *Drugs:* Several classes of drugs have the potential to damage the cochlear structures and therefore cause a sensorineural hearing loss. Drugs that cause hearing loss are labeled **ototoxic**. Ototoxic drugs include certain antibiotics such as gentamicin and streptomycin, some chemotherapy drugs such as carboplatin, salicylates such as aspirin, and some diuretics such as Lasix (furosemide) (Stach, 1998; Weinstein, 2000).
- *Exposure to noise:* Hearing loss resulting from exposure to noise is called noise-induced hearing loss (NIHL). Such loss results when loud noises damage the hair cells in the cochlea. Noise-induced hearing loss can result from sharp sounds such as gunfire or from continuous background noise over a long period of time. According to the National Institute on Deafness and Other Communication Disorders (2008), long or repeated exposure to sounds at or above 85 dB can cause hearing loss. The louder the sound, the shorter the time period before NIHL can occur.
- *Age-related hearing loss:* In addition to those factors listed previously, the aging process may affect hearing ability. Many older persons experience varying degrees of hearing loss. In many cases, this age-related hearing loss reflects a deterioration of portions of the inner ear structures. The term used to refer to age-related hearing loss is **presbycusis**.

Unlike conductive losses, sensorineural losses are usually not reversible. Because different parts of the inner ear respond to different frequencies, sensorineural hearing losses often involve a specific range of frequencies. For example, a person might have normal hearing below 1000 hertz, but sharply reduced hearing ability at higher frequencies. Because speech sounds occur over a wide range of frequencies, the person with a high-frequency loss may hear enough of the speech signal to know someone is talking, but not enough to understand all of what is said. Family members (and in the case of children, teachers) sometimes mistakenly assume that hearing is an "all or none" ability. That is, if anything is heard, it is assumed that everything at that loudness level can be heard. This leads to comments such as, "I know he can hear me, so I guess he is just not paying attention." Such is not the case in a sensorineural hearing loss.

Finally, some individuals have both damaged inner ear structures and obstruction in the middle or outer ear. These people have hearing losses with both sensorineural and conductive components. Such losses are referred to as mixed losses.

To summarize, there are three important differences between a sensorineural and a conductive hearing loss.

1. Conductive losses are often reversible by medication or surgery. Sensorineural losses are generally irreversible.
2. Conductive losses tend to be the same at all frequencies. If speech is made loud enough, the person can understand. Sensorineural losses are variable, with some frequencies worse than others. Even if speech is made louder, the person may not understand all words.
3. Conductive losses typically do not exceed 50 or 60 dB (moderate hearing loss) because after that level, the sound is transmitted directly to the inner ear by vibration of the bones of the skull. Sensorineural losses can be of any severity from mild to profound.

COMMUNICATION PROBLEMS ASSOCIATED WITH HEARING LOSS

Communication problems associated with hearing loss include problems in both speech and language. The speech problems of individuals with hearing loss result from the inability to hear clearly the speech of others and the inability to monitor their own speech through the auditory channel. Most people who have a significant prelingual hearing loss exhibit speech problems. You can only imagine how difficult it must be for a child to learn to produce speech sounds without ever hearing those sounds. Although postlingual hearing losses may also affect speech, the resulting problems are usually less severe.

Speech problems associated with hearing loss may involve speech sound production, voice, resonance, and prosody (e.g., pitch inflections, stress patterns). Speech sound production problems can range from slight distortions of fricative sounds (such as *s*) to multiple substitutions, distortions, and omissions, making speech unintelligible. In the area of voice, pitch may be unusually high, or the pitch may not vary, resulting in a monotone voice. Loudness of the voice also may be affected by hearing loss. An old stereotype associates all speakers with hearing impairment with an excessively loud voice. While many people with sensorineural losses do speak with a loud voice, some with conductive losses may exhibit an excessively soft voice. The quality of the voice may be breathy and weak or harsh and strident. Resonance is another aspect of speech affected by hearing loss. A speaker with a significant hearing loss may be hypernasal (excessive sound in the nasal cavity) or denasal (a "cold-in-the-nose" quality sounding as if the nose were blocked). Speech also may be focused in the back of the throat, giving an unusual quality to the sound of the voice. In addition, persons with hearing loss may also exhibit problems with proper stress and accent patterns. Placing stress on the wrong syllable makes it difficult for listeners to correctly perceive the intended word, especially in connected speech. As mentioned earlier, the nature and severity of these speech problems depend on several factors, including the extent of hearing loss, the type of loss, whether the loss was sudden or gradual, the age at onset, and the amount and type of early training.

With regard to language, it is not possible to provide a specific list of language problems that constitute a "language of those with hearing impairment." As Lahey states,

> To know that a child is hearing-impaired does not tell the clinician what the child needs to know about language. Considerable variability is found among these children . . . variability that is not easily predicted given levels of hearing loss, mean length of utterance, grade in school, nonverbal IQ, or age at onset. (Lahey, 1988, p. 67)

It is, however, reasonable to assume that most children who experience a significant hearing loss early in life will have some language problems. Tye-Murray (1998) identifies some of the more common types of problems exhibited by students with hearing loss in language form, content, and use. These are presented in **Table 10–2**.

TABLE 10–2   Common Language Problems Exhibited by Speakers with Hearing Loss

Problems of Language Form
- Overuse of nouns and verbs with rare use of adverbs, prepositions, and pronouns
- Omission of function words
- Limited number of words per sentence
- Sentences mostly simple subject-verb-object structure
- Omission of plural and past tense markers
- Incorrect ordering of words in a sentence

Problems of Language Content
- Limited vocabulary
- Difficulty with words that have multiple meanings or that can be used as more than one part of speech
- Difficulty understanding idioms
- Difficulty with synonyms and antonyms

Problems of Language Use (Pragmatics)
- Asking inappropriate questions
- Problems with conversational turn-taking
- Failure to acknowledge hearing a message
- Inappropriate shifts in topic

Source: Data from Tye-Murray, 1998.

Dobie and Berlin (1979), through the use of simulated hearing loss, demonstrated that even mild losses of 20 dB could result in the student failing to hear plural and past-tense word endings and inflections indicating a question. The language delay noted in children with hearing loss tends to increase with the degree of hearing loss (Quigley & Thomure, 1968) and with age (Kodman, 1963; Berg, 1986). The latter finding reflects the fact that, as students progress through the grade levels, they face more complex language-based tasks.

Adults who acquire hearing losses later in life tend to have relatively minor changes in voice loudness and quality and some possible distortions of high-frequency sounds such as *s*. Hearing loss acquired in adulthood, however, typically does not have a significant impact on intelligibility (Davis, 1995).

IN MEDICAL SETTINGS

So far, this text has focused on the speech-language pathologist (SLP) as a communication disorders specialist. Although speech-language pathologists have a significant role in working with individuals with hearing loss, the communication disorders specialist most frequently involved with this population in a medical setting is an **audiologist**. Audiologists test hearing, fit hearing aids, provide suggestions for educational management, and help patients improve their communication skills. In addition, audiologists in medical settings may also be responsible for other services such as the assessment and management of vestibular (inner ear) and balance impairments, helping patients deal with tinnitus (ringing or other ear noise), and management of cerumen (ear wax) to prevent obstruction of the external ear canal and of amplification devices (Madell & Montano, 2000; American Speech-Language-Hearing Association, 2004). Do not confuse audiologists with hearing aid dealers who also fit and sell hearing aids but who have considerably less professional training. Audiologists in medical settings often work closely with **otolaryngologists** and other physicians in the prevention, identification, assessment, and treatment of individuals with hearing problems. An otolaryngologist is a physician who treats disorders of the ear, nose, and throat. These physicians are sometimes referred to simply as ENTs (for ear, nose, and throat) or, if they limit their practice to disorders of the ear, **otologists**. The interaction between otolaryngologists and audiologists is so important that many audiologists are based in physician offices or work in departments of otolaryngology in hospital settings.

ASSESSMENT IN MEDICAL SETTINGS

Newborn Screening   Early identification and treatment of hearing loss is critical to the speech, language, and cognitive development of children. Hearing loss in infants is not easy to detect by casual observation. In many cases, severe to profound hearing losses may not be identified until the child exhibits delays in language development. In milder degrees of hearing loss, the problem may not be identified until after the child begins school. For many years, lists of signs or family history factors known as high-risk registers were used to help identify infants who were at risk for hearing problems. These high-risk registers included such items as a family history of hearing loss, high levels of bilirubin (a product resulting from the breakdown of red blood cells that causes the child to appear jaundiced, i.e., yellow), abnormalities of the craniofacial region, birth weight less than 1,500 grams, and maternal disease such as rubella during pregnancy (Fitch, Williams, & Etienne, 1982).

In recent years, technological advances have made it possible to assess more directly the hearing of infants shortly after birth. In its 2007 position paper, the Joint Committee on Infant Hearing indicated that all infants should have access to hearing screening no later than 1 month of age, and that infants who do not pass the hearing screening should have appropriate audiological and medical evaluations to confirm the presence of hearing loss at no later than 3 months of age. Further, all infants with confirmed permanent hearing loss should receive early intervention services as soon as possible after diagnosis but at no later than 6 months of age. You may ask how one goes about testing the hearing of a 1- to 3-month-old infant. Obviously, traditional methods of testing hearing that require subjects to indicate when they hear a sound or to repeat words is not possible with infants. Hearing in infants can be tested by two different methods: auditory brainstem response (ABR) and/ or otoacoustic emissions (OAE). In both cases, what is actually being tested is how well the infant's auditory mechanism is working. OAE is a measure of cochlear function in response to sound. ABR, as the name suggests, assesses the response of portions of the brainstem to sound.

Infants who fail the original screening in the hospital do not always receive the appropriate follow-up testing and treatment. Peterson and Bell (2008) suggest that this failure to follow up on a failed screening may occur as often as 50 percent of the time. Audiologists can help provide more effective services to children and families by making families aware of the services available in their community and by maintaining communication with the primary care physician throughout the process, from screening through intervention (Munoz, Shisler, Moeller, & White, 2009).

Testing Older Children and Adults   Hearing losses that are not identified by a prenatal screening program may be discovered later in life by screening tests or by some behavioral indicators. Severe or profound hearing losses may first be suspected as a result of delayed speech and language development or poor school performance. Hearing losses acquired later in life, especially those losses that progress gradually, may be first noticed when the individual begins to experience difficulty understanding the speech of others (particularly in background noise) or speaks at increased or reduced loudness levels. Because a hearing loss may not be immediately apparent, it is important that school-age children, individuals with family histories of hearing loss or other conditions that place them at risk for hearing problems, and those who are exposed to high levels of noise have their hearing screened periodically. Other adults should have their hearing screened when they begin to have difficulty in verbal situations such as in conversations with others, while talking on the telephone, or when listening to television.

The instrument most frequently used to test hearing is an **audiometer**. There are several different kinds of audiometers, but the type typically used in the initial phase of hearing testing is a **pure tone audiometer**. Pure tone audiometers present "beeplike" tones at various frequencies and loudness levels determined by the examiner. The subject is usually instructed to raise a hand or press a response button when the test tone is heard. Children too young to give a reliable indication of hearing the test tone may be conditioned to look toward a stimulus item (for example an interesting action toy), the appearance of which has been paired with the presentation of the test tone. The test tone is then reduced in intensity and the child is monitored to determine whether there is a head turn toward the toy. In this way, the threshold for sounds can be established.

Pure tone audiometers can be used for screening tests or threshold tests. A hearing **screening test** involves the presentation of tones at a predetermined loudness level at selected frequencies. If a person fails to respond appropriately to the hearing screening, additional tests are indicated. A speech-language pathologist may perform hearing screening tests; however, the additional hearing tests required to determine a person's hearing status must be performed by an audiologist. The audiologist typically begins the hearing assessment by administering a **threshold test** to determine the loudness required for the person to hear a sound at each of several frequencies. The threshold test also can be used to indicate whether a hearing loss is conductive, sensorineural, or mixed by presenting the stimulus tone in two different ways. First, the tone is presented through earphones. This presentation, known as **air conduction**, requires the sound to pass through the outer, middle, and inner ear. If the subject does not hear normally by air conduction, the examiner knows that a hearing problem exists but cannot determine whether it is conductive or sensorineural. To make this determination, sounds are next presented by placing a sound generator on one of the bones of the skull, most often the mastoid bone, directly behind the ear. In this type of presentation, known as **bone conduction**, the inner ear is stimulated directly by vibration of the bones, thus bypassing the outer and middle ear. The results of these tests are represented on a graphlike form known as an **audiogram**. **Figures 10–1** through **10–4** show audiograms that reveal normal hearing, a conductive loss, a sensorineural loss, and a mixed loss, respectively.

Because middle ear problems are so common among early elementary schoolchildren, their middle ear function should be assessed by an additional instrument known as a **tympanometer**. By directly measuring the movement of the eardrum, a tympanometer can reveal the presence of fluid in the middle ear cavity as well as expose a variety of other middle ear disorders. This is not a hearing test per se, but a very helpful assessment of the function of the middle ear.

Because the ability to understand speech is a critical function of the hearing system, several tests are designed to assess how well a person can hear and understand speech. These tests are administered using a speech audiometer that allows the examiner to present spoken words at various loudness levels. The words may be presented by live voice, where the examiner says the words, or via recorded media. These speech-related tests include

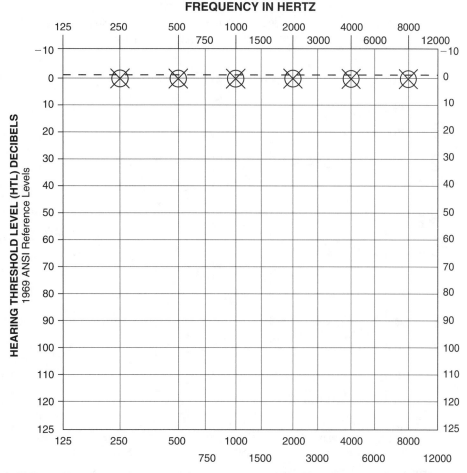

FIGURE 10–1   An audiogram showing normal hearing. 0 = right ear, X = left ear.

speech detection threshold (SDT), which is the lowest level at which a person can detect the presence of speech 50 percent of the time. Speech recognition threshold (SRT) is the lowest level at which a person can understand spoken words 50 percent of the time. SRT is typically assessed using two-syllable words with equal stress on both syllables such as *hotdog* and *toothbrush*. These words are known as spondee words. As mentioned previously, sensorineural hearing losses sometimes make it difficult to understand speech, even when the speech is loud enough to be heard. To test a person's ability to distinguish one word from another when the speech is above threshold level, a test known as a speech discrimination test is administered. Several word lists and some sentence lists are available to be used to assess speech discrimination ability.

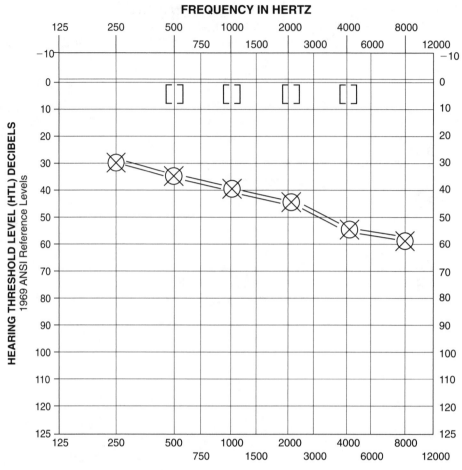

FIGURE 10–2 An audiogram showing a conductive hearing loss. 0 = right ear by air conduction, X = left ear by air conduction, [= right ear by bone conduction,] = left ear by bone conduction. Notice bone conduction thresholds are better than air conduction thresholds.

Young children and other individuals who are unable to respond reliably may have the function of their auditory mechanism tested by the ABR or OAE techniques discussed in the section titled, "Newborn Screening," earlier in the chapter.

INTERVENTION IN MEDICAL SETTINGS

Hearing Aids   For many individuals with hearing loss, a hearing aid is a critical tool in facilitating their habilitation and education. Selecting the best hearing aid for a particular person is an important role for an audiologist in a medical setting. Audiologists can choose

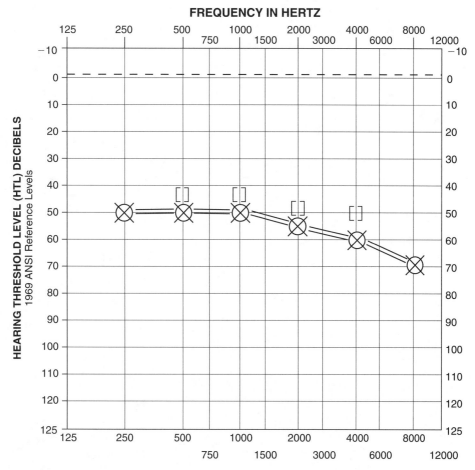

FREQUENCY IN HERTZ

FIGURE 10–3 An audiogram showing a sensorineural hearing loss. Notice that both air and bone conduction thresholds are below normal.

from several styles of hearing aids. Tiny **canal aids** or slightly larger **in-the-ear aids** fit snugly into the outer ear and are quite popular with adults because they are not as noticeable as other styles. Because children's ear canals grow and change dimensions along with the rest of their bodies, hearing aids that fit entirely into the ear are not used frequently for children. The **behind-the-ear aid** has become the aid of choice for most children (**Figure 10–5**). The child wears the instrument, as the name implies, behind the ear and it is connected to the earpiece, or **ear mold**, by a short section of tubing. The ear mold is the part of the aid that fits into the ear and directs the amplified sound into the ear.

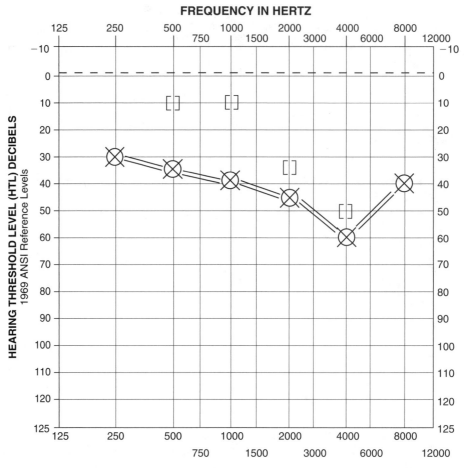

FIGURE 10–4   An audiogram showing a mixed loss. Notice that bone conduction thresholds are below normal but air conduction thresholds are even worse.

Ear molds are custom made to fit the patient's ear and, in the case of a child, are changed as the ear grows. Regardless of the style, all hearing aids include the following components:

Microphone: Sound enters the hearing aid through the microphone. The microphone converts sound into an electrical signal. The microphone should not be covered or blocked by clothing or any other material.

Amplifier: The amplifier, not visible on the outside of the aid, electronically boosts the signal received from the microphone and passes on the strengthened signal to the receiver.

Receiver: The receiver acts like a loudspeaker. It receives the boosted signal from the amplifier, converts the electrical signal back to sound, and passes it on to the ear mold or directly into the ear.

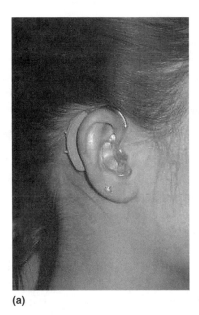

(a)

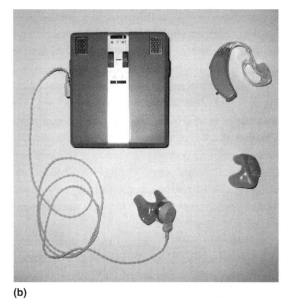

(b)

FIGURE 10–5   A behind-the-ear hearing aid (a) and a body style aid (b).
Source: Courtesy of William Haynes, Auburn University.

Batteries: Hearing aids are powered by batteries. Different hearing aids use different types of batteries. To keep young children from removing the battery inappropriately, some aids come with lockable or tamperproof battery compartments. The patient should know where the battery is located on the hearing aid, how to access the battery, and have a replacement battery kept at school or work.

Many hearing aids also have components such as follows:

Volume control: The volume control is usually set at a specified level. The patient should know the level at which the aid is usually set and should check this level at the beginning of each day and when he or she seems to be having difficulty with the aid. *Telephone switch:* Although this is not part of all hearing aids, many have an additional switch marked "T" and "M." The "T" position is for use on the telephone, and the "M" or microphone position is for all other activity.

Over the past few years, the technology associated with hearing aids has advanced at an impressive pace. The development of innovations such as programmable hearing aids and the application of digital signal processing to these instruments has broadened the choices available to consumers, while at the same time challenging audiologists to keep up-to-date.

Cochlear Implants   Many people with severe or profound hearing loss do not benefit from even the most powerful hearing aids. The cochleas of these individuals are unable to generate neural impulses to be conducted along the auditory nerve (Stach, 1998). An exciting development in the treatment of such conditions has been the ability to directly stimulate the auditory nerve by the use of a surgically implanted device known as a **cochlear implant**. Cochlear implants have internal and external components. The external components resemble a conventional hearing aid. These components include a microphone, a processor, and a transmitter. The microphone, usually worn at ear level, receives the sound from the environment and converts it to an electrical signal. The processor, sometimes worn on the body or at ear level, modifies the signal from the microphone into the type of signal required by the specific instrument. The transmitter, which is attached to the head, transmits the processed signal to the internal components. The internal components, which have been surgically implanted in the skull and cochlea, consist of an internal receiver and an electrode array. The internal receiver picks up the signal from the outside transmitter, and the electrode array stimulates the auditory nerve. Until recently, most people who received a cochlear implant received only one. In recent years, the use of two cochlear implants has been increasing.

It is important to understand that a cochlear implant does not provide normal hearing. The person with an implant is still hearing impaired. Tye-Murray (1998) indicates the performance of children who have received cochlear implants to this time leads us to expect that most children who have prelingual hearing loss achieve some sound awareness and some speechreading enhancement when using their implants. Also, most children show some improvement in their speech and language performance. However, Tye-Murray (1998) goes on to warn that in cautioning parents and teachers to have realistic expectations for children with cochlear implants, hearing professionals should not lead them to expect too little either. Children with implants need to be challenged to develop maximally the hearing ability they do possess. Adults who have suffered postlingual hearing loss benefit greatly from cochlear implants (Davis, 1995).

Parents of children who receive cochlear implants must appreciate the considerable time commitment involved. They must agree to return with the child to the implant center for follow-up testing and monitoring of the cochlear implant. The parents also must be willing to cooperate and work with the child's educators to provide appropriate habilitation.

Aural Rehabilitation   The responsibilities of an audiologist extend well beyond the assessment of hearing ability and the fitting of hearing aids. These professionals are also involved in a broader effort to reduce communication difficulties associated with hearing loss and facilitate successful communication between people with hearing loss and others. These efforts constitute an area known as **aural rehabilitation** (Tye-Murray,1998; Montgomery & Houston, 2000) and may involve both audiologists and speech-language pathologists. Aural rehabilitation may involve some or all of the following:

Hearing aid orientation and training: Even the best hearing aid cannot help a person hear if it is thrown into a drawer and never used because the patient is not comfortable wearing it. Like anything new, hearing aids require some getting used to. Learning how and when to adjust the various settings and some basic maintenance procedures can go a long way toward realizing the benefits of the aid.

Suggesting assistive listening and assistive living systems: Audiologists should make patients aware of the many devices that can help people with hearing loss deal with everyday activities and situations. Devices that cause a light to flash when a doorbell rings or a fire alarm sounds, or instruments that vibrate when a telephone rings, are generally referred to as assistive listening devices. Other devices including amplifiers for traditional telephones and cell phones as well as specially equipped telephone devices known at teletypewriters or TTYs can make life easier and safer for people with hearing loss.

Communication training: The communication abilities of individuals who are deaf or hard-of-hearing can be enhanced by teaching them how to use visual cues to help understand the speech of others. This is sometimes known as **lipreading** or **speechreading**. Also, patients with hearing loss can learn techniques known as **conversational repair strategies** to facilitate communication. Examples of such repair strategies might be to repeat the part of the message that was understood rather than just asking for a repetition of the entire message. For example, it might be more helpful to say, "You are going where?" rather than just saying "What?" In other cases, simply asking, "Could you speak a bit more slowly?" or saying, "Please let me see your face when you talk" might help the patient better understand the message.

For individuals who are unable to attend communication training sessions on a regular basis, an audiologist might suggest several computer-based programs for a patient to use at home. These programs include *Listening and Communication Enhancement (LACE)* (Sweetow & Henderson, 2006) and *Conversation Made Easy* (Tye-Murray, 2002).

Employment counseling: Like many persons with a handicapping condition, individuals with hearing loss often have difficulty finding and keeping employment. With the advent of legislation such as the Americans with Disabilities Act (ADA), employers are more likely to make accommodations that allow people with handicaps to perform the essential functions of many jobs. An audiologist, sometimes in cooperation with a vocational or rehabilitation counselor, can advise persons with hearing impairments of the types of accommodations that are available to allow them to perform well in many occupations.

Arranging peer support groups: An audiologist may be responsible for organizing peer support groups where people with hearing problems can discuss some of the challenges and solutions to the problems they encounter as a result of their hearing impairment. Such groups may also provide opportunities for individuals with hearing loss to learn from invited guests with expertise in many areas including recent developments in the treatment of hearing loss, legislation affecting individuals with hearing impairments, and various aspects of living with a hearing impairment.

In addition to working with individuals with impaired hearing, audiologists or speech-language pathologists can also be a resource for other people in the environment of the person with a hearing loss. These other people may be family members, colleagues at work, or other health professionals. Some simple strategies to aid in communicating with people who have a hearing loss are as follows.

Tips for Communicating with People with a Hearing Loss

- Speak clearly and naturally without shouting.
- Obtain the person's attention before beginning to speak.
- Be sure that the listener can see your face clearly.
- Keeps hands away from your face while speaking.
- Avoid speaking while chewing, eating, or smoking.
- Be sure that the room is well lit.
- Do not stand in front of a light source such as a window.
- Stand approximately 3 to 6 feet from the person.
- Speak at a normal or slightly louder than normal volume.
- Reduce background noise.
- If the person does not understand what you are saying, rephrase what you are saying rather than repeating the same thing over and over.
- If necessary, write down key words.
- Have the person with hearing impairment repeat what you have said to verify the message. (from Tye-Murray, 1998; Weinstein, 2000; Peterson & Bell, 2008)

IN EDUCATIONAL SETTINGS

Perhaps no communication disorder presents a greater challenge to students and professionals in an educational setting than the presence of a significant hearing impairment. At one time, most children with severe and profound hearing losses attended special schools for the deaf. Although these schools still have some proponents, in the years since the implementation of PL 94-142, there has been a dramatic decline in the number of students attending private residential schools and day classes for the deaf (Tye-Murray, 1998). Public schools have assumed more of the responsibility for the education of students who are deaf or hard-of-hearing. This does not mean, however, that all students with hearing impairments are enrolled in regular public schools. The Gallaudet Research Institute survey for the 2007–2008 academic year indicates that of the more than 36,000 students with hearing loss who were included in the survey, 24 percent were enrolled in special schools or centers, 17 percent were in self-contained classrooms in regular education settings, 9.6 percent were in resource room settings, and 39 percent were in a regular education setting (Gallaudet Research Institute, 2008). That same survey also reports the number of hours per week that students with hearing impairments were integrated with students with normal hearing. The survey indicates that approximately one third of students with hearing impairments had no integration with normal-hearing students, one third were integrated from 1 to 25 hours/week, and the remaining one third for 26 or more hours/week.

Although the number of students enrolled in special schools for the deaf has decreased, these schools do have their proponents. Supporters feel that such schools constitute a less restrictive environment than integrated settings. They argue that the child who is deaf is isolated, socially stigmatized, and discriminated against in regular schools. Many regular schools and regular school teachers are not adequately prepared to deal with children who are deaf. In many cases, the major dissatisfaction with regular schools involves the method of communication the child is taught to use. Regular public schools are based on oral communication. Many deaf children and their families use communication systems that incorporate some form of manual signs.

Regular classroom teachers rarely have adequate training or experience to deal effectively with students who are deaf, and support services for the teacher and student may be inadequate or poorly coordinated. Uninformed personnel and poor support services can make school a frustrating situation for children with any significant degree of hearing loss.

CASE EXAMPLE

In addition to their academic burden, students with hearing loss sometimes must deal with insensitivity, misunderstanding, and prejudice. The following excerpt from a newspaper column chronicles the experiences of a student with a severe hearing loss who was "mainstreamed" in a public school system. This touching account points out many of the challenges that children with hearing loss encounter in a school setting, particularly when the school personnel are not adequately trained to prevent such problems.

VIGNETTE 10–1

Marla frequently came home from school crying because other children made fun of her deafness. When Marla was in the 1st grade, there was one day when the children were to dress as if they were from the period on the TV series *Little House on the Prairie*. Marla did not hear the announcement. "You can imagine how she felt when she was the only one of six hundred students who did not show up dressed like that," said her mother.

One day when she was in the 3rd grade, a teacher planned an April Fool's Day joke on another teacher. Marla did not know that it was a joke because she did not hear the teacher tell the class. Somehow Marla gave the joke away and the teacher who instigated the joke scolded Marla.

"The teacher humiliated me in front of the class," said Marla. "I cried." Harassment from the other children increased after that. It was as if the teacher's action was a signal to the students that it was all right to ridicule the child with the hearing impairment.

There were endless incidents, such as children gathering around her at recess and moving their lips while pretending to talk to her. She would turn up her hearing aid and become frightened because suddenly there was no sound at all while the children would break into hysterics at her panic.

"It was the same old thing day after day," she said. "I always wanted friends. There was really nobody. I was alone most of the time."

In the 10th grade, she became so depressed over not having friends that she thought about killing herself.

In the 11th grade, a classmate named Pam began talking to her and persisted in showing Marla that she accepted her. Marla and Pam became close friends. "Some people even told me to stay away from her because she is deaf," said Pam. "I ignored them. She's just deaf. There's nothing wrong with Marla."

A few months ago, Marla started dating, and she has been accepted at a state university. She said her advice to other children with severe hearing impairments who are being mainstreamed is to be strong. "School is very important," she said. "No matter how bad it gets, just keep going." (Nick Lackeos, *Montgomery Advertiser-Alabama Journal*, May 25, 1986. Reprinted courtesy of The Montgomery Advertiser Company.)

SPECIALISTS IN EDUCATIONAL SETTINGS

Several specialists might be involved with children with hearing impairments in educational settings. Three specialists discussed here, in addition to classroom teachers, are audiologists, speech-language pathologists, and teachers of the hearing impaired.

Some school systems employ audiologists who focus specifically on the assessment and treatment of children with hearing loss enrolled in that school system. These individuals are typically referred to as educational audiologists. Most schools, however, do not employ audiologists and students who require hearing testing may be referred to medical settings. Whether audiologists are employed by school systems or act as outside consultants, they may make several contributions to the academic setting other than testing hearing ability. Audiologists may participate in the development of Individual Education Programs (IEPs) for school-age children or Individual Family Service Plans (IFSPs) for children from birth to 36 months old. They may provide inservice programs for school personnel and advise school districts in planning educational programs and accessibility for students with hearing loss and other auditory dysfunction. They may provide recommendations for environmental modifications to reduce the noise level. And they may give advice regarding the selection, installation, and evaluation of large-area amplification systems (American Speech-Language-Hearing Association, 2004).

Speech-language pathologists are far more likely to be employed by school systems than are audiologists. SLPs may administer hearing screening tests, but any further testing must be done by an audiologist. In terms of providing services to students with hearing impairments, SLPs may provide, among other services, treatment for speech and language problems secondary to hearing loss; auditory training for children with cochlear implants and hearing aids; training in speech reading; visual inspection and listening checks of amplification devices for the purpose of troubleshooting, including verification of appropriate battery voltage (American Speech-Language-Hearing Association, 2004).

Teachers of the deaf and hard-of-hearing are teachers with special training to work in academic settings with students who have significant hearing loss. Teachers of the deaf and hard-of-hearing may be certified by the Council on Education of the Deaf (CED) and may be endorsed for the following areas: parent–infant education, early childhood education, elementary education, secondary education and multidisabilities education. Teachers of the hearing-impaired are not one of the two professions in the discipline of communication disorders (those being audiology and speech-language pathology). Therefore, we do not discuss the role of these teachers in any depth in this chapter.

ASSESSMENT IN EDUCATIONAL SETTINGS

Because the communication disorders specialist in the schools is most frequently an SLP, the hearing testing actually performed in the school setting may be limited to screenings. Most states provide guidelines for when and how students should be screened for hearing loss. The American Speech-Language-Hearing Association (2009) provides the following recommendations for screening school-age children.

School-age children should be screened at the following times.

- On first entry into school
- Every year from kindergarten through 3rd grade
- In 7th grade
- In 11th grade
- Upon entrance into special education
- Upon grade repetition
- Upon entering a new school system without evidence of having passed a previous hearing screening

Further, ASHA indicates that hearing screening should be done in other years when indicated by the following situations.

- Parent/care provider, healthcare provider, teacher, or other school personnel have concerns regarding hearing, speech, language, or learning abilities.
- There is family history of late or delayed onset hereditary hearing loss.
- Otitis media with effusion (fluid in the middle ear) recurs or persists for at least three months.
- There are skull or facial abnormalities, especially those that can cause changes to the structure of the pinna and ear canal.
- Characteristics or other findings occur that are associated with a syndrome known to include hearing loss.
- Head trauma occurs with loss of consciousness.
- There is reported exposure to potentially damaging noise levels or to drugs that frequently cause hearing loss.

HOW TEACHERS CAN HELP IN ASSESSMENT

The formal procedures for identifying hearing loss among students are not infallible. The classroom teacher may be the first person to detect behaviors that are associated with a hearing loss. Unfortunately, these behaviors are often attributed to a lack of attention, antisocial attitudes, or learning problems.

School-based SLPs should make teachers aware that the following behaviors may indicate the presence of a hearing loss.

- Lack of attention during classroom discussions
- Noncompliant behavior
- Frequent requests for repetitions of what has been said
- Confusion and unusual errors in following directions
- Responding inconsistently or inappropriately to environmental sounds or spoken communication
- Turning the head to one side when listening to teachers or other students
- Paying close attention to the speaker's face
- Tendency to be withdrawn or isolated
- Appearing uncomfortable or confused in noisy situations
- Earaches and pulling at the ears
- Dizziness
- Problems in speech, language, reading, and/or writing (based on Phillips, 1975; Flexer, 1994)

INTERVENTION IN EDUCATIONAL SETTINGS

Preschool Children   Early intervention can have a positive effect on the school performance of children with significant hearing loss regardless of the type of school setting or the communication method used (Marschark, Lang, & Albertini, 2002). Early intervention here refers to preschool programs and early parental involvement. Marschark et al. describe several types of preschool programs for children with significant hearing impairments. These include programs administered by public school systems, state health and human services departments, and residential schools. Some programs may take the form of home-based intervention involving periodic visits to the home and instruction provided to the parents. Marschark et al. indicate that preschool programs can help to prepare children for school by helping them to develop realistic and flexible social strategies and can promote language growth whether the communication system used is oral or total. Another benefit of preschool programs for children with hearing loss is that they sensitize parents to the need to be involved in the education of their children.

As most teachers would probably agree, parental involvement is often a key to any child's success in school. However, the parents of children with severe and profound hearing losses face unique problems. The presence of any child with a disability places unusual stress on the family (Luterman, 2001). In the case of a child with a severe or profound hearing loss whose parents have normal hearing, one source of stresses may be how to communicate with the child. Because of this uncertainty about communication with the child, "active, hands-on involvement of the parents in deaf children's education is relatively infrequent" (Marschark et al., 2002, p. 150). Parents of children with severe and profound hearing losses may require some additional training and guidance to provide the type of involvement that will benefit the child. In fact, much of the benefit of early intervention for children with hearing loss may be in helping parents understand and cope with the needs of their child. Calderon, Bargones, and Sidman state:

> From a practical perspective, what early intervention programs seem to accomplish . . . is to help parents settle into their role of being a parent of a deaf or hard of hearing child, develop some level of awareness of the child's needs, fitting the child with hearing aids, and developing basic skills for communication with the child. (Calderon, Bargones, & Sidman, 1998, p. 361)

School-Age Children Audiologists, speech-language pathologists, and other educational professionals can facilitate learning for students with hearing loss by focusing on four areas: providing appropriate amplification, managing the listening environment, developing and improving communication skills, and providing appropriate educational accommodations (Johnson, 2000). Briefly, amplification includes personal hearing aids as well as group amplification systems in classrooms. Managing the listening environment includes the reduction of background noise and preferential seating for the student with a hearing loss. Developing and improving communication skills involves many of the activities discussed under the topic of aural rehabilitation in the medical settings portion of this chapter, including communication repair strategies. It also includes choices between oral and manual communication methods. Educational accommodations are specific to the individual student but may include providing various devices or assistive personnel such as note takers or sign language interpreters. A more detailed discussion of each area follows.

Providing Amplification
Hearing Aids   Many students with hearing loss wear one or sometimes two hearing aids. A properly functioning hearing aid enhances the ability of a student with a hearing loss to benefit from classroom instruction. Some students do not like their aids at first. They are not comfortable with them, or they feel that the hearing aid stigmatizes them. There are many stories of expensive hearing aids being thrown on the school roof or flushed down the toilet. As stated in the medical settings section of this chapter, hearing aids that are not worn or that are not in good working order do not benefit the user. Some authorities suggest that on any given day more than 50 percent of amplification devices worn by school students might not be working (Mainstreaming the student who is deaf or

hard of hearing, 2002). An SLP can perform a few simple checks or can instruct teachers on how to perform these checks to ensure that a student's hearing aid is working.

Be sure the hearing aid is present and in place. The best and most sophisticated hearing aids will not work if they are left at home or in a student's locker.

Examine the aid for obvious signs of damage. Dents, cracks, gouges, or missing parts may signal that the aid has been damaged and will not work as intended. With aids such as behind-the-ear aids, wires leading to the ear mold should be inspected for breaks and kinks.

Be sure that the aid is clear of ear wax and dirt particles. Those portions of the aid that fit into the ear (i.e., all or most of the device as with in-the-ear and in-the-canal aids, or the ear mold in cases of behind-the-ear and body aids) may become clogged with ear wax (cerumen). This will prevent the efficient transfer of sound to the ear. The microphone portion of some aids may become clogged with dust or dirt and prevent it from receiving sound.

Create feedback. When turned on and held between two cupped hands, most hearing aids will produce a squealing sound known as feedback. Feedback is the result of the aid reamplifying its own output. The presence of feedback suggests that the device is on and the battery has at least some power.

Check battery levels. Although feedback suggests that the battery has some power, a more specific measure of a battery's strength may be gained from a battery tester, which teachers and SLPs can keep in the classroom or in a central location in the school. Some students may have locked or tamper-resistant battery compartments. Is such cases, the teacher, SLP, or school nurse should work with the parents to learn how to access the battery.

Perform a listening check. The teacher, SLP, or school nurse should have a hearing aid stethoscope and use it to monitor the sound produced by the hearing aid. The sound should be clear and free from any distortion. Adjustments to the volume control should result in differences in the sound coming from the aid.

Know when and where to get help. Given the rapid pace of development in hearing aid technology and the increasing array of amplification devices and components found in today's classrooms, it is quite possible that some students may have hearing aids for which the previous suggestions prove more difficult than expected. The first source for additional information about the care and function of a specific hearing aid should be the student's parents. They have most likely been provided with information regarding how the hearing aid works, how to spot trouble, and how to make simple and appropriate adjustments. If the parents cannot provide the appropriate information, an audiologist should be consulted. If the school system does not employ the services of an audiologist, the audiologist who fit the student with the hearing aid(s) would be an excellent source of additional information. Finally, hearing aid manufacturers typically supply troubleshooting information for each model of hearing aid they produce. This information may be available online at the manufacturer's Web site. Some manufacturers also publish teacher guides that include instructions and/or forms for general daily hearing aid troubleshooting.

Teachers should be reminded that the microphone of a hearing aid is at the student's ear, and the farther away from the teacher the student sits, the lower the intensity of the teacher's voice. Also, hearing aids amplify noise as well as speech. This means that if a child with a hearing aid is seated near a source of noise, and far from the teacher, the amplified noise may overwhelm the speech of the teacher. These conditions can be improved greatly by the use of classroom amplification systems.

Classroom Amplification Systems Several types of amplification systems have been used in classrooms over the years. These systems, at one time referred to as **auditory training units (ATUs)** or auditory trainers, can be used instead of or with a hearing aid during class activity. Today most of the classroom systems employ FM or infrared signals. These classroom systems serve the same purpose as a hearing aid, that is, to amplify sound. The major difference between a hearing aid and a classroom amplification system is that the microphone for the classroom system is worn by the teacher. The advantages of the teacher wearing the microphone are that background noise in the immediate area of the student is not amplified and that the teacher can move more freely around the room without concern about being too far from the student with a hearing loss. The signal is then sent from the microphone to a receiver worn by the student or in some cases built into the student's hearing aid or cochlear implant. In other situations, the signal may be sent from the microphone to a speaker or speakers placed appropriately in the classroom. In this case, all students hear the amplified signal. After a brief orientation from a speech-language pathologist, audiologist, or company representative, most teachers can operate the equipment quite easily. All that is required is a genuine effort on the part of the teacher to use the instrument for the maximum benefit of the student.

The Listening Environment Although classroom amplification systems overcome some of the issues created by background noise, they cannot completely eliminate interference from such environmental noise. Tye-Murray (1998) identifies three noise conditions that negatively affect the ability of students with hearing aids to hear classroom presentations. These conditions are as follows.

> *Ambient noise:* Tye-Murray (1998) defines **ambient noise** as noise that is present in a room when it is unoccupied. Such noise includes that emanating from heating and air-conditioning systems, fluorescent lights, computers, and hallways.
> *Reverberation:* This refers to echoes caused by sound bouncing off walls, ceilings, and floors. Carpeting and heavy draperies tend to reduce **reverberation**, but not many classrooms are "sound treated" in that way. Therefore, reverberation is a common problem in schools.
> *Background noise:* Background noise is the noise made by other students in the room. Background noise may include such sounds as shuffling papers, talking, coughing, tapping a pencil on the desk, and so forth.

Table 10–3 provides a checklist that may help SLPs and teachers identify and reduce sources of noise and other factors that may interfere with communication between teachers and students with hearing loss.

Communication Training Students with mild and moderate hearing loss tend to have better speech and language skills than those with more severe losses. Some speech and language problems are commonly noted in children with these mild and moderate losses that require the attention of an SLP. For example, children with a history of middle ear problems tend to exhibit deletion of initial consonants and substitution of *h* and the glottal stop in the initial position. These children also tend to have more errors on nasal consonants (Shriberg & Smith, 1983). Paden, Matthies, and Novak (1989) suggest that although most children with histories of middle ear problems overcome any speech delays without intervention, some may not. Warning signs for those who may not catch up to their peers,

TABLE 10–3 Checklist for a Listener-Friendly Classroom

Concern	Yes	No	What Can Be Done to Improve the Situation?
Is there noise outside the classroom such as traffic, construction, or playground?			
Is there noise inside the classroom from fans, lights, heating and/or cooling systems, and the like?			
Are there noisy student activities?			
Is there sufficient light in the room to aid students in speech reading?			
Are there bright lights, light from windows, or reflected light that makes speech reading difficult for the students with hearing impairment?			
Is the room arranged to maximize face-to-face contact between teacher and student(s) with hearing impairment?			
Is the room arranged to maximize the use of visual aids (i.e., adequate chalk board space, electrical outlets for slides and transparencies, projection screen)?			
Is there carpeting and other reverberation-reducing features?			

Source: Some of the suggestions in this table are based on those presented in *Teachers Guide to Hearing*, a pamphlet produced by Oticon Corporation, Somerset, NJ.

according to Paden et al., include the presence of velar deviations, cluster reductions, and lack of improvement four months after insertion of ventilating tubes. The techniques involved in working with these students are similar to those used with any children with phonological problems with the exception that greater emphasis on visual feedback may be required. Several instruments and software packages are available that provide such visual feedback regarding the speech signal. In regard to language problems, the SLP should direct attention to the types of problems identified earlier in Table 10–2.

Communication training for students classified as deaf, that is, students with hearing losses of 70 dB or greater, presents quite a different picture than that for students with less severe losses. Students who are deaf use several methods of communication. These can be broadly categorized as **oral** methods and **manual** methods.

In oral methods, students use speech to express themselves and depend on speechreading (lipreading) and maximum use of amplified hearing to receive spoken language. One of the currently popular approaches to teaching oral communication to children with significant degrees of hearing loss is **auditory-verbal therapy**. This program emphasizes beginning intervention as soon as the hearing loss is detected and involves parents and caregivers as critical parts of the treatment plan. The program focuses on optimal acquisition of spoken language through listening. Amplification by hearing aids or cochlear implants is combined with treatment plans carried out by SLPs, audiologists, or teachers of the hearing impaired who have additional certification as auditory-verbal therapists.

Cued speech is primarily an oral method in which the speaker uses various hand configurations next to the mouth to cue the perception of less visible or easily confused spoken sounds. In some cases, cued speech is incorporated into auditory-verbal therapy.

In manual systems, students communicate through sign language and/or finger-spelling. In sign language, a system of hand configurations and gestures is used to represent words. In finger-spelling, words are spelled letter by letter using a manual alphabet. Finger-spelling is commonly used for proper names or words for which no sign exists. The most widely used manual communication system in this country is **American Sign Language (ASL)**, also called **Ameslan**. The proponents of manual systems suggest that the manual signs facilitate language development in children. Opponents point out that students who communicate through sign can communicate only to those who know sign. Another problem associated with the use of sign language is that the syntactic structure of ASL is not the same as that of spoken English. For example, the question: "Do you want to go to the movies?" in sign would have a syntactic structure more like, "Me you movies go." The ASL syntax can result in difficulties when the student is attempting to read and write in standard English; these are very much like the problems experienced by a dialectal speaker. In an effort to deal with this problem, sign language systems have been developed that use the syntax of spoken English. One of the most widely used of these systems is **Signing Exact English (SEE)**. SEE emphasizes standard English word order, marks verb tense, and indicates irregular verb forms.

A modification of traditional manual approaches is **Total Communication**. The Total Communication philosophy attempts to combine sign language with oral communication. Total communication encourages the use of all available avenues of communication. Although it is primarily a manual system, total communication encourages students to use and to develop whatever speech, speechreading, and hearing ability they may have.

Before the advent of public laws mandating services for children with handicapping conditions, students who were deaf and who were mainstreamed in public schools were usually oral students with reasonably good speech and speechreading skills. Schools have been slow in many cases to provide appropriate accommodations for students who use total or manual communication systems.

Educational Accommodations   In addition to the devices listed previously, the Alexander Graham Bell Society, in a pamphlet titled *Mainstreaming the Student Who Is Deaf or Hard-of-Hearing* (2002), identifies the following human resources that might be employed to assist students with hearing loss in the classroom.

Sign language interpreter: Students for whom auditory input is not sufficient may benefit from the presence of a sign language interpreter in the classroom. A sign language interpreter uses a manual communication system to convey the message of the teacher and other speakers in the classroom for the student with hearing impairment. In some cases, the student may respond in sign and the interpreter would then put the student's message into spoken language for the rest of the class. With the use of sign language interpreters, students using total or manual communication are achieving success in the regular classroom setting. Finding a sign language interpreter is not always an easy task. There are local, state, and national registries of such interpreters. Also, local associations for the deaf, state agencies, and universities with training programs for teachers of the hearing-impaired or for sign language interpreters might be helpful sources of information (Hayes, 1984). In classes where students are expected to take notes, if a student is paying attention to a sign language interpreter, the student may need another method to obtain those notes. In such cases, a transcriber or peer note taker might be employed.

Transcriber: Someone may be assigned to provide the student with a full set of notes to which the student may compare his or her own notes.

Peer note taker: Another student who is a good note taker or who has had some training in taking notes may be employed to supplement the notes the student with hearing impairment is able to take.

The Gallaudet Research Institute survey for the 2007–2008 academic year indicates that, in addition to audiological services, the most common support services provided to students with hearing loss are speech therapy (53 percent), itinerant teacher (41 percent), sign language interpreting services (21 percent), classroom assistant or aide (19 percent), occupational therapy (10 percent), counseling (9 percent), and tutor (9 percent) (Gallaudet Research Institute, 2008).

SUGGESTIONS FOR TEACHERS OF STUDENTS WITH HEARING LOSS

Classroom teachers are not expected to be experts on the habilitation of students with hearing loss, and neither should they be expected to provide one-to-one instruction for the child with a hearing impairment at the cost of the other students. There are, however, several suggestions that school-based SLPs can provide to teachers to help meet the needs of their students with hearing loss.

1. *Provide favorable seating.* The student with a hearing loss should be seated close to the teacher and away from background noise, such as the noise from a hallway or a street. Garwood (1987) suggests that movable desks and flexibility in arranging seating during various activities allows the student with a hearing loss an opportunity to observe and participate in classroom activities. However, remember that moving chairs and desks may produce very distracting background noise. Placing felt pads or tennis balls that have been cut in half on the feet of desks and chairs can cut down on noise when the furniture is moved. Students with hearing aids should be seated to make maximum use of the aid. For example, they should not be seated with the aid against a wall (Kampfe, 1984; Northcott, 1973). Also, children with hearing impairments should be seated with their back to windows and bright light sources because many depend on being able to see the face of the speaker clearly.
2. *Remember that group activities may pose special problems for the child with a hearing impairment* (Gildston, 1973). Some students with hearing impairments may not be aware that group members out of the line of vision are talking. Also, group activities can sometimes be associated with higher-than-normal levels of background noise.
3. *Face the student when speaking and be sure that the student is looking at you.* Other children may be able to listen while looking at their work, taking notes, or while you are facing the board, but students with hearing impairments comprehend best when they can see the speaker (Reynolds & Birch, 1988). It is especially important for the teacher to remember not to talk while facing the chalkboard and not to cover his or her mouth with papers and/or books when giving information to the class.
4. *Provide written instructions and summaries.* Written information helps students with impaired hearing keep in touch with lesson content. Teachers can list on the board simple lesson outlines, key vocabulary words, and homework assignments (Harrington, 1976).
5. *Speak clearly but naturally.* Children with hearing loss often depend on facial cues to aid understanding (Harrington, 1976). To help remember critical factors in speaking to students with hearing impairment, Garwood (1987) suggests **S-P-E-E-C-H** as a mnemonic device:

    S = State the topic to be discussed.
    P = Pace conversation at a moderate speed, allowing occasional pauses to aid comprehension.

E = Enunciate clearly without exaggerated lip movements.

E = Enthusiastically communicate, using body language and natural gestures.

CH = Check comprehension before changing topics. Ask the student questions to evaluate understanding. Do not simply ask, "Do you understand?" and rely on a nod or a "yes." The student may not be willing to admit a problem understanding the material. Be alert to signs of confusion, such as a blank stare or unusual errors in following directions.

6. *Rephrase and restate instructions and directions.* This is especially important when it is apparent that the student with impaired hearing is having trouble understanding. Some words contain sounds that are not easily recognized by students with hearing-impairment. Many students with impaired hearing have some delay in language development and may not be familiar with the vocabulary or grammatical structure used (Garwood, 1987).

7. *Use a "preteach-teach-postteach" strategy* (Reynolds & Birch, 1988). In this approach, the classroom teacher discusses upcoming lessons with other professionals who may be working with the student with hearing loss, such as a teacher of the hearing-impaired or a speech-language pathologist. The special teacher or speech-language pathologist then ensures that the student understands key words and concepts to be used in the coming class presentation. The classroom teacher presents the lesson and reports back to the other professionals any apparent difficulties the student with hearing impairment had with the lesson. The special teacher or speech-language pathologist then reviews the concepts with which the student experienced difficulty. This strategy is an excellent way to coordinate the efforts of several professionals and a good example of a consultative model in action.

8. *Establish positive attitudes toward the student with a hearing impairment.* Encourage participation in expressive activities such as reading, "show-and-tell," and creative dramatics (Garwood, 1987). Have the speech-language pathologist or teacher of the hearing-impaired explain hearing loss (and hearing aids if appropriate) to the class (Stassen, 1973; Harrington, 1976; Brill, 1978). Teachers serve as models for the children in their classes. Recall from the story of Marla earlier in this chapter that it was a teacher's ridicule of a deaf student that seemed to trigger the same behavior by other students.

AUDITORY PROCESSING DISORDER (APD)

A problem that should be discussed here, although it is not a problem of hearing acuity, is the condition known as **auditory processing disorder (APD)**. Until recently, this condition was frequently called central auditory processing disorder (CAPD). APD has many manifestations and therefore many definitions depending on the discipline of the person providing the definition. The situation is further complicated by the fact that APD is not universally recognized as a legitimate disorder category. Some feel that the symptoms suggesting APD are really symptoms of a broader language impairment or reflective of ADHD (Cacace & McFarland, 1998). Many definitions are highly technical and esoteric, but basically APD is a problem understanding the meaning of incoming sounds (Flexer, 1994) or as Lasky and Katz (1983) put it, a problem in what one does with what one hears. The ears work well and do their job in getting the signal to the brain, but the problem lies with the way the signal is decoded and interpreted in the central nervous system. Many children labeled as learning disabled may have APD. According to Baran and Musiek (1995), the symptoms of APD may include the following.

- Problems following complex auditory directions
- Problems hearing in noisy backgrounds
- Difficulty determining from where sounds originate (localizing sound)
- Trouble participating in long, quickly spoken conversations
- Distractibility
- More difficulty with verbally based subjects such as reading than with nonverbally based subjects such as mathematics
- Lack of musical appreciation
- Tinnitus (noise in the ear or head)
- Missing subtle acoustic cues
- Unusual difficulty learning foreign languages

It should be readily apparent that children who exhibit various combinations of the preceding symptoms may experience difficulty in a typical classroom setting. These children may be perceived as less intelligent than they really are, inattentive, lazy, disruptive, and/or uncooperative. As with some children with language disorders, children with APD may experience greater difficulty in school as the demands for language processing increase, usually around third grade. Many of the suggestions provided earlier in this chapter for students with hearing impairment would also be effective strategies for children with APD. In addition to those suggestions, Johnson and Danhauer (1999) provide the following suggestions for teachers of children with APD:

1. *Reduce distractions.* Avoid extraneous noise and visual distractions, especially when providing new or important information.
2. *Be sure that you have the child's attention.* Saying the child's name and gently touching his or her shoulder are easy ways to refocus attention. Words and phrases such as *listen, ready*, and *remember this* may be helpful in signaling an important message.
3. *Reduce those noises that cannot be eliminated.* The use of sound attenuation ear plugs or ear muffs may help the child to "tune out" those noises that cannot be eliminated from a school environment.
4. *Use visual aids.* The use of overhead projectors, LCD projectors, and computers likely enhances the learning experience for all children in the class but may be especially helpful to the child with APD.

5. *Avoid auditory exhaustion.* Remember that children with APD must work hard at listening. This can lead to fatigue. The teacher may be able to schedule intensive listening activities early in the day or alternate auditory tasks with nonauditory tasks.

6. *Tape record important information.* A tape may be made of critical information to provide the child with an opportunity to hear the information again at a later time when he or she is more receptive to this type of auditory input.

7. *Assign a "buddy."* Another child who appears to be strong in auditory processing may be assigned to assist the student who is having difficulty. The nature of that assistance will differ with the specific individuals and class material involved.

One additional point should be made before ending the discussion of APD. As stated earlier, this condition is not recognized as a disorder that affects school-aged children (Cacace & McFarland, 1998). Therefore, a diagnosis of APD does not qualify as an eligible condition for treatment in most school systems. Children showing the symptoms of APD are often treated under a diagnosis of receptive language disorder.

Hearing loss can range in severity from mild to profound and can be present at birth or acquired at any age. The degree of severity and the age at which the hearing loss occurs are significant factors in determining its effects on communication, the types of accommodations required in educational and employment settings, and the individual's quality of life. Speech-language pathologists and audiologists, whether working in an educational or medical setting, can facilitate effective communication for individuals with hearing loss by providing appropriate amplification devices, aural rehabilitation activities, and counseling for patients, families, and other professionals in the patient's environment.

Terms to Know

Deaf	Microtia
Hard-of-hearing	Atresia
Hearing threshold	Cerumen
Threshold	Otitis media
Slight hearing impairment	Ventilating tubes
Mild hearing impairment	Otosclerosis
Mild-to-moderate hearing impairment	TORCH infections
Moderate hearing impairment	Ototoxic
Severe hearing impairment	Presbycusis
Profound hearing impairment	Audiologist
Congenital hearing loss	Otolaryngologist
Prelingual hearing loss	Otologists
Postlingual hearing loss	Audiometer
Conductive hearing loss	Pure tone audiometer
Sensorineural hearing loss	Screening test
Mixed hearing loss	Threshold test

Air conduction test
Bone conduction test
Audiogram
Tympanometer
Canal aids
In-the-ear aids
Behind-the-ear aids
Ear mold
Cochlear implant
Aural rehabilitation
Lipreading
Speechreading
Conversational repair strategies

Auditory training unit (ATU)
Ambient noise
Reverberation
Oral methods
Manual methods
Auditory-verbal therapy
Cued speech
American Sign Language (ASL)
Ameslan
Signing Exact English (SEE)
Total Communication
S-P-E-E-C-H
Auditory processing disorder (APD)

Study Questions

1. Identify the parts that all hearing aids have in common. Provide suggestions as to how a teacher or SLP can troubleshoot a faulty aid.
2. Provide specific classroom behaviors or teaching techniques that can be employed to enhance the learning of students with hearing impairment.
3. Why might a student with hearing impairment have difficulty with reading and writing?
4. Discuss the advantages and disadvantages of oral and manual communication methods for the deaf.
5. Identify other professionals who work with students with hearing impairment, and discuss how these other professionals could be of help to the classroom teacher.
6. Discuss accommodations that might be appropriate for individuals with hearing loss in various job settings.

Bibliography

American Academy of Otolaryngology–Head and Neck Surgery. (2009). Fact Sheet: What you should know about otosclerosis. Retrieved June 3, 2010, from http://www.entnet. org/HealthInformation/otosclerosis.cfm

American Speech-Language-Hearing Association. (2004). *Scope of practice in audiology*. Retrieved June 3, 2010, from http://www.asha.org/docs/html/SP2004-00192.html.

American Speech-Language-Hearing Association. (2009). Hearing screening. Retrieved June 3, 2010, from http://www.asha.org/public/hearing/testing.

Anderson, K., & Matkin, N. (2007). Relationship of degree of long term hearing loss to psychosocial impact and educational needs. Retrieved June 3, 2010, from http://www. sifteranderson.com

Baran, J., & Musiek, F. (1995). Central auditory processing disorders in children and adults. In L. G. Wall (Ed.), *Hearing for the speech-language pathologist and health care professional.* Boston, MA: Butterworth-Heinemann.

Berg, F. (1986). Characteristics of the target population. In F. Berg, J. C. Blair, J. H. Viehweg, & A. Wilson-Vlotman (Eds.), *Educational audiology for the hard of hearing child.* New York, NY: Grune and Stratton.

Brill, R. G. (1978). *Mainstreaming the prelingually deaf child.* Washington, DC: Gallaudet College Press.

Cacace, A. T., & McFarland, D. J. (1998). Central auditory processing disorder in school-aged children: A critical review. *Journal of Speech, Language, and Hearing Research, 41,* 355–373.

Calderone , R., Bargones, J., & Sidman, S. (1998). Characteristics of hearing families and their young deaf and hard of hearing children: Early intervention follow-up. *American Annals of the Deaf, 143,* 347–362.

Chorost, S. (1988). The hearing-impaired child in the mainstream: A survey of attitudes of regular classroom teachers. *Volta Review, 90,* 7–12.

Davidson, S. (1995). Hearing aids. In L. G. Wall (Ed.), *Hearing for the speech-language pathologist and health care professional.* Boston, MA: Butterworth-Heinemann.

Davis, L. (1995). Speech and language characteristics of children and adults with hearing impairments. In L. G. Wall (Ed.), *Hearing for the speech-language pathologist and health care professional.* Boston, MA: Butterworth-Heinemann.

Dobie, R. A., & Berlin, C. I. (1979). Influence of otitis media on hearing and development. *Annals of Otology, Rhinology and Laryngology, 88,* 48–53.

Epps, R. E., Pittelkow, M. R., & Su, W. P. (1995). TORCH syndrome. *Seminars in Dermatology, 14,* 179–186.

Fitch, J. L., Williams, T. F., & Etienne, J. E. (1982). A community based high risk register for hearing loss. *Journal of Speech and Hearing Disorders, 47,* 373–375.

Flexer, C. (1994). *Facilitating hearing and listening in young children.* San Diego, CA: Singular.

Friel-Patti, S., & Finitzo, T. (1990). Language learning in a prospective study of otitis media with effusion in the first two years of life. *Journal of Speech and Hearing Research, 33,* 188–194.

Gallaudet Research Institute. (2008). *Regional and national summary report of data from the 2007–2008 annual survey of deaf and hard of hearing children and youth.* Washington, DC: GRI, Gallaudet University.

Garwood, V. P. (1987). Audiology in the public school setting. In F. N. Martin (Ed.), *Hearing disorders in children.* Austin, TX: Pro-Ed.

Gildston, P. (1973). The hearing-impaired child in the classroom: A guide for the classroom teacher. In W.H. Northcott (Ed.), *The hearing-impaired child in the regular classroom: Preschool, elementary, and secondary years. A guide for the classroom teacher/administrator.* Washington, DC: Alexander Graham Bell Association for the Deaf.

Grievink, E., Peters, S., vanBon, W., & Schilder, A. (1993). The effects of early bilateral otitis media with effusion on language ability: A prospective cohort study. *Journal of Speech and Hearing Research, 36,* 1004–1012.

Harrington, J. D. (1976). The integration of deaf children and youth through educational strategies. Why? When? How? *Highlights, 53,* 8–18.

Harrison, C. J., & Belhorn, T. H. (1991). Antibiotic treatment failures in acute otitis media. *Pediatric Annals, 12,* 600–610.

Hayes, J. L. (1984). Interpreting in the K–12 mainstream setting. In R. H. Hull & K. L. Dilka (Eds.), *The hearing-impaired child in school.* Orlando, FL: Grune and Stratton.

Hodgson, W. R. (1978). Disorders of hearing. In P. H. Skinner & R. L. Shelton (Eds.), *Speech, language and hearing: Normal processes and disorders.* New York, NY: Wiley.

Job Accommodation Network. U.S. Department of Labor, Office of Disability Employment Policy. Retrieved June 3, 2010, from Searchable online accommodation resource http://askjan.org/soar/hearing/hearingq.html.

Johnson, C. D. (2000). Management of hearing in the educational setting. In J. Alpiner & P. McCarthy (Eds.), *Rehabilitative audiology: Children and adults* (3rd ed.). Philadelphia, PA: Lippincott Williams & Wilkins.

Johnson, C. E., & Danhauer, J. (1999). *Guidebook for support programs in aural rehabilitation.* San Diego, CA: Singular.

Joint Committee on Infant Hearing. (2007). Year 2007 position statement: Principles and guidelines for early hearing detection and intervention programs. *Pediatrics, 120,* 898–921.

Kampfe, C. M. (1984). Mainstreaming: Some practical suggestions for teachers and administrators. In R. H. Hull & K. L. Dilka (Eds.), *The hearing-impaired child in school.* Orlando, FL: Grune and Stratton.

Klein, J. O. (1991). Prevention of acute otitis media. *Seminars in Hearing, 12,* 140–145.

Klein, J. O., Baker, C. J., Remington, J. S., & Wilson, C. B. (2006). Current concepts of infections of the fetus and newborn infant. In J. S. Remington, J. O. Klein, C. B. Wilson, & C. J. Baker (Eds.), *Infectious diseases of the fetus and newborn infant* (6th ed.). Philadelphia, PA: Elsevier Saunders.

Kodman, F. (1963). Educational status of hard-of-hearing children in the classroom. *Journal of Speech and Hearing Disorders, 28,* 297–299.

Lahey, M. (1988). *Language disorders and language development.* New York, NY: Macmillan.

Lasky, E. Z., & Katz, J. (1983). Perspectives on central auditory processing. In E. Z. Lasky & J. Katz (Eds.), *Central auditory processing disorders: Problems of speech, language, and hearing disorders.* Baltimore, MD: University Park Press.

Leavitt, R. J. (1984). Hearing aids and other amplifying devices for hearing-impaired children. In R. H. Hull & K. L. Dilka (Eds.), *The hearing-impaired child in school.* Orlando, FL: Grune and Stratton.

Luterman, D. M. (2001). *Counseling persons with communication disorders and their families* (4th ed.). Austin, TX: Pro-Ed.

Madell, J., & Montano, J. (2000). Audiologic rehabilitation in different employment settings. In J. Alpiner & P. McCarthy (Eds.), *Rehabilitative audiology: Children and Adults.* Baltimore, MD: Lippincott Williams & Wilkins.

Mainstreaming the student who is deaf or hard-of-hearing: A guide for professionals, teachers and parents. (2002). Washington, DC: Alexander Graham Bell Association.

Marschark, M., Lang, H. G., & Albertini, J. A. (2002). *Educating deaf students.* New York, NY: Oxford University Press.

Montgomery, A. A., & Houston, K. T. (2000). The hearing impaired adult: Management of communication deficits and tinnitus. In J. Alpiner & P. McCarthy (Eds.), *Rehabilitative audiology: Children and Adults.* Baltimore, MD: Lippincott Williams & Wilkins.

Moores, D. F. (1987). *Educating the deaf: Psychology, principles, and practices* (3rd ed.). Boston, MA: Houghton Mifflin.

Munoz, K., Shisler, L., Moeller, M., & White, K. (2009). Improving the quality of early hearing detection and intervention services through physician outreach. *Seminars in Hearing, 30,* 184–192.

National Institute on Deafness and Other Communication Disorders. (2008). Noise-induced hearing loss. Retrieved June 3, 2010, from http://www.nidcd.nih.gov/health/hearing/noise.asp

Newton, L. (1987). The educational management of hearing-impaired children. In F. N. Martin (Ed.), *Hearing disorders in children.* Austin, TX: Pro-Ed.

Northcott, W. H. (1973). A speech clinician as multi-disciplinary team member. In W. H. Northcott (Ed.), *The hearing-impaired child in the regular classroom: Preschool, elementary, and secondary years. A guide for the classroom teacher/administrator.* Washington, DC: Alexander Graham Bell Association for the Deaf.

Northern, J. L., & Downs, M. P. (1984). *Hearing in children* (3rd ed.). Baltimore, MD: Lippincott Williams & Wilkins.

Paden, E., Matthies, M., & Novak, M. (1989). Recovery from OME-related phonologic delay following tube placement. *Journal of Speech and Hearing Disorders, 54,* 232–242.

Patrick, P. E. (1987). Identification audiometry. In F. N. Martin (Ed.), *Hearing disorders in children.* Austin, TX: Pro-Ed.

Paul, R., Lynn, T., & Lohr-Flansers, M. (1993). History of middle ear involvement and speech/language development in late talkers. *Journal of Speech and Hearing Research, 36,* 1055–1062.

Peterson, M. E., & Bell, T. S. (2008). *Foundations of audiology: A practical approach.* Upper Saddle River, NJ: Pearson Education.

Phillips, P. P. (1975). *Speech and hearing problems in the classroom.* Lincoln, NE: Cliffs Notes.

Quigley, S., & Thomure, R. (1968). *Some effects of a hearing impairment on school performance.* Champaign-Urbana, IL: University of Illinois Institute of Research on Exceptional Children.

Reynolds, M. C., & Birch, J. W. (1988). *Adaptive mainstreaming: A primer for teachers and principals.* New York, NY: Longman.

Robb, M., Psak, J., & Pang-Ching, G. (1993). Chronic otitis media and early speech development: A case study. *International Journal of Pediatric Otorhinolaryngology, 26,* 117–127.

Roberts, J. E., Rosenfeld, R. M., & Zeisel, S. A. (2004). Otitis media and speech and language: A meta analysis of prospective studies. *Pediatrics, 113*(3 pt 1), 238–248.

Robin, N. R. (2008). *Medical genetics: Its application to speech, hearing, and craniofacial disorders.* San Diego, CA: Plural.

Schildroth, A., & Hotto, S. (1994). Inclusion or exclusion? Deaf students and the inclusion movement. *American Annals of the Deaf, 139*, 239–243.

Shriberg, L., & Smith, A. (1983). Phonological correlates of middle ear involvement in speech-delayed children: A methodological note. *Journal of Speech and Hearing Research, 26*, 293–297.

Smedley, T. C., & Schow, R. L. (1998). Problem-solving and extending the life of your hearing aids. In R. Carmen (Ed.), *A consumer handbook on hearing loss and hearing aids: A bridge to healing.* Sedona, AZ: Auricle Ink.

Stach, B. (1998). *Clinical audiology: An introduction.* San Diego, CA: Singular.

Stassen, R. A. (1973). I have one in my class who's wearing hearing aids! In W. H. Northcott (Ed.), *The hearing-impaired child in a regular classroom: Preschool, elementary, and secondary years. A guide for the classroom teacher/administrator.* Washington, DC: Alexander Graham Bell Association for the Deaf.

Sweetow, R., & Henderson Sabes, J. (2006). The need for and development of an adaptive listening and communication enhancement (LACE) program. *Journal of the American Academy of Audiologists, 17*, 538–558.

Teele, D., Klein, J., Chase, C., Menyuk, P., & Rosner, B. (1990). Otitis media in infancy and intellectual ability, school achievement, speech and language at age 7 years. *Journal of Infectious Diseases, 162*, 685–694.

Tye-Murray, N. (1998). *Foundations of aural rehabilitation.* San Diego, CA: Singular.

Tye-Murray, N. (2002). Conversation made easy: *Speechreading and conversation training for individuals who have hearing loss (adults and teenagers).* St. Louis, MO: CID Publications.

Weinstein, B. (2000). *Geriatric audiology.* New York, NY: Thieme.

Chapter 11

CLEFT LIP/PALATE AND RELATED CRANIOFACIAL ANOMALIES

NATURE OF THE PROBLEM

Several birth defects are associated with malformations of the skull and/or the face. Such malformations are referred to as craniofacial anomalies. Because the craniofacial area includes the brain, cranial nerves, and the speech and hearing structures, children with craniofacial anomalies frequently exhibit speech, language, and/or hearing problems. The problems encountered by individuals with craniofacial anomalies are sometimes exacerbated by unwarranted beliefs and attitudes of parents and others. Conditions that include facial disfigurements seem to be associated with an unusual number of folk beliefs. These folk beliefs vary from one culture to another. In some cultures, children with craniofacial anomalies are considered to be "witch-babies" and are left to die (Scheper-Hughes, 1990). In other cultures, such birth defects are blamed on some sin, indiscretion, or unkind attitude attributed to one or both parents during pregnancy (Meyerson, 1990; Toliver-Weddington, 1990). Even relatively sophisticated people tend to assume that a facial disfigurement implies reduced intellectual capacity and, therefore, underestimate the abilities of students with craniofacial anomalies. It is important for educational and medical professionals to understand the effects of craniofacial anomalies on communication skills and academic performance, and to draw conclusions about individuals with craniofacial anomalies based on their performance rather than on any preconceived notions about such individuals.

CLEFT LIP AND PALATE

Clefts of the lip and/or the palate are the most common craniofacial anomalies associated with communication disorders. A cleft is an opening or a separation. **Cleft palate** refers to an opening that may involve the soft palate only, or it may extend through both the soft and hard palates. In some cases, the membranous covering of the palate may be intact, but muscles underneath have failed to develop properly, resulting in a **submucous cleft palate**. **Cleft lip** involves a vertical separation of the upper lip on one or both sides. Occasionally, a cleft of the lip may occur at the midline. Cleft lip can exist alone, or it may involve the alveolar ridge as well. In some cases, cleft lip and palate occur together, creating a cleft that extends through the soft and hard palates, the alveolar ridge, and the lip. Such an extensive malformation is referred to as a complete cleft. **Figures 11–1** through **11–4** provide illustrations of various types of clefts.

CAUSATION AND INCIDENCE

Both cleft lip and cleft palate result from a failure of the structures to grow together and fuse properly during embryonic development. This fusion occurs quite early, at about 6 weeks of gestation for the lip and about 8 to 10 or 12 weeks for the palate (Bzoch, 2004; Robin, 2008; Peterson-Falzone, Hardin-Jones, & Karnell, 2010). The causes of cleft lip and palate are not fully understood. It appears that in most cases clefts that are not associated with syndromes result from an interaction of genetic and environmental factors known as

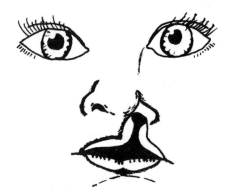

FIGURE 11–1   Unilateral cleft of the lip.
Source: Illustration by Mark J. Moran.

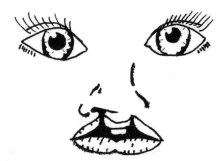

FIGURE 11–2   Bilateral cleft of the lip.
Source: Illustration by Mark J. Moran.

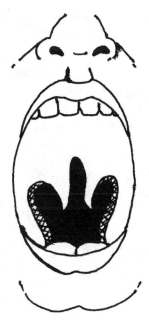

FIGURE 11–3 Cleft of the soft palate.
Source: Illustration by Mark J. Moran.

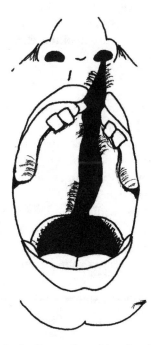

FIGURE 11–4 Complete cleft including soft and hard palates, alveolar ridge, and lip.
Source: Illustration by Mark J. Moran.

multifactorial inheritance (Robin, 2008). Multifactorial disorders tend to follow different and more complex inheritance patterns than do the single-gene inheritance patterns most frequently studied in high school biology classes (Gorlin & Baylis, 2009). According to the Cleft Palate Foundation (2007), 1 in every 600 newborns is affected by cleft lip and/ or cleft palate, making this disorder the most common birth defect in the United States. The incidence of cleft lip varies with race and is higher among Native Americans and Asians and lower among people of African descent. Clefts of the palate do not show such a racial difference. Clefts of the lip occur more commonly in males, and isolated clefts of the palate are more common among females (Robin, 2008; Peterson-Falzone et al., 2010). There is some evidence that the incidence of clefts of the lip and palate is increasing as a result of factors such as increases in teenage pregnancies, pregnancies in older women, and consumption of drugs and alcohol during pregnancy (Slavkin, 1992).

Cleft lip and palate are most often repaired surgically. In the United States, surgery to repair a cleft lip is usually performed early in the first year of life, most typically at about 2 or 3 months of age (Seagle, 2004). The timing of surgery to repair the palate is somewhat more variable and depends on factors such as the extent of the cleft, the general health of the child, and the philosophy of the surgeon. It is generally believed that earlier surgery benefits speech development, but palatal surgery performed at too early an age may interfere with facial growth patterns. Surgery to close a cleft palate in this country is most commonly performed between 6 and 18 months of age (LaRossa, 2000). It must be made clear, however, that surgical closure of the cleft may not eliminate all of the speech, language, and hearing problems associated with this condition. Even after surgery, some children with cleft palates may exhibit any or all of the communication disorders discussed in this chapter and may require follow-up surgery.

SPEECH PROBLEMS

Once repaired, clefts of the lip rarely cause speech problems. A cleft palate affects speech primarily because it prevents the complete separation of the nasal cavity from the oral cavity. Although surgery can usually close the cleft, the soft palate (velum) may be too short or too immobile following surgery to close off the nasal cavity adequately. This condition is called **velopharyngeal insufficiency (VPI)**. Some students with cleft palates require follow-up surgical procedures during the elementary school years to reduce or eliminate VPI.

Speech problems associated with cleft palate are most often problems of resonance and articulation. The most common resonance problem exhibited by cleft palate speakers is **hypernasality**. Hypernasality is what many people refer to simply as a nasal quality, or some may say that hypernasal speakers sound as if they "talk through their nose." Hypernasality is the perceptual result of sound passing inappropriately into the nose. Recall from Chapter 2 that in English, the only sounds that are produced with the nasal cavity coupled with the oral cavity are m, n, and ng. Sound passing into the nose on any other phonemes, especially vowels, causes the speaker to be perceived as excessively nasal.

Articulation problems associated with cleft palate typically involve those consonants that require the speaker to build up oral air pressure, that is, stops (p, b, t, d, k, g), fricatives (f̱, v̱, ṯẖ, s̱, ẕ, s̱ẖ), and affricates (c̱ẖ, j̱ [as in *joy*]). The articulation errors involving these sounds most often take one of two forms: nasal emission, or compensatory articulations. **Nasal emission** refers to air escaping through the nose as a sound is produced. The result is often a "snorting" sound that distorts the target phoneme and reduces intelligibility.

Compensatory articulations refer to changes in the way a sound is produced to adjust for structural inadequacy. Compensatory articulations exhibited by speakers with cleft palate frequently involve moving the place of production farther back in the vocal tract to prevent the loss of air pressure through the nose. For example, rather than producing the s̱ sound at the alveolar ridge, the speaker with a history of cleft palate may attempt to constrict the airflow by placing the tongue against the throat (pharynx), producing a compensation known as a pharyngeal fricative. Another common compensation this population uses is the glottal stop. In this production, which may be substituted for any or all stops, airflow is arrested and then suddenly released at the level of the vocal folds. The result is that words such as *battle* and *button* are produced as "baUHl" and "buUHn." Once learned, these compensatory articulations may be difficult to eliminate. For that reason, early speech training places emphasis on correct placement to prevent the development and habituation of the compensatory productions.

In addition to the articulation problems described here, children with a history of clefting may also exhibit errors on nonpressure consonants such as ḻ and ṟ (Van Demark, 1964; Trost-Cardamone & Bernthal, 1993). Errors on nonpressure consonants may be part of a general delay in speech and language and represent more of a developmental disorder rather than a compensatory or structural problem. How a child's underlying speech sound system is affected by structural deficiencies early in life is not clear but is a subject of ongoing research (Kuehn & Moller,1990; Chapman, 2009).

HEARING PROBLEMS

Another factor that may contribute to communication problems and academic difficulties of students with cleft palate is an extremely high incidence of middle ear disease. This middle ear disease frequently results in a fluctuating mild to moderate, bilateral (both ears) conductive hearing loss (Witzel, 1995). The incidence of middle ear disease in children with clefts has been reported to be as high as 100 percent (Paradise, Bluestone, & Felder, 1969). To be clear, this is a problem in children with clefts of the palate. Children with cleft lip only seem to encounter middle ear problems at about the same rate as children without clefts. The middle ear disease and resulting hearing loss in children with cleft palate most likely result from an inability of the Eustachian tube to properly ventilate the middle ear space, thus causing it to fill with fluid that may become infected. This condition, as you may remember from Chapter 10, is called otitis media. Although surgical repair of the palate does seem to improve the situation in many children, in many others the hearing problems last through most of childhood and beyond (Gerson, 1990). Therefore, children with cleft palate are at risk for hearing loss not only during critical periods of speech and language development, but also during early school years when so much critical information is provided through the auditory channel. As discussed in Chapter 10, mild to moderate conductive hearing losses, especially those that may come and go, do not always have obvious symptoms. The effects of a mild conductive hearing loss on language development have not been proven beyond a reasonable doubt. However, it is certainly a factor that speech and language professionals must keep in mind when discussing language development among children with cleft palate.

LANGUAGE PROBLEMS

It is important to realize that children with clefts cannot be viewed as a homogeneous group when considering language abilities. Golding-Kushner (2001) indicates that there is a wide variety of language abilities among children with clefts and many exhibit normal language development. However, as a group, children with clefts are more likely than their noncleft peers to exhibit delayed language development (Scherer & D'Antonio, 1995; Broen, Devers, Doyle, Prouty, & Moller, 1998; Golding-Kushner, 2001). The reasons for this delay are not clear. Several possible factors may contribute. As mentioned, the conductive hearing loss that is so common among these children may affect language development. Another possible factor is reduced language stimulation. Some children with cleft palates spend a great deal of time in hospitals and at home recovering from surgery. This is not an ideal situation for language stimulation. Some parents do not interact with their handicapped children in the same way as their nonhandicapped children, resulting in reduced language stimulation. Another factor that appears to play a role in language ability is the type of cleft. Children with isolated clefts of the palate with no involvement of the lip tend to exhibit more significant language problems than do children with clefts that involve the lip (Richman, 1980; Richman & Eliason, 1984; Golding-Kushner, 2001).

More than likely, the language delay seen in children with cleft palate reflects an interaction of those and other factors yet to be defined. Regardless of the cause, it appears that many children with clefts would benefit from early language intervention (Brookshire, Lynch, & Fox, 1984; Hahn, 1989). Such early intervention seems to be effective. In one particularly interesting study (Pecyna, Feeney-Giacoma, & Nieman, 1987), it was reported that infants with cleft palate between the ages of 12 and 18 months received higher scores on a test of the concept of object permanence than a control group of noncleft peers. Pecyna et al. suggest that the superior performance by the cleft palate group may have been the result of increased environmental stimulation by their parents.

Parents and teachers should be aware that the potential for language problems exists among children with clefts. As discussed in Chapter 6, many children experience academic difficulty as a result of language problems, even when those problems are too subtle to be identified by standard language tests. Such may be the case with many students with clefts.

SYNDROMES THAT INCLUDE CLEFT LIP/PALATE

In some cases, a cleft lip and/or cleft palate occurs as an isolated condition. In other cases, the cleft may be part of a collection of disorders occurring together called a **syndrome**. There are hundreds of syndromes that include craniofacial anomalies. Peterson-Falzone et al. (2010)

indicate that there are more than 300 syndromes associated with oral-facial clefting. Obviously, it is beyond the scope of the present text to attempt to describe this plethora of conditions. In this chapter, we hope to provide a brief description of some of the more commonly occurring syndromes associated with clefts of the lip and palate, to provide a brief glossary of medical terms used to describe some of the malformations characterizing these syndromes, and to discuss the adjustment of individuals with facial disfigurements. **Table 11–1** lists syndromes that are frequently associated with craniofacial anomalies and provides a brief description of the clinical signs related to each syndrome.

TABLE 11–1 Brief Descriptions of Syndromes That Include Clefts of the Lip and/or the Palate

Abruzzo-Erickson syndrome	Cleft palate, short stature, sensorineural hearing loss, coloboma (a deformity of a part of the eye)
Apert syndrome	Premature closure of the skull resulting in disorders in the shape of skull and face, including excessive distance between the eyes, protrusion of the eyes, down slanting of the eyes, midfacial deficiency or underdevelopment, webbing of the hands and feet, possible conductive hearing loss, and possible cognitive involvement
Crouzon syndrome	Similar to Apert syndrome, but less severe and no webbing of hands and feet
Cornelia de Lange syndrome	Microcephaly, excessive body hair, low-set large ears, small nose, retardation, limb disorders
Fetal alcohol syndrome	Low birth weight, cleft lip or palate or both, microcephaly, and unusual facial features that may include a short nose and an underdeveloped midface area, frequently cognitive delays and ADHD
Nager syndrome	Severe micrognathia (underdeveloped mandible), cleft palate, absent or underdeveloped thumbs, external and middle ear anomalies resulting in conductive hearing loss
Oro-facial-digital syndrome (OFD) Type II	Lobed tongue (the anterior portion of the tongue is divided into two or more roundish projections), more than normal number of digits, cleft lip, underdevelopment of the chin (mandible), malformation of the outer and possibly middle ear, conductive hearing loss
Pierre Robin sequence	Extremely underdeveloped chin (mandible) that causes the tongue to be pushed back into the pharynx possibly resulting in respiratory difficulty, cleft palate, or possible conductive hearing loss; may exist as an isolated condition or as part of several other syndromes
Stickler syndrome	Myopia, retinal changes, early/progressive arthritis, sensorineural hearing loss, cleft palate, Pierre Robin sequence
Treacher Collins syndrome	Down-slanting eyes, defects in the shape of the eye, underdeveloped cheek bones and mandible, defects in auditory canal and middle ear, conductive hearing loss, cleft palate
Velocardiofacial syndrome	Characteristic facial appearance, congenital cardiovascular disease, speech problems, cognitive delays, psychological and behavioral problems, cleft palate (overt or submucosal)

Source: Data from Cohen (1978), Jung (1989), Shprintzen (1997), and Robin (2008).

TABLE 11–2   Selected Medical Terms Used to Describe Various Craniofacial Anomalies

Anencephaly	A condition in which the brain fails to develop.
Anodontia	The absence of teeth.
Atresia	An occlusion of an opening or passage. In communication disorders, it most commonly refers to an underdeveloped pinna, which may result in occlusion of the external auditory canal.
Bifid	Divided into two parts. This most often refers to a divided uvula or tongue.
Brachycephaly	Reduction in the front to back dimension of the skull.
Coloboma	Defect in the shape of the eye that may involve the lower lid, iris, or retina.
Craniosynostosis	A premature fusing together of the bones of the cranium.
Heterochromia iridis	Different color eyes.
Hirsutism	Excessive body hair.
Hypertelorism	Excessive distance between the eyes.
Macroglossia	An excessively large tongue.
Microcephaly	Small head.
Microglossia	A small tongue.
Micrognathia	A severely underdeveloped mandible or chin.
Microtia	Small outer ear.
Oligodontia	Less than the normal number of teeth.
Poliosis	Premature graying of the hair. If limited to a particular area, the term *poliosis circumscripta* may be used.
Proptosis	Bulging eyes.
Synophrys	A growing together or confluence of the eyebrows.

Table 11–2 describes some of the possible malformations of the craniofacial structure that may be seen in addition to the cleft in various syndromes. The purpose of introducing these medical terms is to provide some idea of the variety of facial disfigurements that can occur and to familiarize you with terms that may find their way into patient or student files through reports from various professionals.

OVERVIEW OF ASSESSMENT IN CLEFT LIP AND PALATE

Because children with cleft palate and/or other craniofacial anomalies are at risk for a variety of communication disorders, the assessment of those children should typically include procedures to evaluate speech sound production, voice, resonance, language, and hearing.

ASSESSING SPEECH SOUND PRODUCTION

The assessment of speech sound production ability in a child with a cleft or craniofacial disorder usually begins in a manner similar to any speech sound evaluation. A standardized speech sound inventory and a connected speech sample form the core of the assessment. However, because the speech sound production problems typically associated with cleft palate and craniofacial anomalies tend to involve sounds requiring high levels of oral air pressure, speech-language pathologists (SLPs) use word lists and reading passages that include many stops, fricatives, and affricates to supplement the standardized articulation tests. In addition to determining whether speech sound errors are present, a critical objective of the assessment of speech sound production with this population is to determine the basis for those errors.

As described earlier in this chapter, most speech sound errors in this population have one of three causes. Errors may be related to an inadequate speech structure, they may be compensatory, or they may be developmental. It is important to determine the type of errors because different types of error require different types of intervention. Problems resulting from structural deficits such as hypernasality, nasal emission, and weak pressure consonants indicate the presence of inadequate velopharyngeal function. These problems typically require surgery or other forms of physical management. Speech treatment can remediate compensatory articulations such as glottal stops and pharyngeal fricatives. An SLP can also address any speech sound problems reflecting delayed phonological development. Often the decision as to whether a child requires additional surgery rests on the determination of the basis for the speech sound production errors noted in the assessment.

VOICE AND RESONANCE

In addition to speech sound production problems, the velopharyngeal insufficiency associated with cleft palate also allows sound into the nasal cavity, resulting in excessive nasal resonance called hypernasality. Hypernasality can be assessed both perceptually and through the use of instruments. Various rating scales have been developed to provide SLPs with some guidance in rating the severity of hypernasality. Such scales are usually equal appearing interval scales that provide a numerical rating, allowing the listener to rate the degree of hypernasality as mild, moderate, or severe. Judgments are frequently based on the subject repeating or reading a list of selected words and sentences, some of which contain no nasal consonants, and others that contain many occurrences of nasal consonants. SLPs can use several published word and sentence lists as well as reading passages for this type of assessment. For example, a reading passage called *The Zoo Passage* (Fletcher, 1972), written on a second- to third-grade reading level, tells a story about a zoo using words that contain no nasal consonants. Any nasal resonance heard in this passage would be inappropriate. An old technique that sometimes helps the SLP determine the presence of hypernasality is to have the subject prolong a vowel such as "eee" while the clinician alternately occludes and releases the speaker's nostrils. If hypernasality is present, a very noticeable difference can be heard between the two conditions. This technique has been around for many years and is known by many names including the nasal flutter test (Weiss, 1974) and the cul-de-sac test (Bloch, 1979).

Although a well-trained ear is a valuable tool in assessing nasal resonance, it is quite helpful to have some objective measures to support perceptual impressions. One instrument frequently used to assess hypernasality in a clinical setting is the Nasometer manufactured by KayPEN-TAX Corporation. Briefly, this instrument simultaneously measures sound levels at the nose and the mouth. Then, by means of its accompanying software, the device determines the ratio of nasal sound energy to total sound energy (nasal + oral) multiplied by 100 and displays it as a "nasalance" score. Higher nasalance scores indicate higher levels of nasal sound present.

LANGUAGE

The likelihood and extent of language problems in children with clefts depend on several factors including the type of cleft, the presence and extent of hearing problems, and the child's cognitive abilities. Early identification and treatment of language problems can reduce the impact of these problems on later academic performance. Many of the same language intervention techniques described in Chapter 6 apply to children with clefts and craniofacial disorders. The use of developmental language checklists or parent questionnaires might be an efficient first step in identifying children with language problems. One such parent questionnaire is the *MacArthur Communicative Development Inventory: Toddler* (Fenson et al., 1991). Scherer and D'Antonio (1995) compared the results obtained from the MacArthur with the results of a speech-language screening performed by an SLP. They report that the MacArthur provides a valid estimate of development for language screening of young children with cleft lip and/or palate. With older children, the combination of informal and formal assessment described in Chapter 6 is appropriate.

IN MEDICAL SETTINGS

Cleft lip and cleft palate, whether they occur as isolated conditions or as part of a syndrome, are congenital (present at birth). As a result, some of the most pressing needs of children with these and other craniofacial anomalies are medical in nature and require attention from professionals early in the child's life. Intervention for these children, then, often begins in a medical setting. As described earlier, children with craniofacial anomalies often have multiple problems requiring the attention of several specialists. The most effective way to treat children with clefts and other craniofacial anomalies is through a team approach. The professionals represented on a cleft palate team vary from setting to setting. However, the American Cleft Palate-Craniofacial Association has published standards for the composition of cleft palate and craniofacial teams. According to those standards, both types of teams must include, as a minimum core, professionals from the speech-language pathology, surgery, and orthodontics specialties (American Cleft Palate-Craniofacial Association, 2008). In addition to those core members, teams must have access to a wide variety of professionals to meet the many and varied needs of the patients they serve. Other professionals concerned with communication disorders who are typically part of these teams include otolaryngologists and audiologists because of the high incidence of hearing problems among this population.

Some may incorrectly assume that the role of the SLP on a cleft or craniofacial team does not begin until speech and language problems are identified when a child is 3 or 4 years old. This is not true. Within the first one or two months after the birth of a child, many parents begin to raise questions about how a cleft might affect speech and language development (Chuacharoen, Ritthagol, Hunsrisakhun, & Nilmanat, 2009). SLPs are frequently involved in parent counseling regarding speech and language development as well as the preliminary evaluation of receptive and expressive language skills during the first six to eight months of life (Brookshire et al.,1984; Rampp, Pannbacker, & Kinnebrew, 1984; Golding-Kushner, 2001). In its 2007 publication *Parameters for Evaluation and Treatment of Patients with Cleft Lip/Palate or Other Craniofacial Anomalies*, the American Cleft Palate-Craniofacial Association recommends:

> Each child and family should be seen for discussion of normal speech and language development and assessment of pre-linguistic speech-language development before or by six months of age.
>
> Speech-language evaluations with appropriate documentation should be conducted for each child at least twice during the first two years of life and at least annually thereafter until the age of six years. (p. 23)

In some settings SLPs, because of their expertise in oral functions and swallowing, may also be involved to varying degrees in counseling mothers regarding feeding their newborn from the day the child is born. A brief overview of the responsibilities of an SLP serving on a cleft palate or craniofacial team is provided here.

FEEDING

One of the immediate problems faced by a child born with cleft lip/palate is feeding. Infants feed by sucking on a nipple. To do this the infant must be able to make a seal around the nipple with the tongue and lips, squeeze the nipple between the tongue and palate, and develop negative pressure in the oral cavity. A child with a cleft lip may have difficulty forming the seal around the nipple, but this can usually be overcome by the use of various feeding techniques or devices. A cleft of the palate presents a more difficult challenge because the inability to separate the oral cavity from the nasal cavity makes it difficult or impossible to develop negative pressure in the oral cavity. A sizable cleft of the hard palate provides little or no surface against which the tongue can work the nipple. In some medical centers with large cleft/craniofacial teams, specially trained nurses, dieticians, and lactation consultants are available to help mothers learn to feed their infant with a cleft palate. In other centers, an SLP may be a part of the feeding team.

SPEECH AND LANGUAGE STIMULATION

Speech and language stimulation is particularly important for children with clefts and other craniofacial anomalies because factors such as anatomic differences of the oral structure, the high incidence of middle ear disorders, and early surgeries accompanied by hospital stays all may affect the child's language development. Recall from earlier in this chapter that many children with craniofacial anomalies demonstrate some degree of speech and language delay. Parents should be made aware of normal patterns of speech and language development so that they can identify delays or abnormal patterns exhibited by their child. They should also be given guidance and suggestions as to how they may best facilitate language development. Also, education of parents can help to identify and prevent the development of compensatory articulations (Golding-Kushner, 2001). Speech professionals must consider several practical factors when implementing parent education programs, such as the distance that families must travel from their homes to the medical center, the availability of insurance and other forms of funding for such visits, and the unique structure and scheduling policies of the cleft or craniofacial team. As a result, parent education programs offered by cleft or craniofacial teams can take many forms. A few examples are provided to demonstrate the diversity of such programs.

Brookshire et al. (1984) published a parent–child cleft palate curriculum. This work included a speech curriculum and a language curriculum with the language curriculum divided into areas of content, form, and use. For each curriculum area, specific objectives, activities, and criteria for assessment were provided covering the period from birth to 36 months. This program could be given to the parents with some direction from the clinician and the parent could follow the curriculum at home with scheduled visits to the medical center to evaluate progress.

Hahn (1979) describes a directed home training program for infants with cleft lip and palate. This program consists of three meetings between the SLP and the parents. The first meeting was scheduled at about 3 months of age after closure of the lip. The second was arranged at about 7 months or prior to surgical closure of the palate, and the third meeting at about six to eight weeks following palatal closure. At each of these meetings, the child's current speech and language skills are reviewed, and parents are informed about expected speech and language development over the next few months and are given specific suggestions regarding speech and language stimulation.

The Hospital for Sick Children in Toronto produced a videotape describing its early intervention program. In this program, the clinician meets with parents beginning at about 15 months and discusses topics such as how speech is produced, how to enhance expressive vocabulary, how to encourage oral airflow, production of stop consonants, and recognizing compensatory errors. The SLP demonstrates various activities as a model for the parents, who continue the procedures at home.

Cleft/craniofacial teams may also provide helpful literature. Many teams based in large medical centers produce their own pamphlets and online information for parents. In addition, a number of organizations, such as the American Cleft Palate Foundation (www.cleftline.org), provide extensive information for parents and individuals with clefts in both electronic and printed form.

SPEECH AND LANGUAGE ASSESSMENT IN MEDICAL SETTINGS

One of the most important tasks of an SLP in a medical setting is to determine whether the speech problems exhibited by a child are treatable by speech therapy or whether they require referral for additional surgery or other forms of physical management. In addition to the nature of the speech problems exhibited, treatment decisions also rest on the results of a thorough assessment of the structure of the speech mechanism, particularly the velopharyngeal mechanism and the child's orthodontic status. The SLP may have some indirect indications of velopharyngeal status based on the procedures and instruments described earlier in this chapter. However, more direct measures are also required. One of the great benefits of a team approach is that this information about the structure of the speech mechanism is readily available from other team members. In a cleft palate or craniofacial center, the status of the velopharyngeal mechanism is typically assessed through the use of nasal endoscopy, radiography, or both.

A nasal endoscope consists of a tube containing light-carrying fibers attached to an eye piece. The tube is inserted in the patient's nostril and placed just above the soft palate. Through the eye piece (or via an attached video system) the examiner is able to see the movement of the velum and the pharyngeal walls and determine whether closure is achieved. A physician usually performs this procedure, but an SLP with specialized training may also perform it.

Radiography provides an x-ray view of the velum and pharynx in motion during speech. The structures are often viewed from several angles including a lateral view, a frontal view, and a basal view (looking upward from under the mandible). Once either or both of these procedures have been performed, an SLP can have a better idea of the adequacy of the velopharyngeal structure. When the structure is clearly inadequate, referral for additional surgical management is in order. When the structure is clearly adequate, the SLP should address any existing speech problems. However, in some cases the child's velopharyngeal function may fall into a "borderline" category. Many years ago, Morris (1972) described two categories of borderline velopharyngeal function, "Almost but not quite (ABNQ)" and "Sometimes but not always (SBNA)." In today's highly technical world, these categories may sound a bit simplistic, but they do provide a nice conceptualization of the problem. In the ABNQ category, the velum and pharynx come very close to closing, in some cases even gently touching, but the contact is not sturdy enough to withstand the pressures created during speech. In the SBNA category, closure is inconsistent, occurring on some sounds or in short utterances such as single words, but not on longer utterances such as sentences.

The SLP on the cleft/craniofacial team must be familiar with the terminology and procedures used by other team members and must be able to report speech findings and implications to the rest of the team in a succinct yet thorough manner. Depending on the structure of the particular team, members may report to each other in face-to-face meetings, via written reports, or through dictated notes.

ESTABLISHING AND MONITORING INTERVENTION PLANS

When it is determined that a child with a cleft or other craniofacial anomaly can benefit from speech treatment, the SLP on the cleft/craniofacial team plans an intervention program. In some cases, this treatment may be carried out at the home facility of the team. A model for such team-based care is provided by Blakeley and Brockman (1995). They report on a project involving 41 children to determine whether normal speech and hearing by age 5 was a reasonable goal for children with cleft palate. The project involved "Early and continuing speech and hearing diagnosis, parent education as speech aides, timely professional speech habilitation including use of temporary **speech appliances** and early medical care for ears" (Blakeley & Brockman, 1995, p. 26). They report that this project resulted in normal resonance in 93 percent of the subjects and normal articulation status in 93 percent of the subjects (although not the same subjects) by age 5 years.

In many cases, however, the child may live many miles away from the location of the team and the treatment plan is implemented in the child's community, often by a school-based clinician. D'Antonio and Scherer (1995) state that recommendations from the team SLP to the community-based clinician should include the following.

- Suggested treatment goals
- Recommendation as to the frequency and duration of treatment sessions
- Whether the sessions should be group or individual
- Possibly recommendations regarding the specific techniques to be used in treatment

D'Antonio and Scherer (1995) also suggest that an additional role for the team SLP is to act as an advocate for the child. Despite laws such as the Individuals with Disabilities Education Act (IDEA), it is sometimes difficult for children to obtain all of the services that they require. The influence of a professional working at a major medical center may provide valuable support for parents and school-based SLPs seeking to provide an optimal level of services for a child with craniofacial anomalies.

The SLP structures the treatment plan to address the specific needs of each child. Some objectives commonly found in speech pathology programs for children with clefts are discussed briefly here. **Table 11–3** presents some specific techniques that have been reported in the literature to achieve each of the following goals.

- *Eliminate compensatory articulations.* These articulation errors, described earlier in this chapter, often represent the child's attempt to produce a sound close to the target sound while avoiding problems created by any structural deficit. Because these are learned behaviors, they can be unlearned and are appropriate targets for the SLP. Compensatory errors in children with clefts are frequently errors in place of articulation. For example, the child may substitute a pharyngeal fricative for an alveolar fricative (such as s̲) or a glottal stop for a labial stop (such as b̲). Therefore, a primary goal for the SLP is to achieve the proper placement for the target sound.
- *Encourage oral airflow.* It must be noted that these tasks are designed to encourage an oral direction of airflow. They are not intended to improve or strengthen the velopharyngeal mechanism. Blowing exercises have never proven to be effective for the latter purpose.
- *Reduce hypernasality and nasal emission in borderline cases.* It must be clear that this is a speech-language pathology goal only for borderline cases. When hypernasality and nasal emission are the result of a clearly inadequate structure, they should be treated by surgery or other physical management. In cases of borderline structural adequacy, the treatment should be considered trial treatment and not persist for too long without indications of progress. As shown in Table 11–3, several authors suggest the use of light articulatory contacts to reduce nasal emission. At least one author, Golding-Kushner (2001), suggests the use of strong articulatory contacts to enhance intelligibility. There have been several attempts to reduce hypernasality by working directly on improving velopharyngeal function through behavioral methods. These have included electrical stimulation, establishing control of gagging reflex, and other forms of muscle strengthening. For the most part, these activities have failed to produce better speech (Ruscello, 2004; Glaze, 2009; Peterson-Falzone et al., 2010). In recent years, two techniques, continuous positive airway pressure (CPAP) (Kuehn et al., 2002) and biofeedback via endoscopy (Witzel, Tobe, & Salyer, 1989; Brunner, Stellzig-Eisenhauer, Proschel, Verres, & Komposch, 2005), have shown promising early results. Briefly, CPAP involves introducing a stream of airflow into the nose that offers resistance as the subject raises the velum during specified speech activities. The airflow may be adjusted to offer different levels of resistance. This allows a muscle training principle of resisted motion to be applied to the velum. Biofeedback involves the subject viewing the velopharyngeal mechanism in real time via nasendoscopy and making appropriate adjustments to achieve closure. The reason for the success achieved with these two techniques might be the fact that they are performed during speech.
- *Eliminate any problems not related to the structural deficiencies.* Some children with craniofacial anomalies exhibit speech sound production problems that do not appear to be directly related to structural deficiencies or that are not the typical compensatory

TABLE 11–3 Examples of Activities Reported in the Literature to Achieve Speech Goals for Children with Cleft Palate

Possible Goals	Sample Activities to Achieve Goal	References
Eliminate compensatory articulations	Produce continuous h sound, then stop the flow with the appropriate articulators (for glottal stops).	Golding-Kushner (2001); Kummer (2008)
	Occlude the nares, eliminating any nasal escape and facilitating the correct placement of articulators. Then, release the nares, encouraging the child to keep the appropriate placement.	Golding-Kushner (2001); Kummer (2008)
	Use a mirror, tactile cues, and diagrams to facilitate correct placement of the articulators.	Trost-Cardamone (2009)
	Place a tongue depressor between the child's front teeth. Have the child touch the tongue depressor with his or her tongue while producing t and d (for middorsum palatal stops).	Kummer (2008)
Encourage oral airflow	Blow a Ping-Pong ball across a table, cause a strip of paper to bend by blowing, use a pinwheel or air paddle.	Golding-Kushner (2001); Kummer (2008); Peterson-Falzone et al. (2010)
	Place a straw in front of the patient's mouth so that oral airflow resonates to increase the perceptual awareness of oral airflow.	Riski (1984)
Reduce hypernasality and nasal emission in borderline cases	Use a wider mouth opening.	Wilson (1987); VanDemark & Hardin (1990); Kummer (2008); Peterson-Falzone et al. (2010)
	Use light articulatory contacts.	Kummer (2008); Peterson-Falzone et al. (2010)
	Use feedback device such as the SEE-Scape.	Golding-Kushner (2001); Glaze (2009)
Eliminate any developmental phonological problems not directly related to the structural problems	Activities described in Chapter 4 apply here.	

articulations associated with VPI. These may reflect delayed phonological development or abnormal phonological organization (Chapman, 2009) or may even be the result of a form of apraxia (Kummer, 2008).

Serving as an SLP on a cleft or craniofacial team is challenging and rewarding. To be an effective member of the team, the SLP, in addition to having a working knowledge of the anatomy and physiology of the speech mechanism, some understanding of the various surgical and orthodontic treatment procedures, and mastery of a wide range of speech and language assessment and treatment techniques, must also have excellent communication skills. The team-based SLP must be able to communicate effectively with other team members, community-based SLPs, parents, and patients. SLPs who possess all of these skills know that, as core members of cleft/craniofacial teams, their opinions and suggestions significantly affect the treatment of the children they serve.

IN EDUCATIONAL SETTINGS

In an ideal situation, a child with a cleft lip/palate or other craniofacial anomaly is identified and assessed early in life by a craniofacial team. In such cases, the role of the school-based SLP focuses more on incorporating the treatment objectives established by the cleft/craniofacial team, monitoring the child's progress, and reporting back to the team. If a child has not been seen by a cleft or craniofacial team, the school-based SLP should make such a referral. In addition to the speech and language procedures described previously, the child with a craniofacial anomaly may face many other challenges in an educational setting, many of which involve the SLP.

ACADEMIC PROBLEMS

Students with clefts of the lip and/or palate are at risk for learning disabilities, low school achievement, and grade retention (Richman & Eliason, 1986; Broder, Richman, & Matheson, 1998). In a study of school-age children with clefts and no other associated problems, Broder et al. (1998) report that 46 percent of the children with clefts in their study exhibited learning disabilities, 47 percent demonstrated deficient educational progress as measured by standardized tests, and 27 percent had repeated a grade. One area in which the academic problems of students with clefts can be seen is reading. Richman and Eliason (1986) report that the rate of reading problems among students with cleft palate is approximately 30 percent, as compared to about 5 to 15 percent in the general population. Richman, Eliason, and Lindgren (1988) report that reading problems among students with cleft palate decrease with age. The degree to which the reading problems decrease, however, is related to type of cleft. Students with clefts of the lip and palate exhibit essentially normal reading skills by age 13 years, whereas children with isolated clefts of the palate and no involvement of the lip maintain higher than average levels of reading problems. This, according to Richman et al. (1988), reflects a greater degree of language deficit in children with isolated clefts of the palate. In fact, more recent research (Millard & Richman, 2001) suggests that children with isolated clefts of the palate are not only more likely to exhibit learning problems, but also have more anxiety and depression than children with clefts that involve the lip.

Richman and Ryan (2003) suggest that the reading problems exhibited by students with clefts are not the result of phonemic awareness deficits, but may be related to deficits in short-term automatic memory. Therefore, Richman and Ryan suggest that site word reading approaches should be avoided with this population in favor of phonics-based approaches within the context of meaningful stories.

Because of the language delays and academic problems noted among students with cleft palate, parents, teachers, and SLPs often express concern over the cognitive development of these students. Several early studies report that children with cleft palate, as a group, exhibit slightly lower IQ scores than do their noncleft peers (Means & Irwin, 1954; Lewis, 1961; Estes & Morris, 1970). The results of these studies, however, may be misleading. Many of these early studies often include children with multiple disorders in addition to cleft palate, fail to separate findings for children with varying cleft types, and tend to use tests that rely heavily on verbal skills (Richman & Eliason, 1986; Strauss, 2004; Peterson-Falzone et al., 2010). More recent research views children with clefts as a more heterogeneous group. Endriga and Kapp-Simon (1999) indicate that children with clefts and no other accompanying anomalies (syndromes) are at only a slightly higher risk for mental retardation (4–6 percent as opposed to 2 percent in the general population), but children with clefts as part of a syndrome are at higher risk. With regard to cleft type, it appears that children with isolated clefts of the palate score more poorly on IQ tests such as the Stanford-Binet and the Wechsler Intelligence Scale for Children (WISC) (Richman & Eliason, 1982; Peterson-Falzone et al., 2010). This variation by cleft type prompted Strauss (2004) to suggest that although it is important to periodically screen all children with clefts for cognitive delays, particular attention should be given to those children with isolated clefts of the palate.

Finally, the reduced IQ scores reported in earlier literature reflect the fact that children with clefts tend to do more poorly on tests of verbal IQ than on tests of performance IQ (Richman & Eliason, 1982; Strauss, 2004). This deficit on verbal tests may reflect language problems and specific learning disabilities rather than a generalized cognitive delay.

In addition to difficulties in language-based areas, the classroom performance of students with cleft palate may be affected by social and emotional factors. There has never been evidence of a specific personality type associated with cleft palate, and neither has there been conclusive evidence that people with clefts exhibit psychopathology or severe emotional disturbances at a higher rate than the noncleft population does (Strauss, 2004). There is, however, evidence of more subtle adjustment problems. Students with cleft palate tend to be more withdrawn and inhibited, and tend to participate less in classroom activities than do their noncleft peers (Kapp, 1979; Richman & Harper, 1979; Powers, 1986; Richman & Eliason, 1993; Endriga & Kapp-Simon, 1999). These characteristics reflect the necessity for children with clefts "to adjust and accommodate to a variety of speech-, education-, and appearance-related social and interpersonal challenges in their development" (Strauss, 2004, p. 167). Richman and Eliason (1986) suggest that these social-emotional variables may interact with cognitive variables to produce a greater vulnerability to academic problems.

LEARNING PROBLEMS IN CHILDREN WITH OTHER CRANIOFACIAL SYNDROMES

The learning problems of students with craniofacial anomalies depend to a large extent on the degree of intellectual impairment. Some syndromes typically result in severe intellectual disability, others result in milder degrees of disability, and still others are not associated with any cognitive deficits. Because many of these students have more severe facial disfigurement than those with cleft palate only, social and emotional variables might play a more significant role in their school adjustment.

Students with severe craniofacial anomalies do not appear to exhibit severe psychosocial disorders. Their social and emotional problems, like those of children with cleft palate, tend to be more subtle and seem to be related to coping with social pressures. Pertschuk and Whitaker (1985) report that children with craniofacial malformations demonstrated poorer self-concepts, increased levels of anxiety, and more introversion than a control group of children with normal facial structures. Teachers reported poorer classroom behavior among the craniofacial group, but parents did not observe such behavior problems at home.

One of the more troubling factors for children with craniofacial anomalies is the reaction of others to their appearance. In recent years, movies such as *Elephant Man* and *Mask* have dramatized this problem. The academic performance of children with craniofacial anomalies may be affected by the expectations of parents and teachers. Berscheid and Walster (1974) report that teachers tend to view physically attractive students as having more acceptable behavior and higher mental abilities than less attractive students. This appears to hold true for students with craniofacial disorders. Richman (1979) compared teacher ratings of the intellectual ability of children with facial deformities to the IQ scores of those children. The results indicate that the intellectual abilities of children with noticeable facial disfigurements and above average IQs were underestimated by teachers. Parents also may have lower expectations of children with craniofacial anomalies, resulting in lower academic aspirations (Richman & Eliason, 1982). Children also tend to view students with craniofacial anomalies in a more negative fashion (Schneiderman & Harding, 1984; Tobiason, 1987). It is very difficult for a child to develop a good self-image and to achieve his or her potential when teachers, parents, and peers expect less of that student.

Of all the syndromes listed in Table 11–1, there are two syndromes that, because of the unique speech and language problems as well as the presence of learning problems, merit special attention in this section. Those two conditions are velocardiofacial syndrome and fetal alcohol syndrome.

Velocardiofacial syndrome (VCFS), also known as Shprintzen syndrome, DiGeorge syndrome, and 22q11.2 deletion syndrome (referring to the chromosome abnormality that is the source of the problem), was first described in 1978 (Shprintzen et al., 1978). VCFS occurs in about 1 in every 1800 births (Golding-Kushner, 2001) and is one of the most common syndromes associated with cleft palate (Shprintzen, 2000). The syndrome is characterized by several features including cleft palate (often a submucous cleft), heart anomalies, a long nose with a bulbous tip, puffy eyelids, small ears, learning disabilities, attention deficit hyperactivity disorder (ADHD), and delayed speech and language (Shprintzen, 1997). Also, many children with VCFS unfortunately develop mental illness including bipolar disorder, manic depression, and psychosis later in life (Golding-Kushner, 2001; Peterson-Falzone et al., 2010). As with most syndromes, not every child exhibits every symptom; however, language deficits are almost universal among children with VCFS and the language deficit is present from the onset of language (Scherer, D'Antonio, & Kalbfleisch, 1999). The delays in expressive language are greater than in receptive language, and the expressive speech and language delays are more severe than would be expected compared to their other developmental problems. Some children with VCFS may be essentially nonverbal as late as age 3 years, and some may even be candidates for some form of augmentative (nonvocal) communication such as signing, picture boards, or computer-assisted devices (Scherer et al., 1999; Scherer, 2003). D'Antonio, Scherer, Miller, Kalbfleisch, and Bartley (2001) conclude that young children with VCFS demonstrate speech production that is different from normal and may be specific to the syndrome. For example, children with VCFS often exhibit a high number of glottal stops and have more hypernasality following repair of their cleft palate than do children with clefts not associated with a syndrome (Scherer et al., 1999). Speech and language delays persist through elementary school, however. Children with VCFS appear to narrow the gap somewhat between their language skills and those of their peer age group as they grow (D'Antonio et al., 2001). Golding-Kushner indicates that "the learning curve of children with VCFS may be more stepwise than smooth" (Golding-Kushner, 2001, p. 147). This means that children may have some advances followed by plateaus with no discernable progress. This suggests that parents, SLPs, and teachers should not be discouraged by periodic lack of progress and should continue intervention and stimulation even when the child with VCFS is moving ahead as rapidly as expected of other children. Golding-Kushner (2001) notes that because children with VCFS seem to learn best in frequent short sessions with much repetition, an SLP may want to see these children more frequently than other children on the caseload.

Regarding educational achievement, Golding-Kushner (2001) indicates that although most children with VCFS are of normal or borderline normal intelligence, learning disabilities are common. She states that the learning disabilities exhibited by children with VCFS affect reading comprehension, math concepts, and tasks involving inferential reasoning and abstract thinking. Therefore, the learning problems of children with VCFS may not be apparent until second or third grade when academic tasks become more complex. Because

ADHD is also commonly reported among VCFS children, they are likely to demonstrate many of the problems associated with ADHD described in Chapter 12.

Fetal alcohol syndrome (FAS) is characterized by low birth weight, cleft lip or palate or both, microcephaly, and unusual facial features that may include a short nose and an underdeveloped midface area (Jung, 1989; Shprintzen, 1997). These children also frequently exhibit cognitive delays and ADHD. The problem results, as the name implies, from alcohol consumption by the mother during pregnancy. The severity of the symptoms associated with this syndrome vary widely and may be related to the amount of alcohol consumed and the regularity and timing of the alcohol consumption (Little & Streissguth, 1981; Jung, 1989). FAS is reported to occur at different rates in different parts of the world (Jung, 1989). In North America, the incidence is reported to range from 0.5 to 3 per 1,000 births (Stratton, Howe, & Battaglia, 1996).

The communication abilities of children with FAS vary widely. Some research describes the language of many children with FAS as superficial (Abkarian, 1992; Streissguth, Bookstein, Sampson, & Barr, 1993). This means that a child may appear to have appropriate language in certain social situations, but when pressed to describe or explain more complicated concepts, the child's language skills are inadequate. Such superficial language skills tend to be exposed when increased academic demands are placed on children. This could be seen as early as second or third grade. This description of potential language problems is consistent with the fact that deficits in cognitive performance are beginning to be noted reliably (Stratton et al., 1996).

The habilitative process for students with craniofacial anomalies often is prolonged and typically involves surgeons, orthodontists, and SLPs. Teachers also make a significant contribution to the adjustment and development of these children, yet most teachers have very little training or experience with such students. Moran and Pentz (1995) interviewed members of a parent support group for children with craniofacial anomalies. The parent information was combined with a review of the literature and resulted in the following suggestions.

Suggestions for Teachers of Students with Craniofacial Anomalies

1. *Avoid self-fulfilling prophecies.* Judge the child by his or her performance and objective measures of ability rather than by any preconceived notion based on physical appearance or speech quality.
2. *Consult with the SLP to know what level of speech proficiency to expect.* If the student's oral structure is inadequate, a teacher cannot expect perfect speech. On the other hand, teachers can be of great assistance by reminding the student to use newly acquired speech and language skills in the classroom setting.
3. *Refer any student with hypernasality or nasal emission to the SLP for evaluation.* Some submucous clefts and other forms of velopharyngeal incompetence may have gone undetected during the preschool years.
4. *Be alert to the possibility of language-based learning disabilities.* These problems may surface in reading and writing activities. Although the possibility of learning disabilities is particularly

great in certain craniofacial syndromes such as VCFS and FAS, teachers should be alert to the possibility of such disorders even in children with nonsyndromic clefts of the palate.

5. *Watch for signs of middle ear problems and a mild hearing loss.* See Chapter 10 for specific behaviors that indicate such a hearing loss.

6. *Encourage participation in classroom activities.* Help to foster a feeling of "fitting in" with the rest of the class. Teachers should encourage, but not be overzealous in pressuring, the student with craniofacial anomalies to participate in classroom activities. Teachers must also be alert to any ridicule or teasing that the student with craniofacial anomalies might experience. Although it is not possible to eliminate such behavior completely, teachers must take measures to minimize it. Failure to do so, by default, condones ridicule and permits it to grow.

7. *Be prepared to help the student make up missed work.* Children may miss several classes if secondary surgical procedures or extensive dental work are performed during the school year. An outline of assignments for the various subject areas and a supply of necessary texts and workbooks supplied to the parents would be quite helpful. A brief follow-up by the teacher after the absences can help to identify any deficits that remain.

Clefts of the lip and/or palate constitute the most common birth defect in the United States. Recent research in genetics is shedding more light on the cause of these conditions and improved surgical techniques are providing adequate speech mechanisms in a higher percentage than ever before. However, SLPs are still critical members of cleft and craniofacial teams. They provide speech and language stimulation, parent counseling, and information for other members of the team. The team SLP develops and monitors treatment programs that may be carried out in the child's home community. In educational settings, it should be remembered that, for the most part, children with craniofacial anomalies are just that: children. They may miss somewhat more school than others. They may look a little different. They tend to have a higher incidence of speech, language, and hearing problems than their classmates do. They may struggle a bit with social and academic challenges. However, with a few adjustments and a little extra attention and respect, the overwhelming majority of students with craniofacial anomalies can do just fine in their school routine. A coordinated effort of SLPs, teachers, and parents can do a great deal to build and promote the environment in which a child can earn that attention and respect from both classmates and school personnel.

Terms to Know

Cleft palate

Submucous cleft palate

Cleft lip

Velopharyngeal insufficiency (VPI)

Hypernasality

Nasal emission

Compensatory articulations

Syndrome

Speech appliances

Velocardiofacial syndrome (VCFS)

Fetal alcohol syndrome (FAS)

Study Questions

1. Describe the various speech, language, and hearing problems a child with cleft palate might exhibit.
2. Identify the professions that are required to be represented on cleft palate/craniofacial teams by the American Cleft Palate-Craniofacial Association. Identify other professionals who might also serve on such teams.
3. Describe the possible negative reactions that students with craniofacial anomalies might encounter in a school setting and identify actions that teachers could take to deal with such reactions.
4. Identify several actions that a teacher might do to help the child with a cleft palate in the classroom.

Bibliography

Abkarian, G. G. (1992). Communication effects of prenatal alcohol exposure. *Journal of Communication Disorders, 25*, 221–240.

American Cleft Palate-Craniofacial Association. (2007). *Parameters for evaluation and treatment of patients with cleft lip/cleft palate or other craniofacial anomalies.* Chapel Hill, NC.

American Cleft Palate-Craniofacial Association. (2008). Standards for approval of cleft palate and craniofacial teams. Retrieved June 14, 2010, from http://www.acpa-cpf.org/Standards/index.html.

Berscheid, E., & Walster, E. (1974). Physical attractiveness. In S. Berkowitz (Ed.), *Advances in Experimental Psychology* (Vol. 7). New York, NY: Academic Press.

Blakeley, R., & Brockman, J. (1995). Normal speech and hearing by age 5 as a goal for children with cleft palate: A demonstration project. *American Journal of Speech-Language Pathology, 4*, 25–32.

Bloch, P. J. (1979). Clinical evaluation for the cleft palate team setting. In K. R. Bzoch (Ed.), *Communicative disorders related to cleft lip and palate* (2nd ed.). Boston, MA: Little, Brown.

Broder, H. L., Richman, L.C., & Matheson, P. (1998). Learning disability, school achievement, and grade retention among children with cleft: A two-center study. *Cleft Palate Craniofacial Journal, 35*, 127–131.

Broen, P. A., Devers, M. C., Doyle, S. S., Prouty, J. M., & Moller, K. T. (1998). Acquisition of linguistic and cognitive skills by children with cleft palate. *Journal of Speech, Language and Hearing Research, 41*, 676–687.

Brookshire, B. L., Lynch, J. I., & Fox, D. R. (1984). *A parent–child cleft palate curriculum: Developing speech and language.* Tigard, OR: C. C. Publications.

Brunner, M., Stellzig-Eisenhauer, A., Proschel, U., Verres, R., & Komposch, G. (2005). The effects of nasopharyngoscopic biofeedback in patients with cleft palate and velopharyngeal dysfunction. *Cleft Palate-Craniofacial Journal, 42*, 649–657.

Bzoch, K. R. (2004). Introduction to the study of communicative disorders in cleft palate and related craniofacial anomalies. In K. R. Bzoch (Ed.), *Communicative disorders related to cleft lip and palate* (5th ed.). Austin, TX: Pro-Ed.

Chapman, K. (2009). Speech and language of children with cleft palate: Interactions and influences. In K. Moller & L. Glaze (Eds.), *Cleft lip and palate: Interdisciplinary issues and treatment* (2nd ed.). Austin, TX: Pro-Ed.

Chuacharoen, R., Ritthagol, W., Hunsrisakhun, J., & Nilmanat, K. (2009). Felt needs of parents who have a 0- to 3-month-old child with a cleft lip and palate. *Cleft Palate and Craniofacial Journal, 46,* 252–257.

Cleft Palate Foundation. (2007). About cleft lip and palate. Retrieved June 14, 2010, from http://www.cleftline.org/parents/about_cleft_lip_and_palate.

Cohen, M. M. (1978). Syndromes with cleft lip and cleft palate. *Cleft Palate Journal, 15,* 306–328.

D'Antonio, L. L., & Scherer, N. J. (1995). The evaluation of speech disorders associated with clefting. In R. J. Shprintzen & J. Bardach (Eds.), *Cleft palate speech management: A multidisciplinary approach.* St. Louis, MO: Mosby.

D'Antonio, L. L., Scherer, N. J., Miller, L. L., Kalbfleisch, J. H., & Bartley, J. A. (2001). Analysis of speech characteristics in children with velocardiofacial syndrome (VCFS) and children with phenotypic overlap without VCFS. *Cleft Palate-Craniofacial Journal, 35,* 455–467.

Endriga, M. C., & Kapp-Simon, K. A. (1999). Psychological issues in craniofacial care: State of the art. *Cleft Palate-Craniofacial Journal, 36,* 3–11.

Estes, R. E., & Morris, H. L. (1970). Relationships among intelligence, speech proficiency, and hearing sensitivity in children with cleft palates. *Cleft Palate Journal, 7,* 763–773.

Fenson, L., Dale, P., Reznick, J., Thal, D., Bates, E., Hartung, J., Pethick, S., & Reilly, J. (1991). *MacArthur communicative development inventory: Toddlers.* San Diego, CA: University of California Press.

Fletcher, S. G. (1972). Contingencies for bio-electronic modification of nasality. *Journal of Speech and Hearing Disorders, 37,* 329–346.

Gerson, C. R. (1990). Otologic disease in the cleft palate patient. In D. Kernahan & S. Stark (Eds.), *Cleft lip and palate: A system of management.* Baltimore, MD: Williams & Wilkins.

Glaze, L. (2009). Behavioral approaches to treating velopharyngeal dysfunction and nasality. In K. T. Moller & L. E. Glaze (Eds.), *Cleft lip and palate: Interdisciplinary issues and treatment.* Austin, TX: Pro-Ed.

Golding-Kushner, K. J. (2001). *Therapy techniques for cleft palate speech and related disorders.* San Diego, CA: Singular.

Gorlin, R. J., & Baylis, A. L. (2009). Embryologic and genetic aspects of clefting and selected craniofacial anomalies. In K. T. Moller & L. E. Glaze (Eds.), *Cleft lip and palate: Interdisciplinary issues and treatment.* Austin, TX: Pro-Ed.

Hahn, E. (1979). Directed home training program for infants with cleft lip and palate. In K. Bzoch (Ed.), *Communication disorders related to cleft lip and palate* (2nd. ed.). Boston, MA: Little, Brown.

Hospital for Sick Children (Producer). (1997). *Step by step: Speech pathology techniques for cleft palate speech* [Video]. Toronto, Canada.

Jung, J. H. (1989). *Genetic syndromes in communication disorders.* Boston, MA: Little, Brown.

Kapp, K. (1979). Self-concept of the cleft lip and/or palate child. *Cleft Palate Journal, 16,* 171–176.

Kuehn, D., Imrey, P., Tomes, L., Jones, D., O'Gara, M., Seaver, E., Smith, B., VanDemark, D., & Wachtel, J. (2002). Efficacy of continuous positive airway pressure for treatment of hypernasality. *Cleft Palate-Craniofacial Journal, 39,* 267–276.

Kuehn, D., & Moller, K. (1990). Speech and language issues in the cleft palate population: The state of the art. *Cleft Palate-Craniofacial Journal, 37,* 348–382.

Kummer, A. (2008). *Cleft palate and craniofacial anomalies: Effects on speech and resonance.* Clifton Park, NY: Thomson Delmar Learning.

LaRossa, D. (2000). The state of the art in cleft palate surgery. *Cleft Palate-Craniofacial Journal, 37,* 225–227.

Lewis, R. (1961). A survey of the intelligence of cleft palate children in Ontario. *Cleft Palate Bulletin, 11,* 83–85.

Little, R. E., & Streissguth, A. P. (1981). Effects of alcohol on the fetus: Impact and prevention. *Canadian Medical Association Journal, 125,* 159–164.

Means, B., & Irwin, J. (1954). An analysis of certain measures of intelligence and hearing in a sample of the Wisconsin cleft palate population. *Cleft Palate Newsletter, 4,* 2–4.

Meyerson, M. (1990). Cultural considerations in the treatment of Latinos with craniofacial malformations. *Cleft Palate Journal, 27,* 279–288.

Millard, T., & Richman, L. C. (2001). Different cleft conditions, facial appearance, and speech: Relationship to psychological variables. *Cleft Palate-Craniofacial Journal, 38,* 68–75.

Moran, M., & Pentz, A. (1995). Helping the child with a cleft palate in your classroom. *TEACHING Exceptional Children, 27,* 46–48.

Morris, H. L. (1972). Cleft palate. In A. J. Westin (Ed.), *Communicative disorders.* Springfield, IL: C. C. Thomas.

Paradise, J., Bluestone, C., & Felder, H. (1969). The universality of otitis media in 50 infants with cleft palate. *Pediatrics, 44,* 35–42.

Pecyna, P. M., Feeney-Giacoma, M. E., & Nieman, G. S. (1987). Development of the object permanence concept in cleft lip and palate and noncleft lip and palate infants. *Journal of Communication Disorders, 20,* 233–243.

Pertschuk, M. J., & Whitaker, L. A. (1985). Psychological adjustment and craniofacial malformations in childhood. *Plastic and Reconstructive Surgery, 75,* 177–182.

Peterson-Falzone, S. J., Hardin-Jones, M. A., & Karnell, M. P. (2010). *Cleft palate speech* (4th ed.). St. Louis, MO: Mosby.

Powers, G. R. (1986). *Cleft palate.* Austin, TX: Pro-Ed.

Rampp, D., Pannbacker, M., & Kinnebrew, M. (1984). *Velopharyngeal incompetence: A practical guide for evaluation and management.* Tulsa, OK: Modern Education Corp.

Richman, L. C. (1979). The effects of facial disfigurement on teachers' perception of ability in cleft palate children. *Cleft Palate Journal, 15,* 155–160.

Richman, L. C. (1980). Cognitive patterns and learning disabilities in cleft palate children with verbal deficits. *Journal of Speech and Hearing Research, 23,* 447–465.

Richman, L. C., & Eliason, M. J. (1982). Psychological characteristics of cleft lip and palate: Intellectual, achievement, behavioral, and personality variables. *Cleft Palate Journal, 19,* 249–257.

Richman, L. C., & Eliason, M. J. (1984). Types of reading disability related to cleft type and neuropsychological patterns. *Cleft Palate Journal, 21,* 1–6.

Richman, L. C., & Eliason, M. J. (1986). Development in children with cleft lip and/or palate: Intellectual, cognitive, personality, and parental factors. *Seminars in Speech and Language, 7,* 225–239.

Richman, L.C., & Eliason, M. J. (1993). Psychological characteristics associated with cleft palate. In K. T. Moller & C. D. Starr (Eds.), *Cleft palate interdisciplinary issues and treatment: For clinicians by clinicians.* Austin, TX: Pro-Ed.

Richman, L. C., Eliason, M. J., & Lingren, S. D. (1988). Reading disability in children with clefts. *Cleft Palate Journal, 25,* 21–25.

Richman, L. C., & Harper, D. (1979). Self-identified personality patterns in children with facial or orthopedic disfigurement. *Cleft Palate Journal, 16,* 257–261.

Richman, L. C., & Ryan, S. M. (2003). Do the reading disabilities of children with cleft fit into current models of developmental dyslexia? *Cleft Palate-Craniofacial Journal, 40,* 154–157.

Riski, J. (1984). Functional velopharyngeal incompetence: Diagnosis and management. In H. Winitz (Ed.), *Treating articulation disorders: For clinicians by clinicians.* Baltimore, MD: University Park Press.

Robin, N. (2008). *Medical genetics: Its application to speech, hearing, and craniofacial disorders.* San Diego, CA: Plural.

Ruscello, D. (2004). Considerations for behavioral treatment of velopharyngeal closure for speech. In K. Bzoch (Ed.), *Communicative disorders related to cleft lip and palate* (5th ed.). Austin, TX: Pro-Ed.

Scheper-Hughes, N. (1990). Difference and danger: The cultural dynamics of childhood stigma, rejection and rescue. *Cleft Palate Journal, 27,* 301–307.

Scherer, N. J. (2003, October). *Speech and language development in children with VCFS and children with clefts.* Paper presented at the 16th Annual Cleft Lip and Palate Symposium. Children's Healthcare of Atlanta, Atlanta, GA.

Scherer, N. J., & D'Antonio, L. L. (1995). Parent questionnaire for screening early language development in children with cleft palate. *Cleft Palate-Craniofacial Journal, 34,* 7–13.

Scherer, N. J., D'Antonio, L., & Kalbfleisch, J. (1999). Early speech and language development in children with velocardiofacial syndrome. *American Journal of Medical Genetics, 88,* 714–723.

Schneiderman, C. R., & Harding, J. B. (1984). Social ratings of children with cleft lips by school peers. *Cleft Palate Journal, 21,* 219–223.

Seagle, M. B. (2004). Primary surgical correction of cleft lip and palate. In K. R. Bzoch (Ed.), *Communicative disorders related to cleft lip and palate* (5th ed.). Austin, TX: Pro-Ed.

Shprintzen, R. J. (1997). *Genetics, syndromes, and communication disorders.* San Diego, CA: Singular.

Shprintzen, R. J. (2000). *Syndrome identification for speech-language pathologists: An illustrated pocket guide.* San Diego, CA: Singular.

Shprintzen, R. J., Goldberg, R. B., Lewin, M. L., Sidoti, E. J., Berkman, M. D., Argamaso, R. V., & Young, D. (1978). A new syndrome involving cleft palate, cardiac anomalies, typical facies, and learning disabilities: Velo-cardio-facial syndrome. *Cleft Palate Journal, 15,* 56–62.

Slavkin, H. C. (1992). Incidence of cleft lips, palates rising. *Journal of the American Dental Association, 123,* 61–65.

Stratton, K., Howe, C., & Battaglia, F. (Eds.). (1996). *Fetal alcohol syndrome: Diagnosis, epidemiology, prevention and treatment.* Washington, DC: National Academy Press.

Strauss, R. P. (2004). Social and psychological perspectives on cleft lip and palate. In K. R. Bzoch (Ed.), *Communicative disorders related to cleft lip and palate* (5th ed.). Austin, TX: Pro-Ed.

Streissguth, A. P., Bookstein, F. L., Sampson, P. C., & Barr, H. M. (1993). *The enduring effects of prenatal alcohol exposure on child development: Birth through seven years, a partial least squares solution.* Ann Arbor, MI: University of Michigan Press.

Tobiason, J. B. (1987). Social judgments of facial deformity. *Cleft Palate Journal, 24,* 323–327.

Toliver-Weddington, G. (1990). Cultural considerations in the treatment of craniofacial malformations in African Americans. *Cleft Palate Journal, 27,* 289–293.

Trost-Cardamone, J. (2009). Articulation and phonological assessment. In K. Moller & L. Glaze (Eds.), *Cleft lip and palate: Interdisciplinary issues and treatment* (2nd ed.). Austin, TX: Pro-Ed.

Trost-Cardamone, J. E., & Bernthal, J. E. (1993). Articulation assessment procedures and treatment decisions. In K. T. Moller & C. Starr (Eds.), *Cleft palate interdisciplinary issues and treatment: For clinicians by clinicians.* Austin, TX: Pro-Ed.

Van Demark, D. R. (1964). Misarticulations and listener judgments of the speech of individuals with cleft palates. *Cleft Palate Journal, 1,* 232–245.

Van Demark, D. R., & Hardin, M. A. (1990). Speech therapy for the child with cleft lip and palate. In J. Bardach & H. L. Morris (Eds.), *Multidisciplinary management of cleft lip and palate.* Philadelphia, PA: W. B. Saunders.

Weiss, C. E. (1974). The speech pathologist's role in dealing with obturator-wearing school children. *Journal of Speech and Hearing Disorders, 39,* 155–162.

Wilson, D. K. (1987) *Voice problems of children* (3rd ed.). Baltimore, MD: Williams & Wilkins.

Witzel, M., Tobe, J., & Salyer, K. (1989). The use of videonasopharyngoscopy for biofeedback therapy in adults after pharyngeal flap surgery. *Cleft Palate Journal, 26,* 129–134.

Witzel, M. A. (1995). Communicative impairment associated with clefting. In R. J. Shprintzen & J. Bardach (Eds.), *Cleft palate speech management: A multidisciplinary approach.* St. Louis, MO: Mosby.

Chapter 12

ADULT LANGUAGE DISORDERS

The loss or impairment of language in adults—after years of communicating normally—is socially and emotionally devastating for the patient as well as the family. Communication impairment can be the result of a brain accident, injury, or disease. Impact can be sudden or gradual. The patients' communication symptoms, onset information, case history, and medical findings should suggest a differential language diagnosis (which type of disorder) to the speech-language pathologist (SLP). We advocate consideration of the entire patient in his or her environmental milieu. Adult language disorders include the following communicative diagnostic labels: one of the aphasias, right hemisphere impairment, confusion, and the language of general intellectual deterioration of which there are multiple kinds of dementias.

THE APHASIAS

Aphasia refers to impaired language, not just a total loss of language. (The term *dysphasia*, although more accurate, has never gained popular use outside the medical profession.)

Brain injury from a cerebral vascular accident (CVA), commonly called a stroke or a brain attack, is the most frequent cause of aphasia. Brain tumors and traumatic brain injury (TBI) as from a car wreck or an ammunition injury also can cause adult language disorders of the type known as aphasia. The area of brain damage can be quite localized or more diffuse but encompasses the language centers of the patient's dominant brain hemisphere. For more than 95 percent of the population, the left hemisphere of the brain is dominant for language. **Figure 12–1** depicts the four major lobes of the brain and regions where various language functions are believed to be localized.

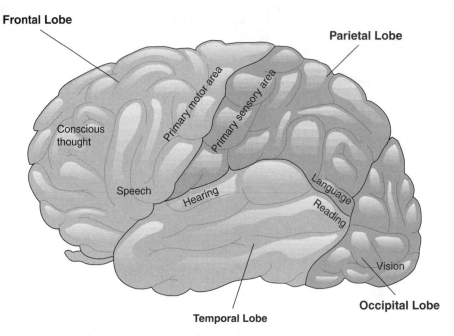

FIGURE 12–1 Lobes of the brain and locations of speech-language functions.
Source: AAOS. (2004). *Paramedic: Anatomy and Physiology* (1st ed., p. 169). Jones & Bartlett Learning. Reprinted by permission.

The term *aphasia* actually refers to a group of different forms of aphasia. It is not a singular impairment, so it is not sufficient to describe a patient as having merely expressive aphasia (difficulty speaking language) or receptive aphasia (difficulty understanding language), though many laypeople do. Symptoms of language impairment are multidimensional. Further, adults with aphasia may write like they speak or comprehend the written word like they understand verbal language. Damage to certain centers of the brain typical in aphasia may also render the patient unable to do simple arithmetic. Clearly, activities of daily living apart from talking and understanding are affected when a person can no longer read the newspaper, sign his or her name, or even count change from a dollar.

Aphasias have been categorized in various ways over the years usually as a result of the diagnostic test used by the speech-language pathologist. Patients' language abilities and disabilities often correspond to the **site of lesion** (place of damage) in the brain because certain functions indeed are localized to certain areas of the brain. Look again at Figure12–1; as you will see in this chapter, the *Boston Diagnostic Aphasia Examination* (Goodglass, Kaplan, & Barresi, 2000) and the *Western Aphasia Battery* (Kertesz, 2006) are both widely used in the assessment of adults with language impairments. Both these assessment tools are based on brain function localization yielding different types of language symptoms.

One common type of language impairment is **Broca's aphasia** with its characteristic site of lesion in the frontal lobe just anterior to the lateral (or Sylvian) fissure in the brain hemisphere dominant for language, usually the left. This area is important for motor function, so a patient may also present with a paralysis or **paresis** (weakness) of the opposite (right) leg, arm, or facial muscles. Motor speech problems and language impairments in patients with Broca's aphasia lead to what is termed **nonfluent expressive output**. This type of patient utters speech in a slow, deliberate fashion, often with omissions of smaller parts of speech. Often there is some degree of articulatory effort noted when speaking; motor speech problems are covered in the next chapter. A person with Broca's aphasia may use automatic speech and stereotypical responses (e.g., "That's it") excessively and display restricted vocal inflection in the voice. Though patients with Broca's aphasia display mild or severe expressive problems, they have relatively good auditory comprehension of language spoken to them.

In direct contrast is a type of aphasia known as **Wernicke's aphasia** where damage occurs primarily in the temporal lobe of the dominant language hemisphere. Damage is posterior to the lateral (Sylvian) fissure, so is in the auditory centers of the brain in the temporal lobe. Damage here results in poor auditory comprehension of language. Indeed, this type of aphasia often is simply called receptive aphasia. The patient may listen to the speaker intently yet show little ability to decode the message just heard. The person with Wernicke's aphasia usually has retained pragmatic language and so responds—often copiously—with a response that is both appropriately timed and with emotion and inflection in the voice. The output, however, is totally or partially **jargon**. The listener has a sense that a story is being told and inflections signal questions, emphatic statements, and occasional humor with chuckles. In patients with less severe jargon, there still is effortlessly **fluent verbal output** that contains **neologisms**, or new words (e.g., "Oh, yes, I know that's a fibiger, yeah, yeah it is" where *fibiger* is actually a coffee cup shown to the patient for naming). These patients often have frequent **paraphasias** that may or may not show some relation to the intended word. For example, some paraphasic error may bear a semantic relationship to the intended word (*spoon* when intending *fork*) or a rhyming, phonetic similarity (*telephone* intending *television*). **Table 12–1** defines some frequently used speech terminology used by speech-language pathologists. Patients with poor auditory comprehension seem oblivious to their own errors and have difficulty self-monitoring their speech output, something that may become the focus of treatment. This is in addition to their poor understanding of what is being said to them or asked of them, which also is central to a language rehabilitation program.

While Broca's and Wernicke's are the two best-known forms of aphasia, there are others. These other forms are apparent through adequate assessment. Most aphasia classifications in use in the United States today divide the types along the lines of how fluent or nonfluent the person's verbal output is and how good or poor the person's auditory

TABLE 12–1   A Brief Glossary of Terms Related to Aphasia

Agrammatism	Language containing grammatical errors such as lack of small parts of speech (articles, prepositions, pronouns) and even verbs; characteristic of nonfluent aphasias such as Broca's
Anomia	Inability to retrieve the word that is intended; often the word is on the speaker's "tip of the tongue" and the person can indicate what letter the intended word starts with or what it means; anomia can occur in all forms of aphasia including a mild aphasia where word-finding difficulties are the sole problem
Jargon	Meaningless connected speech output whether gibberish or interspersed with real words; often in Wernicke's aphasia
Neologisms	An invented word in lieu of a word; often in Wernicke's aphasia
Paraphasia	Substitution of one real word for another word that the brain is not retrieving; often the words are related in semantic meaning or initial sound

---

VIGNETTE 12–1

The wife and adult children visited Mr. Holden in the hospital while the speech-language pathologist was there. The family was very chatty and stated that dad could understand just fine because he could answer most questions as well as nod. The SLP, in the family's presence, engaged Mr. Holder in the following yes–no questions and social dialogue to elicit short replies.

Q: How do you feel today? (with cheery social inflection from the SLP)
A: Oh, yes, yes it is good, yes it is. (nodding constantly)
Q: Have you eaten yet? (with inquisitive inflection)
A: Oh, yes, yes, uh-huh. (nodding constantly)
Q: Are your pajamas on fire? (with inquisitive inflection)
A: Oh, yes, yes, uh-huh. (nodding constantly)

The SLP then talked to the family about the problems of asking yes–no questions and the likelihood of people always answering in the affirmative.

---

comprehension is. Seven types of aphasia and their symptoms are summarized in **Table 12–2**. The sites of lesions that give rise to these aphasic symptoms also are shown.

Because aphasia stems from brain damage, it should be no surprise that, in addition to language expression and comprehension impairments, often patients have to contend with other associated difficulties. We previously mentioned that motor cortex damage in the frontal lobe may lead to limb and facial paresis or paralysis. **Table 12–3** describes other concomitant problems that commonly affect persons with aphasias.

TABLE 12–2   Common Types of Aphasia and Their Symptoms

Type of Aphasia	Fluency of Speech	Comprehension Ability	Repetition Ability	Localization
Broca's	Nonfluent	Good	Good or disordered	Frontal (anterior)
Wernicke's (and jargon)	Fluent	Poor	Poor	Temporal (posterior)
Conductive	Fluent	Relatively good	Poor	Posterior
Global	Nonfluent	Poor	Poor	Widespread
Transcortical motor	Nonfluent	Good	Good	Anterior (surrounding Broca's)
Transcortical sensory	Fluent	Poor	Good	Posterior (surrounding Wernicke's)
Anomia	Fluent	Good	Good	Anywhere

TABLE 12–3   Difficulties That Often Accompany Aphasia

Motor impairment	Paralysis or paresis of body parts opposite the site of lesion, usually of the right leg, arm, or side of the face. Often physical therapy and occupational therapy are provided in addition to speech-language services.
Dysarthria of speech	Paralysis or paresis of speech-related muscles leading especially to articulatory imprecision and reduced speech intelligibility; impairments in respiratory and laryngeal systems also may compromise speech.
Apraxia of speech	Motor control issues of speech systems with articulatory imprecision and groping behaviors most pronounced in nonautomatic speech.
Emotionality	Tendency toward anxiety, generalized depression, situations of crying.
Profanity	Uncontrolled outbursts of cursing (even when the person never cursed before the stroke).
Visual deficits	It is not uncommon for the brain damage to affect parts of the visual pathway connecting the eyes to the back of the brain; loss of half the visual field may be detected in testing where the patient reads part of the page.
Swallowing disorders	Often the muscular issues affect the chewing and swallowing abilities and make choking a hazard (see dysphagia in the next chapter).
Memory deficits	Retrieval of words (anomia) and of recent events most vulnerable.

Sources: Davis (2007) and Tanner (1999).

OTHER LANGUAGE DISORDERS

RIGHT HEMISPHERE IMPAIRMENT

Another type of adult language disorder arises with damage to the nondominant hemisphere of the brain; this is the right hemisphere in more than 95 percent of the population. The right hemisphere, though not the dominant one for language per se, has a very important role in communication in a broader sense. Patients with right hemisphere damage often have adequate receptive and expressive language skills yet display subtle impairments with high-order, complex language tasks or when visual-spatial perception is tapped.

Patients with right hemisphere damage often present with some degree of impaired judgment and impaired self-monitoring skills. Though their expressive and receptive language skills are largely intact, these types of patients apply an overly literal interpretation to figurative language. They, for example, would miss the meaning of "when donkeys fly." Jokes and humor in language might be incomprehensible. Subtle changes in vocal inflection that may convey meaning will likely be missed. These patients appear indifferent to others' emotional vocal tone. There is poor self-expression of their own emotions because of flat intonation patterns, and clinically this is described as a **lack of affect**.

Similar difficulties are mirrored visually. Patients with right hemisphere impairments have trouble with facial recognition. This is in recognizing different faces (persons) but also in tuning into various emotions displayed on faces (sad, happy, and so forth).

Written language impairments also are associated with right hemisphere damage. Patients may exhibit impaired comprehension of written words. Though visual acuity is age appropriate, patients with right hemisphere damage typically have a host of visual deficits that affect language and communicative functioning. The most serious is visual neglect of the left half of space. SLPs working with objects, picture cues, or written stimuli frequently need to remind the patient to "look left" when scanning stimuli. These patients also may show impaired comprehension of written words or difficulty matching words to their pictures. In general, they may exhibit visual memory deficits as well as disorientation to place and space.

LANGUAGE OF CONFUSION

Widespread damage to the brain, especially when traumatic injury extends to both hemispheres, can lead to confused language. Usually there is a clear, swift onset and identifiable injury. Often the verbal output is off-topic and irrelevant to the communicative situation. The confused patient typically has intact grammar and sentence structure but poor topic maintenance. Often the patient can take a topic and weave an elaborate but false story around a theme. This ability is called **confabulation**. There is a general sense that the patient is not thinking clearly. Cognitive problem-solving ability is affected in such patients. Memory may be impaired, though auditory comprehension of language is not.

Confusion, along with other cognitive and perceptual symptoms, may be the result of a traumatic brain injury (TBI). Traumatic injuries to the brain can occur at any age, but most TBIs occur in the teen and young adult years. This seems related to the activities in which this age group participates (e.g., biking without a helmet, trampolining, fast driving, and driving under the influence of alcohol or drugs). TBI presents special challenges to educators, speech-language pathologists, and the medical rehabilitation team, so it is covered separately in Chapter 13.

LANGUAGE OF GENERALIZED INTELLECTUAL DETERIORATION

Though not typical of normal aging, for some adults there is a slow decrement in many abilities, including declines in memory, cognitive thought processes such as judgment and problem solving, language, social skills (including shopping), personal hygiene, and emotional control. Generalized intellectual deterioration forms the basis of a group of disorders known as the **dementias**. Perhaps the most commonly known dementia is that associated with Alzheimer disease, but there are others. In fact, there are characteristic differences in the dementias of Alzheimer disease, Parkinson disease, vascular dementia (e.g., from repeated strokes), advanced Down syndrome, and other diseases (Bayles & Tomoeda, 2007).

The dementias are usually caused by diffuse or widespread subcortical or cortical brain injury or atrophy. In Alzheimer disease, for example, there seems to be the formation of plaques in the brain concurrent with cellular shrinkage. Parkinson disease is linked to chemical changes in the basal ganglia region of the brain. In patients with certain medical diagnoses, the SLP needs to differentiate the communication impairments of aphasia, right hemisphere disability, the language of confusion, and the language of the many dementias.

ASSESSMENT OF ADULT LANGUAGE

The physician who treats the adult for stroke or other brain injury is usually first to recognize aphasia. Frequently, this physician is a **neurologist**. A neurologist specializes in conditions of the nervous system. Or the family physician might be the one to recognize changes in the adult patient over time. Either way, the physician typically asks the adult to follow simple commands, answer questions, name objects, and carry on a conversation. Depending on the adult's performance, if the physician suspects aphasia, the adult often is referred to a speech-language pathologist. The SLP will do a comprehensive assessment of communication abilities (including verbal expressive and receptive language, reading, writing, and swallowing—but more on that in the next chapter).

Assessment of adult language disorders basically ascertains, in detail, the patient's various abilities and disabilities. Armed with this information, and other medical knowledge, the SLP can parse out two things. First, based on the patient's pattern of abilities and disabilities, what is the nature of the problem—in other words, what is the communicative diagnosis? This piece of the puzzle includes differentiating between various disorders and subtypes to achieve a differential diagnosis. Second, based on the patient's detailed abilities, disabilities, and diagnosis, the SLP determines whether treatment is warranted, and if so, how to proceed with treatment. In effect, the SLP formulates a prognosis, treatment goals, and learning objectives.

The milieu of cognition (problem solving), memory, communication, and social pragmatism is a complicated set of intertwined factors. The SLP needs to disentangle the parts to discover answers to the preceding questions. Case history information, standardized testing, and nonstandardized probing are the best ways to proceed.

CASE HISTORY INFORMATION

The SLP, depending on his or her work setting, may have ready access to the patient's presenting complaint. The patient's family and medical records also are a good source. What communication concerns do family members have? Can the patient identify a specific time when speech-language abilities changed? Was there a medical event, and if so, can the SLP explore the evidence? What was speech-language like a month or a year earlier versus now? What has the physician said? Is the patient left or right handed? What is the patient's educational level? What type of work does/did the patient do? What is a typical day now like? What sorts of daily communication occur? What medicines and other therapies are prescribed? The SLP can explore these and many other questions in the case history interview. Inpatient work settings have a history on file that contains much useful information from the admitting physician, nurse, or social services. Imaging studies, such as from a computed tomography (CT) scan or magnetic resonance imaging (MRI), may report site of lesion. Daily chart notes are worthy of a read to ascertain the patient's behaviors displayed in the facility and, if read over time, any progression the patient has made since admission. The SLP is thirsty for any and all information as clues to the patient's problems, abilities, and medical disposition.

Whether the physician had ordered an SLP consult or in another work setting the patient or patient's family had referred, case history information and medical reports are vital clues. The SLP seeks to narrow the field of possible communication disorders to select the most appropriate standardized tests and other assessment tools.

TESTING FOR APHASIA

Many commercial tests for adult language disorders have been developed over the years. They range from simple and quick bedside screening approaches to in depth, multimodality batteries. (See Davis, 2007, or Haynes & Pindzola, 2008, for an overview of commercially available tests suited to various functions.)

If the case history information and the SLP's preliminary indications (perhaps by a screening) are that the patient may have aphasia, the SLP should select a comprehensive test of aphasia. A comprehensive test assesses at a minimum the modalities of speaking, listening, writing, and reading at various levels of complexity. Supplemental tests also are available for related problems. A comprehensive test battery can do many things: diagnose the specific type of aphasia (recall Table 12–1), determine patient strengths and weaknesses for use in designing treatment, establish baseline data from which to judge therapeutic improvements, and some predict probable outcomes.

The *Boston Diagnostic Aphasia Examination* (BDAE 3rd ed.) (Goodglass et al., 2000) comprehensively assesses language skills in 35 subtests. Performance indicators correlate to localized areas of brain damage. A sample of the patient's expository speech (describing an action picture) is rated on six conversational features: melodic line, phrase length, articulator agility, grammatical form, paraphasias, and word finding. The BDAE has become a classic comprehensive assessment tool used over successive decades with only minor revisions. Standardized Z scores and percentile rankings are used in scoring the BDAE, making it useful for reporting data.

The *Western Aphasia Battery* (WAB–Revised) (Kertesz, 2006) is another popular, comprehensive tool for the differential diagnosis of aphasia types. Some 17 subscores and major scores cover a range of expressive and receptive language skills. It includes tasks of written language ranging from matching the written word with a picture to reading comprehension. The WAB, like the BDAE, links language symptoms to cortical lesion sites and the two share similar terms for the various types of aphasia. These types are shown in Table 12–1. Both the WAB and the BDAE are thorough but not necessarily time-consuming tests.

We are aware that clinicians use selected subsets from the BDAE and WAB, but we caution that by doing so, standardized scores lose their utility. Assessment of multiple modalities in subsets covering a range of complexity is the best way to reveal a patient's strengths, weaknesses, and level of breakdown to best design treatment and track subtle changes over time through repeated measures.

RIGHT HEMISPHERE ASSESSMENT ISSUES

For years, assessment of right hemisphere impairments has been a cobbled collection of many small tests and subtests from different sources. SLPs and neuropsychologists pulled from aphasia language tests, linguistic tests, visuospatial perceptual test, and others. Although useful patient information may have been ascertained, standardized testing now is readily available.

The *Right Hemisphere Language Battery* (RHLB) (Bryan, 1995) assesses aspects of higher-level language that often is impaired in subtle ways in such patients. Tasks include metaphor–picture matching, written metaphor choices, inferred meaning comprehension, humor appreciation, lexical semantic recognition, emphatic stress production, and discourse production. The discourse sample has its own 11-parameter rating system.

The *Mini Inventory of Right Brain Injury* (MIRBI) (Pimental & Kingsbury, 2004) is a 27-item screening assessment. Examples include visual scanning, body image, emotion and affective language, and other high-level language skills.

The *Rehabilitative Institute of Chicago Evaluation of Communication Problems in Right Hemisphere Dysfunction* (RICE) (Halper, Cherney, & Burns, 1996) focuses on behavior patterns, visual scanning, analysis of written errors, and pragmatic language violations. In addition, the comprehension of and use of metaphors in language are assessed.

ASSESSING LANGUAGE OF CONFUSION AND OF DEMENTIA

Speech-language pathologists, neuropsychologists, and psychiatrists have either individually or as a professional team endeavored to assess mentally confused patients and those with cognitive-linguistic decline. A myriad of commercial tests is available with varying adequacies of standardized data. The serious reader is encouraged to read summaries elsewhere (Burrows Mental Measurements Yearbook, 2001; Haynes & Pindzola, 2008). Functions assessed may include aspects of cognition, orientation, memory, word fluency (e.g., recalling animals that start with *b*), communicative effectiveness, intelligence, and nonverbal intelligence. An illustrative example of a standardized assessment tool for this clinical population is the *Arizona Battery for Communication Disorders of Dementia* (ABCD) (Bayles & Tomoeda, 1993).

Regardless of the standardized test selected, let it guide treatment decisions. Tests tap into patients' strengths and weaknesses, so help the SLP set goals. Even when treatment is not recommended or is recommended for short-term strategy development only, reassessments done over time provide a useful standardized method for patient monitoring.

ADULT LANGUAGE TREATMENT PRINCIPLES

Comprehensive tests of aphasia cover simple to complex receptive and expressive language tasks, thus giving the SLP detailed analyses of patient abilities and levels of breakdown. The goal of testing is to determine the type and severity of aphasia, but more important to guide the SLP in recommendations, prognosis, and treatment planning to better improve the patient's situation in daily life. Assessment information, together with non-standardized testing, such as cueing or probing into "what might work," helps the clinician design a treatment plan with communication goals and smaller objectives of learning. The plan can be as straightforward as in the following example.

The literature on aphasia therapies is quite robust. World War II saw a marked increase in head wounds, and therapies emerged to meet this need. Advances in health and medicine also allow people to live longer now than at any time in history. With increased longevity have come increases in strokes with survival, as well as other age-related diseases affecting language. The need for effective and efficient treatment approaches is very real.

VIGNETTE 12–2

Mrs. Ferguson's test results suggest a diagnosis of Broca's aphasia, and this is consistent with the site of lesion shown in her MRI. Her treatment goals focus on strategies for word retrieval and on increasing her grammatical length of utterance. The SLP's baseline data should be indicated in the record for gauging progress (or lack of it) in treatment. Testing indicates that currently Mrs. Ferguson easily and fluently can retrieve 23 percent of single words when asked to name objects and pictures. Probes reveal that retrieval is facilitated when the patient is directed to think of the first sound and whisper it slowly. The SLP develops plans for the goal of increasing length of utterance, citing current baseline length, noting absence of articles and other small parts of speech, and stating what approach will be followed in treatment (based on the SLP's knowledge of treatment methods) and the results of nonstandardized trial probes.

Though it is wise to bear in mind that some adults with stroke will not survive or will be in such a severe state that rehabilitation is not warranted, for many patients treatment can lead to full or partial recovery from aphasia. **Spontaneous recovery** can occur even without treatment in some cases. Still, the rule of thumb is for persons with aphasia to seek immediate services within days, weeks, or a few months following stroke. This is the prime time for rehabilitation to be effective, though improvements can often span a two-year interval. A patient motivated to practice treatment activities also is important.

Aphasia treatment seeks to improve the adult's ability to use speech and language so as to function in the daily environment with as much communicative independence as possible. Strategies when practiced can retrain, maybe restore, or perhaps offer compensation. Therapies might target word retrieval strategies; formation of long, fluent, and more complex utterances; enhanced auditory comprehension; monitoring and cessation of jargon, neologisms, or runaway speech; comprehension of written words; or a host of other objectives. Davis (2007) provides a good description of identifying treatment goals and how to track outcomes.

Similar principles hold for high-level-functioning patients with right hemisphere damage and even for lower functioning adults with dementia. The SLP should assess strengths and weaknesses and design intervention strategies and considerable practice around these lines. Although we acknowledge that the disease cannot fully be reversed or that any progressive deterioration can be halted, we do advocate that with good principles of management, overt practice of language skills, and compensatory strategies, the SLP can help enhance the adult's communicative situation within the given daily circumstances. The writings on dementia by Bayles and Tomoeda (2007) and by Ripich (1991) are particularly useful.

TIPS FOR EDUCATIONAL AND DAY CARE SETTINGS

Because traumatic brain injuries (TBIs) of school-aged students is addressed in Chapter 13, the issue of adult language disorders in educational settings can be dismissed unless the concept is broadened to include the settings of family care and adult day care facilities. We have chosen to place adult day care here rather than as a medical setting.

Community adult centers may serve adults with aphasia, but most certainly are populated with adults that have Alzheimer disease or other issues with intellectual deterioration. What is expected of these centers? They are not only to give the primary caregiver of the home a motivational break, but they are to afford a structured social and educational environment for the affected adult. It is important that day care providers offer safe and consistent care that supports the patient's communication skills, cognitive abilities, and social interactions. SLPs as well as other social workers, mental health specialists, cognitive neuropsychologists, and gerontology physicians may form a team in support of the adult day care. The following tips may help, and they are useful to the affected family as well.

1. Use short, simple sentences.
2. Repeat the message as needed (and remain even-tempered).
3. Keep distraction to a minimum (turn down the television when talking to the adult with brain damage).
4. Include the adult in the conversation; do not ignore the person.
5. Engender a need to talk; do not tend to the person's every need without encouraging some language participation.
6. Encourage any type of communication (e.g., speech, gesture, pointing, drawing).
7. Involve the adult in outside activities (e.g., grocery shopping, church, adult day care, visiting friends).

TIPS FOR ALLIED HEALTH PROFESSIONS

Ideally, medical allied health professionals such as gerontologists, neurologists, nurses, social workers, neuropsychologists, respiratory therapists, physical and occupational therapists, and speech-language pathologists can work as an integrated team with a hospital inpatient or clinical outpatient in the assessment and treatment of adult language disorders. During the acute stage of a CVA or a tumor resection, for example, the patient may have difficulty expressing or comprehending language. An early SLP consult is important to begin monitoring the type and severity of aphasia for a more reliable prognosis. Sometimes the type of aphasia evolves into other types with improvement.

The SLP also can assess what communication modalities are more reliable and give communication information to the patient, family, and entire medical team. Some tips for interacting with inpatients and early outpatients with adult language disorders include the following.

1. Do not assume the patient comprehends "yes" or "no" even if the patient speaks the words or nods to questions. Patients with aphasia often are aware of questioning intonations and invariably reply in some fashion in the affirmative. Families especially think Grandma understands everything because she nods yes. Try asking, "Are your fingers chocolate?" and see what responses you get!

2. When seeking information that is also trustworthy, avoid asking yes/no questions. Rather than asking, "Do you feel okay today?" ask "How does your head feel?" Even if the person's reply is brief or struggled, it is of more use than an unreliable nod.

3. Review the tips given in the previous section because they apply here as well.

VIGNETTE 12–3

Jim Curley, a burly, retired factory worker, had a CVA three weeks ago. Since his stroke, he has had difficulty talking in connected sentences of two to three words, and he has some mild word-finding difficulty. Following the stroke, he also was paralyzed on his right leg and right arm. Function in his arm has returned, though it is still weak. His comprehension of language is good. In addition to speech-language therapy, he is getting daily physical and occupational therapies in the rehabilitation hospital. In the team meeting, the OT and PT comment on Mr. Curley's difficulty speaking and how his frustration that follows is disruptive to his sessions. The SLP comments on how pleased she is with Mr. Curley's progress with melodic intonation therapy. The SLP observes the PT and OT sessions and instructs all to intone (with a syllable beat) and to have Mr. Curley intone his attempted replies. The advice not only aids communication, it serves to generalize a therapeutic setting to outside of speech treatment.

Terms to Know

Aphasia	Neologisms
Site of lesion	Paraphasias
Broca's aphasia	Lack of affect
Paresis	Confabulation
Nonfluent expressive output	Dementias
Wernicke's aphasia	Neurologist
Jargon	Spontaneous recovery
Fluent verbal output	

Study Questions

1. What are the typical speech-language characteristics in a patient with Broca's aphasia?
2. What are the typical speech-language characteristics in a patient with Wernicke's aphasia?
3. After a right hemisphere stroke, the physician may not detect any language deficits with a simple aphasia screening of a few questions. Why not? What sorts of issues might the SLP need to explain to healthcare professionals to help them understand the characteristic problems?
4. If dementia is a progressive disease, when is language treatment appropriate? How can you tell?

Bibliography

Bayles, K., & Tomoeda, C. (1993). *The Arizona Battery of Communication Disorders of Dementia.* Tucson, AZ: Canyonland Publishing.

Bayles, K., & Tomoeda, C. (2007). *Cognitive-communication disorders of dementia.* San Diego, CA: Plural.

Bryan, K. L. (1995). *The Right-Hemisphere Language Battery* (2nd ed.). London: Whurr Publishers.

Buros Institute. (2001). *The fourteenth mental measurement yearbook.* Lincoln: University of Nebraska Press.

Davis, G. A. (2007). *Aphasia disorders and clinical practice.* Boston, MA: Allyn & Bacon.

Goodglass, H., Kaplan, E., & Barresi, N. (2000). *The assessment of aphasia and related disorders.* Hagerstown, MD: Lippincott Williams & Wilkins.

Halper, A., Cherney, L. R., & Burns, M. S. (1996). *Rehabilitation Institute of Chicago clinical management of right hemisphere dysfunction* (2nd ed.). Gaithersburg, MD: Aspen.

Haynes, W., & Pindzola, R. (2008). *Diagnosis and evaluation in speech pathology* (7th ed.). Boston, MA: Allyn & Bacon.

Kertesz, A. (2006). *Western Aphasia Battery—Revised.* New York, NY: Psychological Corp.

Pimental, P. A., & Kingsbury, N. A. (2004). *Mini Inventory of Right Brain Injury* (2nd ed). Austin, TX: Pro-Ed.

Ripich, D. (1991). *Handbook of geriatric communication disorders.* Austin, TX: Pro-Ed.

Tanner, D. (1999). *The family guide to surviving stroke and communication disorders.* Boston, MA: Allyn & Bacon.

13

SPECIFIC NEUROLOGICALLY BASED IMPAIRMENTS

Speech and language deficits may be part of a more global condition in which the student or adult has motor impairments, perceptual difficulties, cognitive deficits, behavioral problems, and the like. Problems of these types may be subtle or highly noticeable to peers, teachers, healthcare professionals, or the public at large. They most certainly are educationally or vocationally handicapping and necessitate teamwork among school personnel and healthcare professionals. Conditions discussed in this chapter, although not communication disorders per se, do have neurologic foundations that affect the person's speech-language skills and, ultimately, academic or workplace performance. We provide an overview of neuromuscular problems in children such as cerebral palsy, dysarthria, and dysphagia (swallowing disorders), and then the neuromuscular problems typical in adults. This chapter also covers the neurologic and behavioral sequelae to traumatic brain injury that can occur at any age. Finally, we present the multifaceted problems associated with the condition termed attention deficit disorder. Along the way, we highlight assessment and treatment roles of the speech-language pathologist (SLP) and provide tips for the teacher and healthcare professional.

Students with these neurologic problems may need special education support services, yet most will be mainstreamed into regular classrooms. These students may present a challenge to the classroom teacher and require adaptation of physical facilities, knowledge of special equipment, use of technology, and modification of curricular activities. The conspicuousness of the student's condition also may strain social relations among peers. The teacher's understanding of a student's medical condition is paramount to structuring an optimal learning environment. This chapter discusses some of the medical conditions affecting communication that a classroom teacher is likely to encounter. Adults, whether in the workplace, retired, or in medical care facilities, pose similar issues and are covered in this chapter as well.

THE NATURE OF NEUROLOGIC PROBLEMS IN YOUNG STUDENTS

Damage to the nervous system may render muscular problems of weakness, incoordination, slowness, or even paralysis. The location and extent of nervous system damage are, of course, important, but the essence of the person's **neuromuscular problem** is movement based. If the damage to the brain occurred before, during, or after birth (during childhood), the person is diagnosed as having cerebral palsy. If the affected muscles include those involved in speech production or are limited to those involved in speech production (i.e., muscles of respiration, phonation, and articulation), the speech-language pathologist may refer to the condition as dysarthria. Actually, there are many types of dysarthria; the term simply means a **motor speech disorder**.

    Dysarthria is a collection of motor speech disorders resulting from neurologic abnormalities in strength, speed, range of motion, steadiness, tone, or accuracy of movement (Duffy, 2005). Dysarthria, particularly in adults and adolescents, may exist in the absence of cerebral palsy. In such cases, the dysarthria (motor speech condition) is usually caused by some trauma (e.g., automobile wreck, stroke, near poisoning) or disease state (e.g., muscular dystrophy, myasthenia gravis, tumor invasion, multiple sclerosis, encephalitis, inherited degenerative disorders). The neuromuscular problems of cerebral palsy are discussed followed by brief mention of a form of dysarthria (not associated with true cerebral palsy) that may be seen in school-aged students.

CEREBRAL PALSY

    Cerebral palsy is a static encephalopathy, meaning there is nondegenerative damage to the brain. Cerebral palsy (CP) often is classified on the basis of at least two factors: the type of neuromuscular involvement, and the distribution of injury. **Table 13–1** outlines the six major types of CP with respect to neuromuscular involvement: **spasticity**, **athetosis**, **ataxia**, **tremor**, **rigidity**, and **mixed**. Spasticity is by far the most common form of CP, whereas tremor and rigidity are infrequent in children. At the risk of oversimplification, physical therapists, occupational therapists, speech-language pathologists, and special educators often design intervention programs and handling techniques for these students based on the amount of muscle tone generally present (i.e., whether the student has high tone, low tone, or fluctuating tone). Classification based on the distribution of injury reflects the underlying extent of brain damage. Many classifying terms exist; three common forms of CP are hemiplegia, paraplegia, and quadriplegia. **Hemiplegia** is the most common type of CP and often occurs with spasticity. The arm and leg on the same side of the body are involved; the side of involvement is opposite to the side of brain damage. **Paraplegia** is the term used to describe involvement of both legs but with the arms

TABLE 13–1 The Major Types of Cerebral Palsy as Classified by Neuromuscular Involvement

Type	Neuromuscular Characteristics
Spasticity	Muscles of the limbs feel tight; increased muscle tone; hyperactive reflexes.
Athetosis	Limbs have involuntary purposeless movements; purposeful movements are contorted.
Ataxia	A lack of balance sensation; a lack of position sense in space; uncoordinated movements.
Tremor	Shakiness of the involved limbs; tremor might be noticed only in the attempt to use the limb (intention tremor). Continuous tremor at rest is not common in children but often accompanies brain disease in adults.
Rigidity	Perhaps a severe form of spasticity; in movement the rigid limb gives way as if it were a lead pipe or a cogwheel.
Mixed	A combination of neuromuscular symptoms; often spasticity and athetosis appear in children with quadriplegia.

usually unaffected. Brain damage is confined to a particular region within both hemispheres. When all four extremities are involved, the CP is called quadriplegia. The degree of motor involvement may or may not be equal in the extremities. **Quadriplegia** results from a wide area of brain damage.

The causes of cerebral palsy are many and varied. Suffice it to say that CP can result from brain damage occurring at any time during the developmental period (prenatal, natal, postnatal). Causes include faulty genetic factors, maternal infections, anoxia (lack of oxygen), trauma during delivery, childhood traumatic injuries, and infectious diseases.

The individual with CP often is multiply handicapped. The classroom teacher most certainly needs to know the student's strengths and weaknesses. Frequently occurring disabilities associated with cerebral palsy include those discussed in the following subsections.

Epileptic Seizures   Massive convulsions with or without the loss of consciousness are known as grand mal seizures, whereas minor and fleeting seizures are petit mal or other partial types (Brumback, Mathews, & Shenoy, 2001). Persons with cerebral palsy have a propensity for epileptic seizures. It may be wise to check with the school nurse regarding what to do or not to do if a seizure occurs in the classroom. Also it is desirable to find out whether the student is on medication for seizure control and what the side effects of medication are likely to be, especially regarding activity level and attention span.

Orthopedic Problems   Abnormal muscle stresses may cause deformities and dislocations for which the student may need bracing, compensatory postures, or even surgery. Correct positioning of motorically involved students is critical for the educational environment. Teachers should consult with the appropriate school system personnel to learn optimal positioning and handling techniques for each individual student. The physical therapist, occupational therapist, special education teacher, school medical personnel, or even the SLP might be contacted in this regard. The Individualized Education Program (IEP) meeting provides an optimal time for the various disciplines to interact and discuss an appropriate course of action, including positioning and handling, for the student. Each team member should become familiar with the student's braces, wheelchair, restraint systems, and/or other specialized equipment to best work with the student.

Feeding and Nutritional Problems   Incoordination of muscles involved in chewing and swallowing may lead to feeding or nutritional problems. Often, with infants, specialized feeding programs must be developed, incorporating the use of special postures, techniques, utensils, and exercises. Throughout the child's growth and development, nutrition may continue to be a concern because of reduced food intake (resulting from problems in chewing and swallowing) and the fact that much caloric energy is consumed with involuntary movements. We touch on dysphagia (swallowing disorders) again later in this chapter.

Communication Disorders   Cerebral palsy may encompass any or all of the speech production processes, leading to problems with air control (e.g., able to speak too few words per breath), voice production (e.g., phonatory spasms causing vocal strain or other quality changes), prosody (e.g., difficulty controlling pitch inflections and proportional stressing of syllables), and articulation (e.g., speech sounding slurred or imprecise). Solomon and Charron (1998) espouse that breathing problems are central to most forms of CP and warrant attention from the SLP. They advocate techniques for improved speech breathing and exhalatory control. In general, speech treatment seeks to normalize muscle movements, when possible, or to train compensatory movements to their best potential for improved intelligibility. Individuals with CP and very severe motoric involvement, however, may not be candidates for learning speech. In such cases, therapy is directed at training in the use of an augmentative or alternative communication mode, as discussed later in this chapter.

In addition to speech problems, the student may have delayed language abilities, perhaps resulting from the brain damage itself or from the restricted environmental exposure afforded the child when young. Language intervention programs are likely parts of the total educational needs of the student with CP. Intervention strategies and collaborative learning, as discussed in the early chapters of this book, certainly apply to this type of student.

Cognitive Deficits   Deficits in cognition may parallel language delays. Presumably the brain damage that produces the motor movement problems also reduces the person's ability to assimilate stimuli and to organize it meaningfully (i.e., to think intelligently). However, it has been estimated that about 30–40 percent of individuals with CP are of average or above average intelligence (Mirenda & Mathy-Laikko, 1989), so: Teachers should never underestimate the academic potential of a motorically involved student!

Perceptual Deficits   Perceptual deficits are many and varied. Visual defects stem from problems of eye movement; hearing loss also occurs frequently in cerebral palsied individuals. Often there is difficulty organizing sensory stimuli into some kind of meaning. Students may have figure-ground problems, visual-motor problems, and inabilities shifting to abstract forms of behavior (staying instead at concrete, stereotyped, and predictive responses). Teachers should realize that perceptual problems may necessitate some adaptations in the classroom learning environment.

DYSARTHRIA

As mentioned at the beginning of the chapter, motor speech disturbances often accompany certain disease states and/or may result from trauma to the peripheral nervous system, central nervous system, or both. In particular, dysarthria refers to an impairment in neuromuscular function of the respiratory, phonatory, and/or articulatory processes of speech. The degree of impairment can be so minimal that dysarthria would be difficult to detect during conversational speech or the degree of impairment can be so severe that any speech produced is completely unintelligible. In such severe cases, alternative communication systems often are necessary. Muscular dystrophy is one disease encountered in school-aged youth that eventually results in severe dysarthria.

Television telethons, often broadcast on Labor Day weekends for the past few decades, have made **muscular dystrophy** a household term. As a group of diseases, muscular dystrophy (MD) is anything but simple. There is progressive atrophy, or wasting away of the skeletal muscles throughout the body, without damage to the nerves. Onset is usually at an early age; often a waddling gait appears when a child begins to walk or first starts school. Muscle deterioration can progress rapidly, leaving the youngster on a bracing system for ambulation or confined to a wheelchair by the teenage years. MD seems to be a familial disease, and it occurs more frequently in males than in females. The widespread deterioration of muscles not only interferes with locomotion ability but also affects the muscles involved in respiration. Obviously, speech becomes impaired as these muscles atrophy, but there is major concern for breathing adequacy. Treatment is multidisciplinary and directed toward relieving symptoms and slowing the progress of the disease. Unnecessary immobilization may accelerate the rate of deterioration (Jones, 1985). The student should be encouraged to lead as normal a life as possible.

AUGMENTATIVE AND ALTERNATIVE COMMUNICATION MODES

Speech-language pathologists have a responsibility to help motorically involved persons develop **augmentative or alternative communication (AAC)** strategies when the cerebral palsy or dysarthria is too severe to permit intelligible, conversational speech. The SLP may train the student to use an alternative communication method to speech or the SLP may train the student augmentatively, using a combination of spoken output and a communication device. According to the American Speech-Language-Hearing Association

(2004) and others (Silverman, 1989; McCormick & Wegner, 2003), this responsibility includes the following aspects.

1. Identifying appropriate candidates for AAC
2. Selecting the communication mode or modes that will meet the student's communication needs
3. Securing necessary hardware and software (through school purchasing or leasing)
4. Teaching the student how to use the mode selected for encoding and transmitting messages
5. Developing intervention plans to promote the student's maximal functional communication
6. Working with the education team, especially the classroom teacher, to implement the intervention plan in a school settings (e.g., lunch, gym, art)
7. Periodically reassessing the student's cognitive, motor, sensory, and communication abilities to ensure that the mode selected and semantic choices provided initially continue to meet the student's communication needs

In introducing an augmentative or alternative communication system, the SLP often encounters resistance from a variety of sources. It is important for families and school personnel to recognize that an augmentative and alternative communication system does not interfere with speech acquisition. To the contrary, many reports describe increased speech following implementation of such systems. This substantial literature, reviewed by Abrahamsen, Romski, and Sevcik (1989), documents that users of augmentative and alternative communication demonstrate positive gains in (1) speech production and comprehension, (2) attention span, (3) task orientation, and (4) social skills.

Legislative provisions for assistive technology have been included in the Individuals with Disabilities Education Act (IDEA) and the Americans with Disabilities Act (ADA-PL101-336). As stated by McCormick and Wegner (2003), both laws require that individuals with disabilities obtain whatever assistive devices they need, including items such as battery-powered toys, hearing aids, wheelchairs, computers, eating systems, augmentative communication devices, special switches, and a wide range of other devices that have the potential to improve an individual's ability to learn, compete, work, and interact with others. School districts are required to foster education by providing assistive technology devices and services to eligible children.

Communication may be achieved through a variety of high-tech and low-tech augmentative or alternative systems, such as pointing to picture boards, using sign language, accessing a symbolic code (manually or electronically), typing a message on a computer screen, or using a machine that produces a synthetic or digital voice. The past few years have also seen an explosion of technological advances and miniaturized systems such as palmtop, handheld, and tablet devices. **Table 13–2** lists some Web sources for viewing what is commercially available; it also provides some basic sites for resources on the general subject of augmentative and alternative communication.

TABLE 13–2 A Sampling of Commercially Available Augmentative and Alternative Communication Devices and General Subject Information

1. Palmtop, handheld, tablet, or e-talk Dynavox systems are shown in the products section of www.dynavoxtech.com.

2. Assorted augmentative communication products, such as picture-word boardmaker for the personal computer, a talking picture and word processing program with more than 8000 pictures, or a tool for creating talking interactive activities for the class, are shown at www.mayer-johnson.com.

3. The American Speech-Language-Hearing Association provides basic information on augmentative and alternative communication at the following site: www.asha.org/public/speech/disorders/AAC.htm. In particular, teachers and parents may be interested in the primer of terminology and articles on team approaches to evaluation and management.

4. The AAC Institute provides resources for people who rely on augmentative and alternative communication, their families, friends, educators, and professionals. The education/training information may be of particular interest through www.aacinstitute.org.

5. Low-tech and high-tech products at www.communicationaids.com include the Crestwood line of communication boards, mounting kits, picture kits, talking aids, switches, amplifiers, and more.

6. Full-service hardware and software systems and support are provided by the Prentke Romich Company at www.prentrom.com.

It may be helpful to think of all augmentative/alternative communication systems as having four primary components: symbols, aids, strategies, and techniques (American Speech-Language-Hearing Association [ASHA], 2004). Depending on the student's cognitive and physical skills, the symbols used may range from actual objects, pictures of objects, universal icons (e.g., Minspeak's icons of thumbs up, thumbs down, stop sign, and so forth) (Van Der Merwe & Alant, 2004), and traditional orthography (pictured word). Teachers and classroom peers need to become familiar with the symbols used by a particular student for communication to occur. Aids are devices used to transmit or receive messages. These vary from the very simple and basic to complex technological systems. Strategies are ways in which symbols can be conveyed efficiently. Techniques refer to the various ways messages can be transmitted, either through direct selection or scanning.

Classroom teachers must work with the SLP to understand the communication system and the ways to interact with the student. Teachers also need to be familiar with the device used by a particular student in case the teacher needs to make quick repairs to limit the student's downtime (Daniel, 2004). Although it is beyond the scope of this text to explain the intricacies of the alternative devices (Glennen & DeCoste, 1997, is a thorough source), the SLP should be able to provide detailed assistance on the use of any student's particular system. **Table 13–3** presents roles and responsibilities suggested for the classroom teacher on the AAC team.

TABLE 13–3 Suggested Roles for the Classroom Teacher on the AAC Team

- Adapt the curriculum for the student using an AAC system.
- Write goals and objectives for the student user and maintain documentation.
- Assess, and frequently reassess, cognitive abilities of the student.
- Act as a liaison with the family and between all educational team members.
- Assess, and frequently reassess, the student's social capabilities.
- Provide for ongoing skill development.
- Identify vocabulary to be provided in the student's AAC system.
- Provide information about the student's motivation and attitude toward the AAC system.
- Determine the student's communication needs, working closely with the speech-language pathologist.

Source: Adapted from McCormick & Wegner (2003).

Augmentative and alternative communication has become a vast subject and most all school systems have had or will have students needing such accommodations. It must be remembered that the primary role of AAC systems is to facilitate active participation and engagement in meaningful events in the daily lives of students with handicaps. And it is in this light that teachers and classroom peers must take the responsibility to become true conversational partners.

According to Beukelman and Mirenda (1992), participation is a prerequisite to communication; without participation, there is no one to talk to, nothing to talk about, and no reason to communicate. Consider the following students.

VIGNETTE 13–1

Maria, age 3 years, is in a wheelchair and has limited use of her hands and semi-intelligible speech. The preschool teacher and SLP wish to enhance Maria's participation in small-group playtime. At present, she just sits in her wheelchair and watches peers play in the toy kitchen or with blocks and other manipulable toys. Together the teacher and the SLP plan intervention strategies so that Maria's lap tray becomes a play surface; some toys have been adapted with Velcro so that she can pick them up wearing a Velcro glove, and a small toy stove and sink have been purchased for use on the lap tray (instead of the large play kitchen furniture). Also, the battery-operated blender has been adapted for switch activation. These adaptations to the play situation are generating two-way communication among Maria and her peers, allowing for much-needed speech and language practice. The context-based communication is also aiding peers' understanding of Maria's speech as she simultaneously manipulates toys and real objects.

VIGNETTE 13–2

Tyrone's cerebral palsy has meant that he has long needed AAC systems for communicative interactions, but now, in the second grade, his experiences with symbols and iconic encoding (such as Minspeak) are about to change. The AAC team, especially the speech-language pathologist and the classroom teacher, are transitioning Tyrone to learn orthography for reading and writing development. The vocabulary of the curriculum is becoming more diverse (in language arts, math, science, music, social studies) and Tyrone's thirst for knowledge and participation are growing too. The AAC team is supplying and training Tyrone with computer-based options involving an orthographic keyboard with speech synthesis, screen-reader software (for reading enlarged print text entered into the system), and written literacy software (for Tyrone to compose and write). His typing skills, though slow and laborious, are sufficient for his total communication and educational advancement.

TEACHER TIPS FOR STUDENTS WITH NEUROMUSCULAR PROBLEMS

Students with neuromuscular problems, such as cerebral palsy, dysarthria, and dysphagia, present with multiple handicaps. In the past, the majority of these students were placed inappropriately into residential institutes or special day schools. With the advent of PL 94-142, IDEA, and the ADA, students with dysarthria and cerebral palsy are now educated in regular and special classes within public school systems. Many have sufficient intellectual capacity for education in the normal classroom setting. Classroom teachers, however, may need to provide these students with extra attention, practice understanding, and be willing to modify or adapt academic assignments. The following suggestions are adapted from Eisenson and Ogilvie (1983), Phillips (1984), and Sexson and Dingle (2001).

1. Help the student adjust to the group and instill a sense of belonging. Being socially accepted by classroom peers is difficult for the student who may look different, talk with slurred and labored speech, and walk with a staggered gait or not at all. Social adjustment problems may amplify during adolescence. School dances, first dates, sports, learning to drive a car, and acceptable speech are just some of the ways students with neuromuscular problems are left out. Feeling depressed, discouraged, resentful, and rebellious is common to youth with handicaps. As a teacher, recognize the need for referral to a counselor when a student's feelings become too negative.
2. Provide understanding, not sympathy or pity.
3. Encourage and provide opportunities for classmates to maintain contact and communication with the student.
4. Expect the student to perform tasks that are within his or her capabilities. Do not allow the handicapping condition to become an "excuse."

5. Speech is best when the student is relaxed. Set a casual, relaxed classroom atmosphere. Tasks that frustrate also tend to cause deterioration of speech intelligibility.

6. Support any specific educational accommodations needed, such as test conditions, note taking, large print, and so forth.

7. Modify the environment to suit the motorically involved student. For example, consider placing the student's desk (or other apparatus) in the most accessible location. With young children using augmentative communication devices, positioning of the device with other manipulables (crayons, clay, lunch, maps, globes) is critical and must be learned by teachers.

8. Frequently review the child's learning capabilities and formally evaluate (or refer for evaluation) as needed.

9. Help the child break assignments into discrete tasks to facilitate an organized and successful approach.

10. Be aware of any chewing or swallowing dysfunctions and, when appropriate, assist with safe intake approaches during classroom parties, snacks, and lunch.

11. Encourage participation in all regular classroom activities, yet allow for special considerations. For instance, a student who cannot hold a pencil well or write legibly may do much better typing class work on a typewriter or computer.

12. Be willing to assist the speech-language pathologist in providing speech and language stimulation or assistance in communicating with alternative systems frequently throughout the school day. Students on an augmentative communication system often need much encouragement to use the device in the classroom and to interact with peers. A teacher's assistance is invaluable here.

THE NATURE OF NEUROLOGIC PROBLEMS IN ADULTS

Adults of all ages may experience speech changes as a precursor to and as a result of neurologic damage or disease. Disturbances stemming from neuromotor planning, programming, control, or execution of speech constitute motor speech disorders. The cause of the disturbance can be a number of factors, including cerebrovascular accidents (CVA, stroke, brain attack), brain tumor, or a disease—often a degenerative type of disease (e.g., Parkinson disease, muscular dystrophy, amyotrophic lateral sclerosis). Motor speech disorders in adults are often classified into two main types: the dysarthrias and apraxia of speech.

DYSARTHRIAS AND APRAXIAS

Dysarthrias is a collective name for a group of neurologic speech disorders that result from abnormalities in the strength, speed, range, steadiness, tone, or accuracy of movements required for control of the respiratory, phonatory, resonotory, articulatory, and prosthetic aspects of speech production (Duffy, 2005). The disturbances are the result of central or peripheral nervous system abnormalities and most often reflect weakness, spasticity, incoordination, involuntary movements, or variable muscle tone. At its simplest, the dysarthrias involve weak or poorly coordinated speech movements.

This is contrasted with Duffy's (2005) definition of **apraxia of speech**. Apraxia of speech is a neurologic disturbance reflected as impaired capacity to plan or program sensorimotor commands necessary for directing movements that result in phonetic or prosodic changes in speech. It can occur in the absence of dysarthria and in the absence of a language disturbance. Apraxia of speech, then, reflects a central breakdown in planning or programming speech movements and, in "pure" cases, does not involve dysarthric weakness. A controversy exists as to whether such pure cases exist or the two groups of motor speech disorders are on a single continuum.

ASSESSMENT ISSUES

For nearly 40 years, the assessment of apraxia of speech in adults was accomplished through a battery of aphasia subtests, oral peripheral examination, and simple-to-complex articulatory maneuvers. Standardized tests are now available commercially. The classic *Motorspeech Evaluation* (Wertz, LaPoint, & Rosenbek, 1984) is still in use, as is the *Apraxia Battery for Adults* (ABA-2) (Dabul, 2000).

Typical tasks asked of patients include utterances of increasing length and complexity (*zip-zipper-zippering*), diadochokinetic rates, repetition trails, analysis of articulatory errors, and other automatic versus volitional movements. The SLP needs to differentiate apraxia of speech from conductive aphasia and from dysarthria in the diagnostic assessment, but admittedly this can be easier said than done. For example, patients with conductive aphasia may have significant articulatory sequencing errors but show easier speech imitation than do patients with apraxia of speech.

Dysarthric speech typically shows articulatory errors of simplification and distortion whereas apraxic speakers may transpose syllables and struggle with articulations. We have but scratched the surface of issues involved in apraxia of speech in adults. **Table 13–4** provides an overview of the adult dysarthrias. Commercially available tests of dysarthria include the *Frenchay Dysarthria Assessment* (Enberby, 1983), the *Assessment of Intelligibility of Dysarthric Speech* (AIDS) (Yorkston & Beukelman, 1981), and the *Dysarthria Examination Battery* (DEB) (Drummond, 1993).

TREATMENT ISSUES

The SLP's goal is to help the person with a motor speech disorder to better manage his or her communication difficulties. And, though not a cure per se, many techniques and strategies do indeed improve communication. The SLP probes or experiments with treatment techniques during the assessment session. The SLP endeavors to discover the patient's psychoemotional motivation to improve as well as what techniques mitigate motor speech symptoms. Treatment, often termed symptomatic therapy, targets improved communication, which, in turn, enhances the patient's quality of life.

TABLE 13–4 Types of Adult Dysarthrias, Areas of Neurologic Damage, and Key Features

Types of Dysarthria	Neural Conditions	Key Features
Flaccid	Injury or dysfunction of one or more cranial or spinal nerves, including neuromuscular junction area	Weakness, hypotonia, diminished reflexes, atrophy, fasciculations
Spastic	Bilateral damage to direct (pyramidal) and indirect (extrapyramidal) tracts of the central nervous system	Pyramidal: Loss of fine movements, hypotonia, weakness, hyporeflexia Extrapyramidal: Hypertonicity, spasticity, clonus, hyperreflexia
Ataxic	Damage to cerebellum	Articulatory and prosody changes such as imprecise consonants, irregular articulation, excess/equal stress, mono pitch and loudness, slow movements
Hypokinetic	Basal ganglia pathology (e.g., Parkinson disease)	Resting tremors, rigidity, hypokinesia (including articulators), and freezing of movement
Hyperkinetic	Basal ganglia pathology leading to either slow or fast involuntary movements (e.g., tics, chorea, dystonia)	Varied but may include imprecise articulation, monopitch, voice difference
Mixed	Distributed over two or more of preceding forms, for example, multiple sclerosis, amyotrophic lateral sclerosis, and others	Variable combinations
Unilateral upper motor neuron	Unilateral lesion; features appear on side of body opposite the lesion; lesion may affect pyramidal and extrapyramidal tracts	Hemiparesis/weakness, possible spasticity

Therapeutic techniques are tailored to the patient's needs and presenting disorder. Some general approaches, suggested by Duffy (2005), include the following.

1. State, in concrete terms, the behaviors that the patient exhibits. Examples include saying the person speaks too slowly, grimaces the face, runs out of air, or displays generalized tension.
2. Suggest that such behaviors tax speech attempts, and some changes might improve overall communication.
3. Elicit some normal sounds (e.g., grunts, sighs, prolonged vowels, singing syllables) to positively reinforce the patient's potential to change.

4. Explain the purpose of treatment, including getting the patient on the right track for better communication. Eliminate counterproductive behaviors and maximize helpful behaviors, regardless of medical circumstances.
5. Touch and physical manipulation can be helpful. Examples include laryngeal manipulation and massage to reduce vocal tension.
6. Maintain enthusiasm over speech improvements.
7. Use reading passages and interrupt frequently to discuss how speech "feels" and discuss "before and after" improvements. This conscious insight is important for long-term maintenance and self-monitoring.

TIPS FOR HEALTHCARE PROFESSIONALS WORKING WITH NEUROLOGICALLY IMPAIRED ADULTS

1. Interact with the patient as a valuable human being regardless of any distracting movements and spasms.
2. Endeavor to listen attentively to what the person has to say.
3. Motivate and instill confidence in the patient to counteract tendencies to quit and shy away from society.
4. Ask for repeats because what a patient has to say is important.

OVERVIEW OF SWALLOWING DISORDERS

Swallowing is a complex set of actions that occur sequentially to transport food and liquids from the mouth to the stomach. In the oral stage, food is bitten and chewed in preparation for swallowing. Speech articulators (tongue, jaw, lips, and teeth) need to work in a strong, coordinated, and bilateral fashion to pulverize food and mix it with saliva. In the next stage of swallowing, the morsel of food or liquid is pushed posteriorly, triggering a swallowing reflex at the back of the mouth to send the morsel on its downward journey. At this time, there is velopharyngeal closure to separate the nasal cavity from the oral cavity, and with this, respiration momentarily ceases. This helps keep food out of the lungs and airway. Other safety maneuvers assist: The larynx moves forward, tucking itself under the chin in a less direct pathway of the oncoming food. The vocal folds and the false vocal folds close (adduct) as a further barrier to food, liquids, and saliva entering the airway. Should food particles or liquid seep into the airway, the sensors in the larynx detect this and trigger a cough reflex to expel it and prevent choking, even death. In the last stage, the food or liquid enters the esophagus, which carries it automatically into the stomach. Now imagine an adult or child with a neuromuscular problem typical of those covered in this chapter. Difficulty chewing and swallowing safely can arise at many points as a result: What if the person has some sort of muscle weakness, paralysis, incoordination, poor timing, uneven muscle abilities on the right versus the left side? Things can get difficult, even life-threatening, when an adult or child has dysphagia.

The role and scope of practice in speech-language pathology include the burgeoning area of evaluation and treatment of swallowing disorders, alternately called **dysphagia**

(ASHA, 2002). Although adult and pediatric swallowing and feeding are not communication disorders per se, they do share some of the same anatomic structures and issues of neuromuscular control. Students with cerebral palsy or adults with dysarthria (especially following stroke or neck cancer) are likely to present with dysphagia as well.

With medical referral, the speech-language pathologist assesses the person's swallow via an imaging technique. This might entail the SLP and radiologist having the patient perform a barium swallow. Also in widespread use is a fiber-optic endoscopic examination of swallowing (FEES) (Logemann, 2007). Imaging allows observation of swallowing maneuvers and visualization of where small amounts of food and liquids trickle. Other background information and trial testing with various types and textures of food are part of the SLP assessment. Nutrition of the person is paramount as is a reliable and safe swallow. Treatment decisions may include that the patient should not be an oral feeder (opting for tube feeding or other methods) or that with control of food size and consistency and some learned techniques the patient can again swallow safely. In treatment, the SLP may opt for electrical stimulation of face and neck muscles, teach a double swallow or other strategy, train an optimal head or tongue lateralization for swallowing, and the like.

Dysphagia presents another opportunity for the healthcare professional, classroom teacher, and speech-language pathologist to work collaboratively. Indeed, as in the following vignette (Logemann & Sonies, 2004), the classroom teacher may be the person to suspect a problem and make a referral to the SLP.

VIGNETTE 13–3

A 5-year-old child was referred to the SLP in a public school because he refused to eat snacks with the other children and was noted to be uncoordinated and small for his age. On investigation with the family, it was discovered that the child had anoxia at birth, was diagnosed with mild cerebral palsy, and at one time had been diagnosed through imaging studies to have oropharyngeal dysphagia and gastroesophageal reflux. A feeding tube had once been used and later a private clinician had worked with the child on oral feeding. It was said that the child did not like to brush his teeth, would refuse certain foods, and generally was a picky eater. He often made nonnutritive chewing motions and sucked on clothing and soft toys. He was "floppy" and ill-coordinated during playtime at school and so was not included in some tasks. At parties for children, he did not put anything into his mouth, preferring to smell or lick items rather than taste them. Upon evaluation of the child's strengths and weaknesses, the SLP determined that this student was a candidate for services, noting on the Individualized Education Program (IEP) how the disabilities affected the child's participation in appropriate school activities. The parents obtained an updated swallowing study at the local medical facility and all parties involved determined that intervention was both safe and educationally necessary. The school SLP focused on oral (tactile) desensitization, behavior modification, and restructuring the environment at home (with the parents) and at school (with the classroom teacher).

STUDENTS WITH TRAUMATIC BRAIN INJURY

Youth and young adulthood represent age groups that are extremely vulnerable to **traumatic brain injuries (TBIs)**. Potentially dangerous pastimes these ages enjoy include bicycling, skateboarding, trampolining, driving all-terrain vehicles, cruising in a car, gang activities, and so forth. The term **closed head injuries (CHIs)** is used when the brain has been damaged in an accident, yet the skull has not been penetrated. In contrast, a bullet penetrates the skull and destroys a specific path through brain tissues. The resulting neurologic deficits from such an **open head wound** may be surprisingly minor if the bullet entered a not-so-critical area of the brain. Closed head injuries, on the other hand, often result in widespread damage and the neurologic disability often is quite extensive. Imagine the areas of widespread damage that might occur when a person's head impacts the dashboard or windshield of a car. The brain, suspended within the bony skull, continues its forward momentum despite impact, hitting the front of the bony skull (causing what is known as *coup* damage), and then rebounding with great force to hit the back of the bony skull (causing *contrecoup* injury). Damage also may occur as the brain moves and bends over rough bones at the base of the skull. All of this rotary movement of the brain tears or shears many blood vessels and nerve fibers. Unconsciousness, either brief or prolonged, may result from disruption of nerve fibers going to the brain stem. Loss of consciousness occurs in about 50 percent of children with brain injuries (Segalowitz & Lawson, 1995). Closed head injuries are the more common type of TBI and often are the result of motor vehicle accidents, falls, sports injuries, or abuse. Children and young adults tend to be involved in such injuries, with junior and senior high-school-aged students most vulnerable.

Following an accident, doctors initially work to control bleeding, maintain oxygen supply, and treat shock. There may be associated injuries in the abdomen, pelvis, and chest that need immediate attention. The brain damage sustained during the accident may be worsened by secondary complications such as brain swelling and bleeding into or around the brain. These complications, too, may result in death or may directly affect later neurologic function in a recovering patient. Predicting long-term outcomes and degree of disability is difficult. However, recovery tends to be good, though not necessarily complete, following most brain injuries (Brumback et al., 2001).

Once the patient is out of immediate danger, the rehabilitation team at the medical facility begins the rehabilitation program in earnest. Acute hospitalization often lasts a few weeks to a few months; some patients are discharged to specialized rehabilitation hospitals or centers for continued therapies. As soon as the student returns home, the public school system is responsible for ensuring that a homebound teacher is provided as well as speech-language services, physical therapy, and other support services as needed. Counseling is often a very important aspect of the initial adjustment for the student and family. The emotional state of the student and severity of injury are extremely important factors. Eventually, the decision regarding the appropriateness of a return to school is made, and the student may begin with only one or two classes per day. Reintegration of a student with a head injury into the school is a challenge for the student, the family, and the entire educational system. The TBI student is likely to present with a myriad of problems. It has often been said that no matter how serious the physical disabilities are following an injury, the neuropsychological and behavioral abnormalities are the most limiting factors in recovery and the major reason for stress within the family.

According to Brumback and colleagues (2001), studies of the long-term effects of brain injury on cognitive functioning in children following even mild brain injury have found that the most consistent impairments involve visuospatial skills and verbal abilities. Other reported effects include sleep disturbances, social difficulties, altered handedness pattern, attention disturbances, depression, and reading disorders.

The widespread nature of the brain damage may cause unusual kinds of behavior and learning patterns in the student. School systems typically have no specific programs for students with head injuries and, therefore, place them back into the same class schedule as before the accident. Such an inappropriate placement often results in emotional distress and academic failure. At other times, school systems place students with head injuries into learning disability programs or classes for those with mental retardation. Again, placement often is inappropriate. Each student with TBI who returns to school presents with a unique combination of deficits. The educational team should be aware of the student's deficits and be prepared to plan for them with flexibility. **Table 13–5** lists possible deficit areas of

TABLE 13–5 Neuropsychological and Behavioral Deficit Areas Often Present in Students with TBI Returning to School

Physical	Impairments can exist in mobility, strength, coordination, vision, and/or hearing.
Communication	Problems may include deficits in processing and sequencing information; use of "confused" language; dysarthric articulation; prosody abnormalities; and word-finding (anomia), reading, writing, computation, and abstraction difficulties.
Cognitive	Difficulties can be found with long- and short-term memory, thought processes, reasoning, conceptual skills, problem solving, abstraction level, learning abilities, and mental fatigue.
Perceptual motor	Involvement can include visual neglect, visual field cuts, motor apraxia, motor speed, motor sequencing, distractibility, reduced hand–eye coordination, and spatial disorientation.
Behavioral-emotional	Problems can account for impulsivity, poor judgment, disinhibition, dependence, anger outbursts, displacing aggressive behavior or bizarre/psychotic behavior, denial, depression, emotional lability, apathy, lethargy, poor motivation, poor initiative, inability to make decisions, and poor attention span.
Social	Impairments can result in the student not learning from peers, not generalizing from social situations, behaving like a much younger child, withdrawing, becoming distracted in noisy surroundings, and becoming lost or disoriented even in familiar surroundings.

returning students, compiled from the writings of Blosser and DePompei (1994), DePompei and Blosser (1987), Griffith (1983), and from the definition of TBI provided by the federal Division of Special Education (Traumatic brain injury, 1992).

The following list of TBI characteristics may sound similar to other handicapped conditions, yet their interactions produce some unique needs and the necessity for specialized teaching strategies. The TBI student is not like the typical student with learning disabilities or multiple handicaps, and the educational plan should reflect an understanding of the differences. (For example, the reading teacher must not assume that teaching reading skills to a TBI student is like teaching to a student with developmental reading problems.) Blosser and DePompei (1994), Cohen, Joyce, Rhodes, and Welks (1985), and Rosen and Gerring (1986) cite some of the characteristic and frustrating differences between the TBI student and those with other handicaps.

1. Students with TBI have previous successful experiences in academic and social settings; they may retain the premorbid self-concept of being perfectly normal.
2. Discrepancies in ability levels may be more extreme. Learning problems may exist even though some skills remain relatively unaffected. For example, the level of reading comprehension may be four years lower than spelling ability.
3. There may be inconsistent patterns of performance. Uneven progress can occur because of continuing recovery. Programs must maintain flexibility to accommodate sharp and frequent improvements.
4. Students with TBI often learn more rapidly than do students with learning disabilities. To "relearn" material, a reacquaintance with the process or concept may be all that is necessary.
5. Students with TBI may have more extreme problems with generalizing, integrating, or structuring information. More individualized instruction may be necessary. They may not be able to process even limited amounts of information; comprehension deteriorates markedly as the quantity and complexity of material increase.

The educational setting can be an ideal situation in which to continue the student's rehabilitation toward relearning and new learning. Structure is vitally important and must encompass social and academic activities. For such coordination to take place, all disciplines must work closely together. To assist in a student's smooth transition, the rehabilitation team members from the medical facility should be invited to participate with the educational team and the parents in the multidisciplinary evaluation and formulation of the IEP. A typical team for a student with TBI includes an SLP, physical therapist, occupational therapist, vocational rehabilitation counselor, parents, special education teacher, and classroom teacher(s). Much can be gained for the student when such open communication exists. Discussion about skills, needs, and problems related to reentry should be encouraged. For students who are junior high or senior high school age, vocational evaluation and training may become priority goals. If the student is no longer ambulatory, special transportation skills may become a need.

The SLP should be an active participant in planning for the reintegration of a student with a head injury into the school. This is true because the SLP possesses an understanding of language and learning problems as well as other specific skills that will benefit the reentry process. These skills, as cited by DePompei and Blosser (1987), include the following.

1. In-depth understanding of anatomy and physiology as they relate to language processing
2. Ability to observe and diagnose subtle communication deficits and hidden inadequacies of the communication system
3. Proficiency in objective evaluation procedures
4. Ability to establish remediation goals based on hierarchical approach, working on a simple to complex continuum
5. Understanding of the process for teaching judgment, organization, planning, and problem solving
6. Understanding of the communication requirements necessary for task performance at various academic levels
7. Awareness of the impact communication deficits can have on school success
8. Awareness of the pragmatic skills necessary for social interaction and communication
9. Understanding of physical environmental factors that can interfere with learning and communication

Blosser and DePompei (1994) provide excellent examples of cognitive-communicative interventions using functional outcome–based plans. Both SLPs and classroom teachers may find these plans useful. Concrete examples are provided for goals such as developing cognitive skills for math, adapting amount of auditory information for enhanced receptive language, increasing ability to respond to questioning and engage in concise conversations (expressive language), taking turns and self-monitoring aspects of pragmatic language, and so forth.

TEACHER TIPS FOR STUDENTS WITH TBI

As discussed by Cohen (1991) and by Cohen and his colleagues (1985), strategies are procedures that help a student clarify, organize, remember, and express information. Strategies help structure and emphasize parts of the learning process that a student with a head injury previously performed automatically. Snow and Hooper (1994) also endorse this treatment approach. It is suggested that the teacher spend time teaching the student *how* to use these strategies and *why* they should be used. At first, the teacher uses strategies to structure the environment or the student's behavior (e.g., blocking out everything but the sentence the student is to read). The teacher then cues the student to apply the compensatory strategies in specific situations. The ultimate goal is for the student to use the strategies independently (e.g., to take out a marker and use it to keep the place when reading). Thus, programming should progress from the point at which the teacher implements strategies to the point at which the student is expected to use them independently. **Table 13–6** presents some of the cognitive-communicative problems that a student with

TABLE 13–6   Compensatory Strategies for Cognitive Problems in a Classroom Setting

Attending problems: Student may be unable to attend to auditory and visual information. He or she may do such things as talk out of turn or change the topic, be distracted by noise in the hall, fidget, or poke others. It is important to note that the student may maintain eye contact and appear to be listening and actually not be attending.

Strategies:

- Remove unnecessary distractions such as pencils and books. Limit background noise at first and gradually increase it to more normal levels.
- Provide visual cues to attend (e.g., have a sign on student's desk with the word or pictured symbol for behaviors, such as *look* or *listen*). Point to the sign when the student is off task.
- Limit the amount of information on a page.
- Adjust assignments to the length of the student's attention span so that he or she can complete tasks successfully.
- Focus the student's attention on specific information: "I'm going to read a story and ask who is in the story."
- Both partners in a communication dyad should reduce utterance length, reduce sentence complexity, reduce rate of speech (or increase pause time), and vary intonation patterns to emphasize key words.

Difficulties with language comprehension or following directions: Student may have difficulty understanding language that is spoken rapidly, is complex, or is lengthy.

Strategies:

- Limit amount of information presented, perhaps to one to two sentences.
- Reduce rate of delivery.
- Use more concrete language.
- Teach student to ask for clarification or repetitions or for information to be given at a slower rate.
- Give prompts and assistance such as using pictures or written words to cue students or pairing manual signs, gestures, or pictures with verbal information.
- Act out directions: If the student is to collect papers and put them in a designated spot, demonstrate how this should be done.
- Use cognitive mapping: Diagram ideas in order of importance or sequence to clarify content graphically. This also helps students to see part–whole relationships.
- See also strategies listed under memory and attending that can be used to improve language comprehension.

Memory problems: Student may be unable to retain information that he or she has heard or read and may not remember where to go or what materials to use.

Strategies:

- Include pictures or visual cues with oral information because this multisensory input strengthens the information and provides various ways to recall it.

(continues)

TABLE 13–6 Compensatory Strategies for Cognitive Problems in a Classroom Setting (Continued)

- Use visual imagery. Have student form a mental picture of information that is presented orally. Retrieval of the visual images may trigger the recall of oral information.
- Use verbal rehearsal. After the visual or auditory information is presented, have the student "practice" it (repeat it) and listen to himself or herself before acting on it.
- Limit the amount of information presented so that the student can retain and retrieve it.
- Provide a matrix for the student to refer to if he or she has difficulty recalling information (such as a number fact chart).
- Have the student take notes or record information on tape.
- Underline key words in a passage for emphasis.
- Provide a log book to record assignments or daily events.
- Provide a printed or pictured schedule of daily activities, locations, and materials needed.
- Role-play or pantomime stories or procedures to strengthen the information to be remembered.
- Write down key information to be remembered, such as who, what, and when. Help the student develop note-taking skills.

Information retrieval challenges: The student may have difficulty retrieving information that has been stored in memory and may exhibit word-finding difficulties.

Strategies:

- Have student gesture or role-play. He or she may be able to act out a situation that has occurred but not have adequate verbal language to describe it.
- Provide visual or auditory cues: "Is it _ or _?" or give the beginning sound of a word.
- Include written multiple-choice cues or pictures in worksheets.
- Teach the student to compensate for word-finding problems by describing the function, size, or other attributes of items to be recalled.

Difficulties organizing and sequencing information: Student may have difficulty understanding, recognizing, displaying, or describing a sequence of events presented orally or visually.

Strategies:

- Limit the number of steps in a task.
- Present part of a sequence and have student finish it.
- Show or discuss one step of the sequence (lesson) at a time.
- Give general cues with each step: "What should you do first? Second?"
- Have student repeat multistep directions and listen to self before attempting a task.
- Present information in chunks or help student group it.
- Provide pictures or a written sequence of steps to remember: Tape a cue card to the desk with words or pictures of materials needed for a lesson, and then expand original written directions. For example, if the direction was "Underline the words in each sentence in which <u>ou</u> or <u>ow</u> stands for the vowel sound. Then, write the two words that have the same vowel sound," change it to "(1) Read the sentence; (2) underline <u>ou</u> and <u>ow</u> words; (3) read the underlined words; (4) find the two words that have the same vowel sounds; (5) write these two words on the lines below the sentence."

TABLE 13–6 Compensatory Strategies for Cognitive Problems in a Classroom Setting (*Continued*)

- Introduce information with attention-getting words.
- Tell student how many steps are in a task: "I'm going to tell you three things to do." (Hold up three fingers.)
- Act out a sequence of events to clarify information.
- Provide sample items describing how to proceed through parts of a worksheet.
- Number the steps in a written direction and have the student cross off each step as it is completed.
- Teach student to refer to directions if he or she is unsure of the task.

Thought disorganization: Student has difficulty organizing thoughts in oral or written language. Students may not have adequate labels or vocabulary to convey a clear message; he or she may tend to ramble without getting to the point.
Strategies:

- Attempt to limit impulsive responses by encouraging the student to take "thinking time" before answering.
- Have student organize information by using categories, such as who, what, when, and where. (Emphasize each of these separately if necessary.) This strategy can be used in an expanded form to write a story.
- Teach student a sequence of steps to aid in verbal organization: Have the student use cue cards with written pictured steps when formulating an answer.
- Focus on one type of information at a time (e.g., the main idea).
- Decrease rambling by having student express a thought "in one sequence."

Problems with generalization: Student learns a skill or concept but has difficulty applying it to other situations (e.g., may count a group of coins in a structured mathematics lesson but not be able to count money for lunch).
Strategies:

- Teach the structure or format of a task (e.g., how to complete a worksheet or mathematics problem).
- Maintain a known format and change the content of a task to help student see a relationship: Two pictures are presented and student must say if they are in the same category, or have the same initial sound; a worksheet format requires filling in blanks with words or numbers.
- Change the format of the task: Have student solve mathematics facts on a worksheet as well as on flash cards.
- Have completed sample worksheets in a notebook serve as models indicating how to proceed.
- Demonstrate how skills can be used throughout the day. For example, discuss how the student relies on the clock or a schedule to get up in the morning, begin school, or catch a bus.
- Role-play situations that simulate those that the student may encounter, emphasizing the generalization of specific skills taught; for example, completing school assignments and going to the store may involve the same strategies of making a list or asking for help.

Source: Data from Blosser & DePompei (1994); Cohen (1991); Cohen, Joyce, Rhoades, & Welks (1985).

a head injury demonstrates and strategies that can be used to compensate for them. The SLP and teacher should work collaboratively on identifying problems and useful strategies for each particular TBI student.

The following list of techniques and classroom adaptations also can be implemented to help the student (DePompei & Blosser, 1987; Blosser & DePompei, 1994). Educators working with a TBI student should use as many of these techniques as possible during classroom activities.

1. Plan many small group activities to facilitate learning of appropriate interaction skills.
2. Clarify verbal and written instructions in the following ways:
   a. Alert the student to the important topic or concept being taught ("I'm going to tell a story, and then we'll discuss where it takes place").
   b. Accompany verbal instructions with written instructions.
   c. Repeat instructions and redefine words and terms.
   d. Verbally explain written instructions or assign a "classroom buddy" to do so.
3. Privately ask the student to repeat information and/or answer a few key questions to be sure that important information presented has been understood. Care should be taken, however, not to cause stress in students who have difficulty responding to direct questions.
4. Use pauses when giving classroom instructions to allow time for processing information.
5. Because response time is often delayed, provide the student with ample time to respond verbally and to complete in-class and home assignments.
6. Avoid figurative, idiomatic, ambiguous, and sarcastic language when presenting lessons (Example: "You're a ham").
7. Select a classroom buddy to keep the student aware of instructions, transitions, and assignments.
8. Permit the student to use assistive devices such as a calculator, tape recorder, and/or computer.
9. Help the student formulate and use a system for maintaining organization. Require the student to carry a written log of activities, schedule of classes, list of assignments and due dates, and room locations. Frequently monitor the student's use of the organization system.
10. Schedule a specific time for rest and/or emotional release. Encourage the student to share any problems being experienced.
11. Plan extracurricular activities based on the student's physical and emotional capabilities as well as interests.
12. Structure the physical environment of the classroom to decrease distractions and permit ease of movement by carefully planning seating and furniture arrangements.
13. Modify and individualize the student's assignments and tests to accommodate special needs. Examples of modifications include reducing the number of questions to be

answered or amount of material to be read, permitting the student to tape record the teacher's lectures or responses to test questions, and changing the format of a task.

14. Develop resources to accompany textbook assignments. For example, use pictures and written cues to illustrate important information and concepts. Assign review questions at the end of chapters. Write new vocabulary. Present a summary of a chapter on tape or paper. Go over errors made on tests to let the student know where and why errors occurred.

15. Establish a system of verbal or nonverbal signals to cue the student to attend, respond, or alter behavior (examples include calling the student's name, touching, written signs, or hand signals).

Above all, access the team of specialists who are serving the student (SLP, occupational therapist, physical therapist, vocational rehabilitation counselor, and course or special education teachers). As a teacher, ask for these consultants to come and help work through problems, especially in the early phases as the student is adjusting. Also, it is important to remember to keep in close contact with the parents regarding the student's attitude, stamina, emotional ability, self-concept, perceptions of peer relations, use of medication (many students are seizure prone), and other important but frequently changing characteristics of the student.

ATTENTION DEFICIT/HYPERACTIVITY DISORDER

An increasing number of children who exhibit learning and behavior problems are being diagnosed as having **Attention Deficit Hyperactivity Disorder (ADHD)** (Taylor, Smiley, & Richards, 2009). ADHD results in a complex pattern of interrelated problems in attention, behavior, organization, peer interactions, and social competence that affects a child's ability to perform many of the tasks expected in educational settings as well as in other situations that require the child to stay focused and pay attention. Other situations include speech-language and hearing testing and treatment sessions. Although not a communication disorder as such, the problems associated with ADHD may cause a child to have difficulty communicating effectively with peers and adults. This is particularly true in the area of pragmatics (appropriate use of language). Barkley (2005) identifies several language-related characteristics of children with ADHD including the following.

- Delayed onset of language (in some cases)
- Excessive conversational speech
- Poor organization and expression of ideas
- Impaired verbal problem solving
- Poor rule-governed behavior
- Diminished development of moral reasoning

Although mostly associated with children, ADHD can continue through adolescence and adulthood. It is not our purpose here to provide a detailed discussion of the neurologic research on this disorder. However, it is important that teachers, parents, and other individuals who work with children realize that the condition of ADHD stems from a neurologic basis.

The *Diagnostic and Statistical Manual of Mental Disorders, Fourth Edition, Text Revision* (*DSM-IV-TR*) indicates, "The essential feature of Attention-Deficit/Hyperactivity Disorder is a persistent pattern of inattention and/or hyperactivity-impulsivity that is more frequently displayed and more severe than is typically observed in individuals at a comparable level of development" (American Psychiatric Association [APA], 2000, p. 85).

PREVALENCE

The prevalence of Attention Deficit Hyperactivity Disorder has been estimated at 3–7 percent in school-age children (APA, 2000; DuPaul & White, 2005). One factor that may cause some confusion in recognizing ADHD is that not all children with this condition demonstrate the same set of signs and symptoms. The *DSM-IV-TR* (APA, 2000) recognizes three types of ADHD: (1) predominantly hyperactive-impulsive, (2) predominantly inattentive, and (3) combined hyperactive-impulsive and inattentive. Also, behaviors associated with ADHD may be somewhat different for boys than for girls. Boys are more likely to be hyperactive, whereas girls tend to be inattentive. Girls who have trouble paying attention often daydream, but inattentive boys are more likely to play or fiddle aimlessly. Boys tend to be less compliant with teachers and other adults, so their behavior is often more conspicuous (APA, 2000; Mayo Foundation for Medical Education and Research, 2009).

ADHD is often not well understood by classroom teachers and parents, and the children exhibiting this disorder are even less well understood. Almost 20 years ago, Jordan made the following observation, which is, unfortunately, still true in many cases: "It would be accurate to say that most persons who have AD/HD are among the most seriously misunderstood individuals within our culture. They live most of their developmental years being misunderstood and failing to understand the world around them" (Jordan, 1992, p. 42).

Children with ADHD have, over the years, been assigned to a number of different diagnostic categories including learning disabled, hyperactive, and children with minimal brain dysfunction (Taylor et al., 2009). These children also have been, and in many instances still are, frequently accused of being lazy, inattentive, disobedient, or having below normal intelligence. Even when a diagnosis of ADHD has been made, many teachers and parents fail to understand that this is a neurologic disorder. Scolding, detention, or other punishments are no more likely to make students with ADHD improve their attention and memory than they are to make children in wheelchairs walk. Children with ADHD usually have average or above average intelligence. But these students are likely to experience difficulty in the classroom as a result of problems in the following areas.

- Failure to pay close attention to details, resulting in careless mistakes in schoolwork or other activities
- Poor organization and memory
- Difficulty maintaining on-task behavior because they are easily distracted by external and internal stimuli
- Problems with time management
- Rigidity
- Difficulty waiting for their turn
- Inappropriate and out of proportion reactions to negative events
- Problems establishing and maintaining peer relationships
- Frustration resulting from failed socialization and academic difficulties
- General immaturity

Children with ADHD tend to operate on their own schedules, which are different from those of their age peers and certainly different from those that adults try to impose on them. This is true in terms of maturation and readiness to deal with various concepts as well as in the time required to complete tasks. When no accommodations are made for their disorder, students with ADHD experience a myriad of difficulties in educational settings. Some of the problems frequently encountered by students with ADHD in educational settings are described as follows.

Inability to follow verbal directions: Because of an inability to process connected speech quickly, to focus attention on the spoken message, to separate important information from less important information, and to remember a sequence of instructions, students with ADHD frequently have difficulty doing what they are asked to do. As a result, these children are often confused about what they are to do. Some may ask for instructions to be repeated. Many students with ADHD, however, do not admit to the teacher and their classmates that they did not understand the instructions because of the emotional sensitivity that accompanies this disorder and because of past negative experiences with an exasperated teacher or the snickering of classmates. These students simply go ahead and do the wrong thing.

Inability to finish assignments: Because of an inability to stay on task, students with ADHD typically cannot complete many tasks as quickly as their peers can. This is true of tests as well as written assignments and class projects. Unfortunately, instead of providing more time for the student with ADHD, teachers frequently respond to unfinished tasks with punishment such as detention or missed rewards, which does nothing more than increase the student's frustration.

An interesting pattern noted in the work of many students with ADHD is deterioration in performance as the task progresses. It is not unusual to see a student with ADHD make the majority of errors on the second part of a spelling or math test. It seems that they can focus their attention for a while, but not for the duration of the test.

Other reasons for problems with timed tasks include the inability to hold one piece of information in memory while processing another part of the problem, having to rely on finger counting or other manipulatives to perform basic addition and subtraction, and agonizing over choices in multiple-choice or true-false test formats.

Poorly organized and messy assignments: Assignments prepared by students with ADHD frequently reflect the lack of organization and scattered attention that characterize the disorder. Any assignment that requires a certain orderly progression will be extraordinarily challenging for these students. Whether it is placing in logical sequence the events that led to the Revolutionary War, conducting and/or describing a science project, or solving a multistep mathematics problem, the student with ADHD will have difficulty with the organization and execution. Written work is typically characterized by numerous erasures with resulting ripped and crinkled papers, misspelling, and punctuation errors (see **Figure 13–1**). Artwork often resembles that of a much younger child. These students often have notebooks and desks that are in such disarray that they cannot find the materials needed to complete assignments. Sometimes they cannot find the assignments they have completed to turn in to the teacher.

Difficulties with homework: Homework is a particularly challenging part of school for students with ADHD. First, there is the formidable task of remembering exactly what it is they are to do. Even when they can remember what the task is, they frequently forget to bring home the texts or other materials required to complete the task. A typical dialogue between parent and a child with ADHD might go something like this:

> **Parent:** How was school today?
> **Child:** OK.
> **Parent:** Do you have any homework?
> **Child:** We have a test tomorrow.
> **Parent:** In which class are you having a test?
> **Child:** I forget.
> **Parent:** Well, which teacher told you that you were having a test?
> **Child:** I think it was Mrs. Smith.
> **Parent:** Well, Mrs. Smith teaches social studies. Is your test in social studies?
> **Child:** I guess.
> **Parent:** Where is your social studies book?
> **Child:** I left it at school. Oh, Mrs. Jones says I have to miss story time tomorrow because I didn't do my chapter summary.
> **Parent:** We did your chapter summary last night. Why didn't you hand it in?
> **Child:** I couldn't find it.
> **Parent:** AAAGGHH!

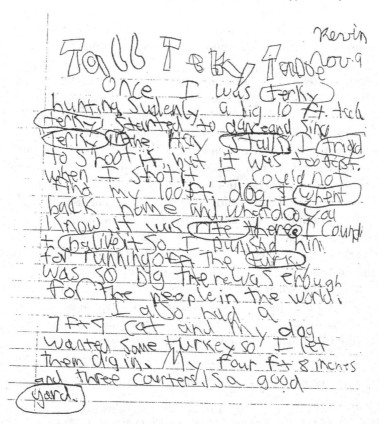

FIGURE 13–1   A story written by a fifth-grade student with ADHD. Notice the writing phonetic spelling and incomplete erasures. The story is supposed to be as follows.

Tall Turkey

Once I was turkey hunting. Suddenly a big 10 ft. turkey started to dance and sing, "Turkey in the Straw." I tried to shoot it, but it was too fast. When I shot it, I could not find my 100 ft. dog. I went back home, and what do you know, it was right there. I couldn't believe it, so I punished him for running off. The turkey was so big there was enough for the people in the world. I also had a 7 ft. 7 cat and my dog wanted some turkey so I let them dig in. My four ft 8 inches and three quarters is a good guard.

Additional problems related to homework include that it often takes children with ADHD far longer than other students to complete the homework assignments. What might be a half-hour homework assignment for most students may take two hours or more for the student with ADHD. Also, many children with ADHD take medication such as methylphenidate (Ritalin) or amphetamine and dextroamphetamine mixed salts (Adderall) to help them focus attention. In some cases, the effects of the medication may wear off just as it is time to begin homework. Parents are then faced with the choice of giving the child more medication so that he or she can do the homework, or trying to get an unmedicated child to focus attention on the assignment, which may be only partially understood to begin with. These homework issues contribute to the child's frustration with school-related activities and can create unhealthy tension between parents and child.

Interpersonal skills: Many students with ADHD have difficulty relating to peers and, sometimes, interacting appropriately with adults. These students tend to be less mature than students of similar chronological age and are often more comfortable and more successful when interacting with younger children. As a result, students with ADHD are frequently social outcasts among their age peers. Many students with ADHD are very sensitive and react to this social ostracism in a negative and often inappropriate or immature fashion. Their reaction then tends to reinforce their status as an outsider. Because they have difficulty with impulse control, students with ADHD are also prone to lash out in both a verbally and physically aggressive manner against those whom they feel are treating them unjustly. To make matters worse, students with ADHD, once committed to a course of action, are often unable to alter that course regardless of the circumstances. For example, most students know better than to retaliate against another student when a teacher is looking. Students with ADHD, however, seem unable to suppress their behavior and are more likely to be "caught in the act." This social frustration combines with academic difficulty experienced by many students with ADHD to make school a very unpleasant place.

ACCOMMODATIONS TO HELP THE STUDENT WITH ADHD

Students with ADHD are entitled to accommodations under a variety of federal laws, including the Rehabilitation Act of 1973, the Individuals with Disabilities Education Act of 2004 (IDEA), and the Americans with Disabilities Act of 1992 (ADA). The effects of ADHD on academic performance vary among individuals. As a result, many children with ADHD may not qualify for services under IDEA. Those students, as indicated in Chapter 1 of this text, may still be eligible for services under section 504 of the Rehabilitation Act of 1973. Section 504 is a civil rights statute that requires that schools not discriminate against students with disabilities and that they provide students with reasonable accommodations. If a student is eligible for accommodations under section 504, the school must develop a 504 plan. One significant difference between a 504 plan and an IEP is that regulations governing 504 plans do not specify the frequency with which a plan should be reviewed and do not specify the rights of parents to be involved in the development of the plan (National Resource Center on AD/HD, 2007).

Structure and routine are very important for children with ADHD (Taylor et al., 2009). Appropriate techniques of behavioral and environmental management are a critical part of intervention for these children (DuPaul & White, 2004). Some possible accommodations that may prove helpful to students with ADHD whether they are covered by federal legislation or not are included in the following lists.

Homework

1. Provide an assignment notebook that is *checked daily by the teacher.*
2. Check to ensure that appropriate books and materials are taken home.
3. Textbooks and other materials can be supplied to the parents.
4. Establish a "buddy system" where a reliable student is assigned to help remind the student with ADHD what the assignments are and which materials need to be taken home.
5. Notify parents of upcoming tests and assignments.
6. Establish a voice mail system at the school, where parents call to check on assignments.
7. Reduce the amount of homework for students with ADHD. Perhaps every other math problem or answer half of the questions at the end of the chapter.

Classroom Activities

1. Check to see if the student with ADHD is on task and gently remind him or her when attention wanders.
2. Remember that physical proximity to the teacher often serves as a reminder for the child to stay on task.
3. Provide additional time to complete tasks.
4. Check to be sure that the student understands directions. Do not simply ask, "Is that clear?" but say something like, "Show/tell me how you are going to do this."
5. Help older students to develop note-taking skills.
6. Help the student to maintain an organized notebook. Notebooks with dividers and pockets may help students with ADHD to organize assignments and notes.
7. Allow students to tape record lectures.
8. In schools where students change classrooms, attempt to keep these changes to a minimum for students with ADHD.
9. Consider alternative test methods:
   a. Consider allowing the student with ADHD to take tests alone rather than with the rest of the class.
   b. Avoid computer scan sheets.
   c. Avoid writing test items on the blackboard.
   d. Avoid using faded or poor quality copies of tests.
   e. Print or type test questions; avoid using cursive.
10. Be aware of potential difficulty with multistep tasks.
11. Do not assume that students with ADHD will draw appropriate conclusions.
12. Identify the best learning avenue. Some children may be better visual learners than auditory, some better auditory than visual.

A speech-language pathologist may be able to assist students with ADHD and their teachers by incorporating classroom material in the speech-language treatment process.

For example, an SLP could ask teachers if there is a task in class that seems to be giving the student with ADHD particular difficulty. The SLP could then incorporate vocabulary or language tasks that reflect that subject matter in the speech-language treatment sessions.

In addition to the preceding general suggestions, Kline, Silver, and Russell (2001) provide the following suggestions that are specific to children who exhibit predominantly inattentive type ADHD and those who exhibit predominantly hyperactive-impulsive type. For children who have problems with inattention and distractibility, Kline, Silver, and Russell suggest the following.

1. Shorten the task or break one task into several smaller parts.
2. For rote tasks, use shorter more frequent sessions rather than fewer longer sessions.
3. Use hand signals to remind the student to refocus.

For children who exhibit the predominantly hyperactive-impulsive type ADHD Kline, Silver, and Russell (2001) make these suggestions.

1. When possible, allow nondisruptive, directed movement in the classroom or standing during seat work.
2. Use activity as a reward.
3. Teach substitute verbal or motor responses that the child may use while waiting his or her turn.
4. Allow the student with ADHD to doodle with paperclips or other items while waiting or listening to instructions.

Socialization and Behavior

1. Be aware of the behavior problems that may result from ADHD:
   a. Inability to inhibit responses
   b. Overreaction
   c. Immaturity
2. Avoid situations that tend to exacerbate behavior problems:
   a. Boisterous group activities.
   b. Use preferential seating on the school bus, in the cafeteria, at assemblies, and so forth.
3. Help students manage peer relations:
   a. Students with ADHD are often "easy marks" for teasing and bullying.
   b. Students with ADHD tend to retaliate without regard for consequences.

Medications   As mentioned earlier, many students with ADHD may take one of several available medications to help control the symptoms of ADHD. Despite what many people think, these medications are not designed to sedate these children. Instead they are intended to increase the production or decrease the absorption of certain chemicals in the brain known as neurotransmitters (Kline et al., 2001). In general, stimulants used for ADHD are methylphenidate (Concerta, Focalin XR, Metadate, Ritalin, and Daytrana [a Ritalin patch worn by the child]) or amphetamines (Adderall XR and Vyvanse). These medications stimulate the production of neurotransmitters. In other cases, nonstimulants such as atomoxetine (Strattera) are prescribed to block the absorption of the neurotransmitter, making it last longer in the child's system (Taylor et al., 2009). All medications have potential side effects and all must be given in the appropriate dosage. Teachers should be aware of any children in their class who are taking medication on a regular basis and should be aware of the possible side effects of those medications. Some behaviors that teachers may be able to notice as well as or better than others in the child's environment are signs that the medication is wearing off too soon, irritability (sometimes a rebound effect associated with the wearing off of the medication), appetite suppression, sluggishness, drowsiness, stomach pain, and behavior change when child forgets medication. Teachers should report the presence of any possible side effects to the parents or the school nurse (in schools where a nurse is on staff). Such reports by teachers can be quite helpful to the physician in determining the best medication and the most appropriate dosage.

Terms to Know

Neuromuscular problem	Quadriplegia
Motor speech disorder	Muscular dystrophy
Dysarthria	Augmentative/alternative communication
Cerebral palsy	(AAC)
Spasticity	Apraxia of speech
Athetosis	Dysphagia
Ataxia	Traumatic brain injury (TBI)
Tremor	Closed head injury (CHI)
Rigidity	Open head wound
Mixed cerebral palsy	Attention Deficit Hyperactivity Disorder
Hemiplegia	(ADHD)
Paraplegia	

Study Questions

1. Why are many persons with cerebral palsy multiply handicapped? Discuss some of the most frequent types of handicapping conditions, especially as may affect the educational process.

2. Speech may or may not be affected in neuromuscular disorders. Discuss the speech characteristics and problem areas typically noted in these individuals when speech is moderately to severely affected.

3. Speech may be so severely affected in neuromuscular disorders that intelligible speech is not a reasonable expectation. Discuss as many alternative methods of communication as you can.

4. Discuss why placing a student with closed head injured back into the class schedule held before the accident often is not appropriate. Why is placement in special classes for those with learning disabilities or mental retardation also inappropriate?

5. Discuss some specific strategies and techniques that classroom teachers can employ in working with students with closed head injuries.

6. Describe accommodations that would be appropriate for a student with Attention Deficit Hyperactivity Disorder, and discuss how such accommodations might be implemented in a regular classroom setting.

7. Identify signs and symptoms that indicate that a child may have ADHD.

8. Discuss some similarities and differences in the speech of adults with apraxia and with dysarthria following a stroke.

9. Swallowing is neither speech nor language so explain why SLPs perform dysphagia assessment and treatment.

Bibliography

Abrahamsen, A. A., Romski, M. A., & Sevcik, R. A. (1989). Concomitants of success in acquiring an augmentative communication system: Changes in attention, communication, and sociability. *American Journal on Mental Retardation, 93*(5), 475–496.

American Psychiatric Association. (1994). *Diagnostic and statistical manual of mental disorders* (4th ed.). Washington, DC.

American Psychiatric Association. (2000). *Diagnostic and statistical manual of mental disorders* (4th ed., Text Revision). Washington, DC.

American Speech-Language-Hearing Association. (2002). Roles and responsibilities of speech-language pathologists with respect to evaluation and treatment for dysphagia. *ASHA Supplement, 22,* 73–87.

American Speech-Language-Hearing Association. (2004). Roles and responsibilities of speech-language pathologists with respect to augmentative and alternative communication: Technical report. *ASHA Supplement, 24,* 93–95.

Barkley, R. A. (2005). *Attention deficit hyperactivity disorder: A handbook for diagnosis and treatment* (3rd ed.). New York, NY: Guilford Press.

Beukelman, D., & Miranda, P. (1992). Augmentative and alternative communication: Management of severe communication disorders in children and adults. Baltimore: Paul H. Brooks.

Blosser, J., & DePompei, R. (1994). *Pediatric brain injury: Proactive intervention.* San Diego, CA: Singular.

Brumback, R., Mathews, S., & Shenoy, S. (2001). Neurological disorders. In F. Kline, L. Silver, & S. Russell (Eds.), *The educator's guide to medical issues in the classroom* (pp. 49–64). Baltimore, MD: Paul H. Brooks.

Cohen, S. B. (1991). Adapting educational programs for students with head injuries. *Journal of Head Trauma Rehabilitation, 6*, 56–63.

Cohen, S. B., Joyce, C. M., Rhodes, K. W., & Welks, D. M. (1985). Educational programming for head injured students. In M. Ylvisaker (Ed.), *Head injury rehabilitation: Children and adolescents*, San Diego, CA: College-Hill Press.

Dabul, B. (2000). *Apraxia Battery for Adults*. Austin, TX: Pro-Ed.

Daniel, D. (2004). AAC in the schools: Moving students along a communication continuum. *ASHA Leader, 9*, 10, 16–17.

Denckla, M. (1991). *Brain behavior insights through imaging*. Paper presented at the Learning Disabilities Association National Conference, Chicago, IL.

DePompei, R., & Blosser, J. (1987). Strategies for helping head-injured children successfully return to school. *Language, Speech, and Hearing Services in Schools, 18*, 292–300.

Drummond, S. S. (1993). *Dysarthria Examination Battery (DEB)*. San Antonio, TX: Communication Skill Builders.

Duffy, J. (2005). *Motor speech disorders*. St. Louis, MO: Elsevier Mosby.

DuPaul, G. J., & White, G. P. (2004). An ADHD primer. (Counseling 101 column). *Principal Leadership Magazine, 5*, 11–15.

DuPaul, G. J., & White, G. P. (2005, November/December). Intervention strategies for children with ADHD. *Principal*, 27–29.

Eisenson, J., & Ogilvie, M. (1983). *Communicative disorders in children* (5th ed.). New York, NY: Macmillan.

Enderby, P. (1983). The standardized assessment of dysarthria is possible. In W. R. Berry (Ed.), *Clinical dysarthria*. San Diego, CA: College Hill.

Glennen, S. L. & DeCoste, D. C. (1997). *Handbook of augmentative and alternative communication*. San Diego, CA: Singular.

Griffith, E. R. (1983). Types of disability. In M. Rosenthal, E. R. Griffith, M. R. Bond, & J. D. Miller (Eds.), *Rehabilitation of the head injured adult*. Philadelphia, PA: F. A. Davis.

Jones, H. R. (1985). Diseases of the peripheral motor-sensory unit. *Clinical Symposia, 37*(2), 22–25.

Jordan, D. R. (1992). *Attention deficit disorder*. Austin, TX: Pro-Ed.

Kline, F. M., Silver, L. B., & Russell, S. C. (2001). *The educator's guide to medical issues in the classroom*. Baltimore, MD: Brookes.

Logemann, J. (2007). Dysphagia: Basic assessment and management. In Johnson, A. & Jacobson, B. *Medical speech-language pathology: A practitioner's guide*, 131–147. New York, NY: Thieme.

Logemann, J., & Sonies, B. (2004). Grand rounds dysphagia. *ASHA Leader, 9*(13), 4–5, 18–19.

Mayo Foundation for Medical Education and Research. (2009). Attention-deficit/hyperactivity disorder in ADHD in children. Retrieved June, 2010 from www.mayoclinic.com/health/adhd/DS00275.

McCormick, L., & Wegner, J. (2003). Supporting augmentative and alternative communication. In L. McCormick, D. F. Loeb, & R. L. Schiefelbusch (Eds.), *Supporting children with communication difficulties in inclusive settings* (2nd ed.). Boston, MA: Pearson Education.

Mirenda, P., & Marhy-Laikko, R. (1989). Augmentative and alternative communication application for persons with severe congenital communication disorders: An introduction. *Augmentative and Alternative Communication, 5,* 3–13.

National Resource Center on AD/HD (2007). *Educational rights for children with AD/HD in public schools.* What We Know Fact Sheet 4. Retrieved June 2010 from http://www.help4adhd.org/documents/WWK4.pdf.

Phillips, P. P. (1984). *Speech and hearing problems in the classroom.* Lincoln, NE: Cliffs Notes.

Rosen, C. D., & Gerring, J. P. (1986). *Head trauma: Educational re-integration,* San Diego, CA: College-Hill Press.

Segalowitz, S. J., & Lawson, S. (1995). Subtle symptoms associated with self-reported mild head injury. *Journal of Learning Disabilities, 28,* 309–319.

Sexson, S. B., & Dingle, A. D. (2001). Medical disorders. In F. Kline, L. Silver, & S. Russell (Eds.), *The educator's guide to medical issues in the classroom* (pp. 28–48). Baltimore, MD: Paul H. Brooks.

Silverman, F. H. (1989). *Communication for the speechless* (2nd ed.). Upper Saddle River, NJ: Prentice Hall.

Snow, J., & Hooper, S. (1994). *Pediatric traumatic brain injury.* Thousand Oaks, CA: Sage.

Solomon, N. P., & Charron, S. (1998). Speech breathing in able-bodied children and children with cerebral palsy: A review of the literature and implication for clinical intervention. *American Journal of Speech-Language Pathology, 7*(2), 61–78.

Taylor, R. L., Smiley, L. R., & Richards, S. B. (2009). *Exceptional students: Preparing teachers for the 21st century.* Boston, MA: McGraw-Hill.

Traumatic brain injury. (1992). *Federal Register, 57*(189).

Van Der Merwe, E., & Alant, E. (2004). Associations with Minspeak icons. *Journal of Communication Disorders, 37*(3), 255–274.

Wertz, T., LaPointe, L., & Rosenbek, J. (1984). *Apraxia of speech in adults: The disorder and its management.* New York, NY: Grune and Stratton.

Yorkston, K., & Beukelman, D. (1981). *Assessment of intelligibility of dysarthric speech.* Tigard, OR: C. C. Publications.

Zametkin, A. J., Nordahl, T. E., Gross, M., King, A. C., Semple, W. E., Ramsey, J., & Cohen, R. M. (1990). Cerebral glucose metabolism in adults with hyperactivity of childhood onset. *New England Journal of Medicine, 323,* 1361–1367.

Chapter 14

COMMUNICATION DISORDERS AND SUCCESS: ACADEMIC, OCCUPATIONAL, AND QUALITY-OF-LIFE ISSUES

Thus far, we have talked a lot about the nature, assessment, and treatment of individual disorders of communication. Our discussion may have been more "clinical" in nature and not focused as much on the person who has the disorder. But make no mistake, these disorders affect far more than just communication. They affect the daily lives of children and adults in very dramatic and far-reaching ways. This chapter addresses how communication disorders have been shown to affect a person's academic and occupational success and overall quality of life.

Academic success can be defined as a child's or adolescent's ability to effectively achieve curricular goals such as reading, spelling, writing, mathematics, and knowledge in various content areas (e.g., history, language arts, science, sociology). Academic success also involves earning a good grade point average so that the student is promoted to the next higher grade level. Ultimately, a student is academically successful if he or she attains the educational preparation for either vocational placement or postsecondary studies in a college or university. As you see in this chapter, students with language and phonological impairments are at high risk for academic problems. They often earn poor grades and have difficulty with learning to read, write, and spell. Thus, you might say that their academic success is threatened by their communication disorder.

Occupational success typically involves adults and is often measured by obtaining/maintaining a position in a desired vocation and the ability to advance appropriately through promotion. For an adult who acquires a communication disorder later in life, there is a distinct possibility that his or her occupational success might be at risk. Although many adults can successfully continue in the working world after acquiring a communication disorder, some may not have a realistic chance to do so. For instance, if a high school teacher has a stroke and develops aphasia, he or she might not be able to resume teaching without considerable accommodations in the workplace. It is possible that certain communication disorders can be "career enders" for some individuals in occupations that rely on rapid and precise use of speech and language.

Quality-of-life issues include, among other things, the ability of a person to be independent, to establish and achieve personal goals, to communicate needs and desires, to maintain social networks, and basically to enjoy life. Such activities are taken for granted in children with normally developing communication, but they are often compromised in those with communication disorders. Severely involved children may depend heavily on others (parents, aides, peers) for assistance in the most basic tasks. They may have trouble communicating even basic needs and may have few friendships and opportunities for social interaction. Thus, the more the speech-language professional can move them toward independence, realistic goals, effective communication, and social relationships, the better their quality of life.

Similarly, you might naturally assume that adults with normal communication can effectively navigate the social and occupational domains using efficient speech and language skills. It goes without saying that normal adults can make their needs known to others in any environment. Adults with communication disorders (e.g., aphasia, laryngectomy, vocal disorders, motor speech disorders) are often left with conditions that create difficulties in performing the activities of daily living (ADLs). These ADLs include such basic skills as feeding, dressing, hygiene, and walking, among others. Communication is also an activity of daily living because a person must be able to make his or her needs known to others. Social interaction can also be considered a basic function of living beyond merely expressing wants and desires. Thus, it should not be surprising that most medical settings measure "success" in terms of comparing functional ADL outcomes that a patient can accomplish at the beginning and the end of remediation. It should be clear that a severe medical disorder (e.g., stroke, cancer) can affect elemental functions such as eating, grooming, and ambulation. If a person needs assistance with these, he or she is no longer completely independent and quality of life changes for the worse. You should also remember, however, that an impairment in communication can have a significant effect on the quality of a person's life. The inability to make one's needs known efficiently or to participate in social interactions can be almost as penalizing as severe medical problems and certainly affect a person's quality of life.

It is important for speech-language pathologists (SLPs), teachers, and health professionals to know how academic and occupational performance can be affected by a communication disorder and how quality of life can be affected in the children and adults that they see in treatment. This information influences their daily interactions in therapy, goal setting in treatment, and the counseling they do with clients and their families.

COMMUNICATION DISORDERS AND ACADEMIC SUCCESS

If education were a monetary system, the currency would no doubt be language. SLPs encounter certain groups of students that have a weakness in the area of language. The obvious ones, of course, are those students who had language disorders during their preschool years, and these linguistic difficulties have simply persisted into the early grades. Other groups that may not be as obvious are those children with phonological disorders, learning disabilities, hearing impairment, attention deficit disorder, and students who have experienced traumatic brain injury. Specific chapters in this book deal with all of these groups, but we devote a single portion here to how these language-based disorders affect a student's academic performance. Also, this chapter illustrates some recent research that suggests working on language goals and metalinguistic abilities may play a significant role in a student's academic achievement, especially in terms of reading.

STUDENTS WITH LANGUAGE PROBLEMS: THE HIGH-RISK GROUPS

It is important to emphasize that certain groups of school-age students have a tendency to exhibit problems with language. If the teacher and speech-language pathologist carefully examine these "high-risk" groups, they can detect the bulk of older students with language disorders and serve them appropriately. Certainly, however, this does not mean that a student who is not included in these groups is immune to a language disorder, and anyone who manifests symptoms of language disturbance should be referred for evaluation. Sometimes the underlying language problems of students are overlooked, and teachers may tend to focus their efforts on symptoms rather than the underlying problems. For instance, a student who has difficulty learning to read and write may also have subtle problems with producing spoken language and comprehension of complex sentences uttered by others. If teachers know that research shows that certain groups of students exhibit more pervasive language problems than simply those seen in one modality (e.g., reading, writing), they can make appropriate referrals. This allows the SLP to address any underlying language problem that exists. These major groups are discussed next.

Students with a History of Preschool Language Delay   If a student had a language delay as a preschooler, sometime after school entrance the child is at high risk to experience difficulties with language-based tasks. This does not occur because the SLP has done a poor job of treatment during the preschool period. In fact, many of these students may have been dismissed from treatment because they have remediated all of the symptoms that they were enrolled to correct. In many cases, they were enrolled for problems with semantics, syntax, phonology, and morphology, and when the problems no longer exist, they are dismissed. In other cases, the student is not dismissed from treatment but simply continues therapy upon school entrance because he or she has not reached the goals that have been set. Remember that these students, for want of a better word, exhibit a "weakness" in the area of language. They had trouble learning to talk and using language rules appropriately.

When the SLP completes treatment on such a child, you might think that the problem has been solved. Perhaps the problem would have been solved if the young child were in an environment where his or her linguistic system was not taxed any further by forcing the use of more and more complex language operations. But when a child enters school, the emphasis is on learning to read, write, and speak in far more complex ways than the child dealt with prior to school entrance. Much of the teaching–learning process is done through the use of language, with the teacher explaining ideas and facts, and the students listening and trying to understand. We address some of the stresses and strains of typical school curricula in a later section, but for now it is enough to mention that, upon school entrance, students are subjected to significant increases in the complexity, speed, and expectations with which they use language. For a student with a history of language problems, these increased expectations and complexities may be inordinately difficult. The very language rules with which the student experienced weakness as a preschooler are emphasized and prized in early elementary grades.

Several longitudinal investigations attempt to follow up on students with a history of preschool language disorders. In essence, these studies examine clinical records to determine the students who received treatment for language impairment as preschoolers, and then locate these students when they reach school age. For example, Strominger and Bashir studied 40 such students and state that "no child was found without residual deficits" (Strominger & Bashir, 1977, p. 3). Most of the students had difficulties with spoken and written language and reading. The authors state, "The child who evidences early disruption of language acquisition is at the highest risk for future educational failure or difficulty in reading and written language" (Strominger & Bashir, 1977, p. 4). They emphasize that the language problems do not disappear, but simply become more subtle and manifest differently when a student becomes older. This, of course, is a result in part of the concomitant increases in the complexity of the educational curriculum coupled with the weakness in the language area.

Aram and Nation (1980) examined 63 students who had a history of preschool language problems. Four to five years after their initial evaluation, problems persisted in 80 percent of the group. About half of the students had persisting speech-language problems, while the other half demonstrated normal language but had difficulties in reading and math. King et al. (1982) did a 15-year study of 50 preschool students with language disorders who ranged in age from 13 to 20 years at follow-up. The majority had histories of academic problems (failed grades, special placements, and so on), and almost half of them had persisting communication problems. Hall and Tomblin (1978) found that 50 percent of the preschool children with language impairments that they studied longitudinally showed persistent language problems into adulthood. Many other studies show that children with language problems often experience academic difficulties throughout their time in school (Bashir, Kuban, Kleinman, & Scavuzzo, 1983). Parents of children with a history of language disorders should be routinely counseled regarding the increased possibility of language-based academic difficulties as the child progresses through the educational system.

Students with Speech Sound Disorders   Three academic skills, reading, writing, and spelling, each require that students have a degree of mastery of the sound system of their language. Therefore, you might expect that students who exhibit speech sound disorders would be likely also to exhibit problems with reading, writing, and spelling. Most of the research investigating the relationship between speech sound errors and academic performance focuses on reading. The results of this research, especially earlier research, are somewhat equivocal. For example, some studies reported a significant relationship between reading problems and speech sound disorders (FitzSimons, 1958; Ham, 1958; Winitz, 1969). On the other hand, Everhart (1953), Flynn and Byrne (1970), and Hall (1938) reported no significant differences in the speech sound production abilities of good and poor readers.

One possible reason for the lack of consensus among these early studies is the fact that the investigators failed to take into account the difference between articulation problems and phonological problems. Remember that speech sound production has two aspects: the motor-based aspect of speech sound production known as articulation, and the linguistic rule-based aspect generally referred to as phonology. The inability of a student to make correct motor movements to produce speech sounds may not have a significant effect on reading, writing, or spelling. However, if a student's phonological disorder reflects an underlying problem in the organization of the sound system, it would be reasonable to expect this underlying problem to surface in one or more of the academic skills related to the sound system.

Stackhouse (1982) investigated the distinction between the possible effects of structurally based articulation disorders and phonological disorders on reading. She compared the reading and spelling abilities of children exhibiting articulation problems related to cleft lip and palate with those of children with expressive phonological problems not related to structural anomalies. Stackhouse reports that the children with cleft lip and palate did not differ significantly in reading and spelling ability from a group of normally developing children. However, the children with expressive phonological impairments performed significantly more poorly in reading and spelling than did the normally developing control group. In a later work, Stackhouse (1997) states that it appears that children who exhibit an isolated articulatory difficulty relating to a physical abnormality may be no more likely to have reading impairments than do those with normally developing speech. Catts and Kamhi (2005) discuss the relationship between reading problems and the broader area of phonological processing, which includes phonological awareness, memory, and production and retrieval. They state that there is much evidence to suggest that a phonological processing deficit is at the core of the reading problems in dyslexia.

Another confounding factor in the research exploring the relationship between speech sound disorders and reading, writing, and spelling is the presence of coexisting language disorders. Catts (1991) reports that children with phonological and language impairments are much more likely to exhibit reading problems than are children with phonological problems only. The relationship between phonology and the other components of language is complex. Many, but not all, children with phonological disorders also exhibit language disorders. Several studies indicate that about 60 percent of preschool children with speech sound disorders also have co-occurring language problems (Tyler & Waterson, 1991; Shriberg & Kwiatkowski, 1994; Shriberg & Austin, 1998).

It would seem that research designed to investigate the relationship between reading and phonology must take into account the presence of coexisting language disorders. A word of caution, however; because language disorders are frequently more subtle and less obvious than phonological disorders are, SLPs and teachers must be aware of the potential for a language disorder in any child who exhibits a moderate to severe disorder of phonology. Therefore, a child with a phonological disorder should be considered at risk for problems in reading and spelling.

There is a growing body of research that suggests that **phonological awareness** may be yet another link between phonological disorders and reading ability. As described in Chapter 3, phonological awareness is the explicit understanding of the sound structure of language, including the awareness that words are composed of syllables and phonemes (Catts, 1991). The link between phonological awareness and reading has been well established (Adams, 1990; Blachman, 1991; Catts, 1991; Muter, Hulme, Snowling, & Stevenson, 2004; Olson & Byrne, 2005). Several studies have indicated that many children with phonological problems perform more poorly on phonological awareness tasks than do children of similar age with normal phonological skills (Magnusson & Naucler, 1990; Webster & Plante, 1992; Cowan & Moran, 1997). Bird, Bishop, and Freeman (1995) report that children with persisting speech sound disorders often have literacy and phonological awareness problems.

Several types of tasks have been used to assess phonological awareness. These tasks include rhyming activities, segmenting words into phonemes or syllables, producing words after the first or last sounds have been changed or deleted (e.g., "What does *fat* become if we take away the f̲ sound?"), and comparing the length of spoken words (e.g., when asked, "Which word is longer, *whale* or *mosquito*?" children with poor phonological awareness may respond that *whale* is longer because the object it represents is longer). All of these measures, to one extent or another, appear to be predictors of reading ability (Blachman, 1991; Catts, 1991; Magnusson, 1991). That is, children who have difficulty on the phonological awareness tasks also frequently prove to be poor readers. Catts and Kamhi (2005) state that children with more severe phonological disorders, who have broad-based language impairments and who perform poorly on tests of phonological awareness, are most at risk for reading disabilities. Preston and Edwards (2009), after reviewing the literature in this area, indicate that children with speech sound disorders most at risk for literacy problems include those who exhibit the following characteristics.

- Coexisting language impairment
- Childhood apraxia of speech
- Persisting speech problems (speech sound problems in children 6 years and older)
- Low nonverbal IQ
- Speech perception deficits
- Many atypical speech sound errors

Certainly the research on the possible relationships among phonology, phonological awareness, and reading should hold some interest for classroom teachers, reading specialists, and SLPs. However, of even more importance are reports demonstrating that training in tasks designed to develop phonological awareness appears to facilitate learning to read (Blachman, 1991; Ehri et al., 2001). The relationship of phonological awareness to reading has resulted in schools reevaluating the way reading is taught. Several years ago, many school systems incorporated so-called whole-language approaches to teaching reading. Whole-language approaches tend to deemphasize or eliminate specific training in awareness of sounds (Hall & Moates, 2002). Mounting evidence that training in phonological awareness may greatly facilitate learning to read has resulted in reading programs that place greater emphasis on the awareness of sounds. Adams, after reviewing the literature on this subject, concludes, "The evidence is compelling: Toward the goal of efficient and effective reading instruction, explicit training of phoneme awareness is invaluable" (Adams, 1990, p. 331). Ehri et al. (2001), after conducting a meta-analysis of existing literature, conclude that phonemic awareness instruction improves word reading as well as comprehension. Ehri et al. also report that both normally developing children as well as children with reading disabilities benefit from phonemic awareness instruction. This is certainly one area in which speech-language pathologists, classroom teachers, and reading teachers can engage in a mutually beneficial collaborative effort to improve both the phonological and reading skills of students.

Blachman (1991), Blachman, Ball, Black, and Tangel (2000), Goldsworthy (1998), and Lindamood and Lindamood (1998) provide several approaches to teaching phonological awareness to kindergarten and first-grade students. These interventions include techniques based on categorizing words according to the sounds they contain, segmenting words into their phonemic components, and rhyming activities. Such techniques have been demonstrated to result in improved reading and/or spelling skills (Blachman, 1991; Ehri et al., 2001). There have been no studies to date, however, that demonstrate whether children with phonological disorders perform better in one type of reading instruction than another.

The relationship between phonological disorders and spelling is even less clear than with reading. Intuition says that a child who has problems processing sounds for speech production may have problems processing sounds for written production. Research, however, has not conclusively proved or disproved the prevailing clinical intuition.

One reason may once again be the concept of phonological awareness. Extensive recent literature demonstrates a relationship between phonological awareness and spelling (Ball & Blachman, 1991; Tangel & Blachman, 1992; Lombardino, Bedford, Fortier, Carter, & Brandi, 1997; Ehri et al., 2001; Apel, Masterson, & Hart, 2004). Clarke-Klein (1994) suggests that children who have phonetic errors (e.g., spell *candle* as "candol" or *square* as "skwar") likely do not have phonological awareness problems and are no more likely than other children to have phonological problems. However, children who show nonphonetic or "bizarre" spelling patterns (i.e., spell *smoke* as "scoteser," or *crayons* as "carinsteds") are more likely to have phonological awareness problems. Clarke-Klein suggests that children who have histories of severe expressive phonological deviations are at risk for these unusual or bizarre types of spelling errors. Lombardino et al. (1997) suggest that children who do not exhibit expected spelling patterns should be provided with phoneme awareness training.

In summary, there appears to be a significant relationship between speech sound disorders and reading, writing, and spelling. However, the exact nature of that relationship is not entirely clear. It would appear that children with a phonological disorder as opposed to a simple motor-based articulation disorder are at risk for reading, writing, and spelling problems. This is particularly true in situations where the phonological problem is accompanied by a language problem. A critical link between phonology and reading and spelling might be phonological awareness. Poorly developed phonological awareness is characteristic of many students with phonological problems as well as of students with reading problems. The assessment and development of phonological awareness skills in young children provide many marvelous opportunities for collaborative efforts among speech-language pathologists, classroom teachers, and reading specialists.

Students with Hearing Loss   Many of the effects of hearing loss on classroom performance should be obvious. If a student cannot hear instructions, examples, or assignments, his or her performance will likely be incorrect or inappropriate. As discussed in Chapter 10, students with a sensorineural loss may hear some sounds but not others so that they hear the teacher's speech as garbled or distorted. Speech and hearing professionals can address these obvious problems using the technology and suggestions provided in Chapter 10. Students with hearing impairments, however, also experience more subtle academic problems. These problems are determined largely by the extent to which the hearing loss disrupts the student's ability to process language. Sometimes this critical link between language skills and academic achievement is not apparent to teachers, who are unaccustomed to working with the population of children with hearing impairments.

Because a language problem underlies most of the academic difficulty of a student with hearing impairment, it is not surprising that the greatest problem with most of these students is with language-based skills, especially reading and writing (Jensema, 1975; Allen, 1986; Berg, 1986; Marschark, Lang, & Albertini, 2002). Allen (1986) reports that the average reading and writing level of deaf high school students is at the third- or fourth-grade level. Quigley and Thomure (1968) report that elementary and secondary students with hearing impairments demonstrate scores of one to three years below those of normal-hearing peers on the word meaning, paragraph meaning, and language subtests of the Stanford Achievement Test. Marschark et al. (2002) indicate that although the literacy skills of students with severe and profound hearing impairments have improved in more recent years, a large discrepancy between hearing and deaf peers remains. They indicate that many deaf students graduating from high school are reading at levels comparable to hearing students who are five to nine years younger.

Davis (1974) reports a "discouragingly low performance" on the Boehm Test of Basic Concepts by children who are hard-of-hearing. Several studies report that children with hearing impairment demonstrate delays in syntactic ability (Pressnell, 1973; Wilcox & Tobin, 1974; Davis & Blasdell, 1975; Quigley, Wilbur, Power, Montanelli, & Steinkamp, 1976). There is evidence that even mild hearing loss can affect language development and, therefore, academic skills. Holm and Kunze (1969) administered a battery of language development tests to children ages 5 to 9 years. One group had fluctuating mild hearing losses resulting from persistent otitis media. The other group was a matched peer group of children with no history of middle ear problems. The authors report that the otitis media group received lower scores than the control group on all tasks involving the reception or processing of auditory information or the production of a verbal response. In recent years, early identification and early intervention (in the form of language stimulation and amplification) have resulted in dramatic improvement in the educational achievement of students with hearing impairment. Paul and Quigley (1987) state that recent studies suggest that the academic lag reported for children with impaired hearing is not as great as that indicated earlier. Such improvement, as a result of early language training, underscores the fact that the academic deficit experienced by these students reflects their language difficulties rather than any generalized intellectual deficit.

Although early identification and intervention make the picture considerably brighter for the students with impaired hearing in the classroom, the teacher must continue the momentum with certain practices such as ensuring that the student's hearing aid is in working order, making maximum use of assistive listening devices, incorporating slight modifications in teaching style to accommodate the student, and making the best use of the support personnel available in any particular school system.

Students with Learning and/or Reading Disabilities   Maxwell and Wallach state: "Research and clinical data from a variety of sources and orientations continue to suggest that the largest percentage of learning and reading-disabled children have language problems" (Maxwell & Wallach, 1984, p. 25). Wiig and Semel (1976) have said, after reviewing the literature in this area, that 75–85 percent of students with learning disabilities have experienced language delays and that some of these perpetuate into adulthood. As these references indicate, the research is quite clear about the occurrence of language problems in populations with learning and reading disabilities. Some publications refer to such students as "language-learning disabled," a nomenclature that reflects the far-reaching effect of language on the disorder (Wallach & Butler, 1994). In school systems, the speech-language pathologist is most interested in screening the students who are receiving special services for learning or reading disabilities because there is a reasonable chance that their problems in the areas of reading and writing may stem from an underlying difficulty with language in general.

Students Who Are Academically At Risk If through formal testing a student is not found to have a language problem, learning disability, or reading disturbance, typically the school system provides no special services. In early elementary grades, of course, there are different levels of reading instruction and some special services (the "Chapter One" reading programs, for example), but as children become older, less emphasis is placed on teaching basic skills such as reading. Simon (1985) refers to students who have significant academic difficulties but who do not qualify for special services in learning disabilities, reading, or speech-language as students who have "fallen between the cracks" in the educational system. Simon further indicates that if these students are given in-depth testing for language abilities, a significant percentage (about 50 percent) exhibit gaps in their ability to perform age-appropriate linguistic tasks.

Hill and Haynes (1992) studied fourth-grade children who were rated by their teachers as "academically at risk." These children repeatedly earned grades below C in their academic coursework and were in the low reading group. The children had no history of speech-language problems and were currently receiving no remedial services of any kind. Hill and Haynes administered three language tests to the academically at-risk children and their normally achieving peers. The tests focused on pragmatics, metalinguistics, and the language typically used by teachers in giving classroom directions. They found that more than 50 percent of the academically at-risk children scored low enough on the three language tests to warrant enrollment in treatment.

Thus, the third major population in the school system that is at risk for language problems is the group that is often earning poor grades, experiencing grade retention, and who may be receiving no special services. Perhaps their language problems are subtle enough that they are either not referred or not identified by routine screenings and evaluation techniques.

CURRICULUM AND TEACHING IMPACT ON STUDENTS WITH LANGUAGE PROBLEMS

Using language in the home environment is quite different from communication in a school setting. Even children who have gone to day care facilities prior to school entrance have not been subjected to the pressure of using the level of language demanded in most kindergartens. This section attempts to bring to a conscious level the types of communication used in classroom settings. It is through an understanding of the typical communicative milieu in the classroom that teachers might appreciate the profound disadvantage this setting presents to a student with borderline or deficient language skills.

THE SCHOOL CULTURE

Prior to school entrance, children have a limited number of daily routines with which they are familiar. These routines allow the child to understand events in the environment and even help the child to determine how to act in certain situations (Tattershall & Creaghead, 1985). Many of these routines, however, are not an integral part of the school experience, and the child entering school must make the appropriate adjustments to existing routines and learn new ones. Although the preschooler knows routines such as going to the store, visiting grandma, dinnertime, bedtime, discipline, and party behaviors, new school routines such as following directions, asking questions, taking turns, and such may be foreign to the child. Also, the child may be accustomed to routines that include no other children or only one or two peers. The preschool child lives in a supportive environment where family members and friends are familiar with the child's abilities, accomplishments, preferences, and behavioral tendencies. Many times, familiarity with the child can compensate for any language deficiencies of the child. In the classroom, however, there are many other potential interactants and different rules for interaction. In addition, the child, the child's history, preferences, and abilities are virtually unknown to the teacher and other students. The student must learn the classroom routine and the teacher must learn about the new children in the classroom. Creaghead and Tattershall state, "A sixth grade teacher was asked the following question in early September, 'What is the hardest thing about starting school?' Her answer was, 'teaching the children my routine'" (Creaghead & Tattershall, 1985, p. 12). This is even more difficult with younger students. Another complication is that teachers' expectations change from year to year, which makes the adjustment to school even more difficult for students. Tattershall and Creaghead (1985) quote a study by Baron, Baron, and MacDonald (1983) in which teachers of various grades were asked about the skills children should possess for kindergarten and first grade. Prerequisite skills for kindergarten are as follows.

1. Say his full name, his parents' full names, his address, and his phone number
2. Talk loud enough
3. Recognize his name in print
4. Listen and sit quietly while others are talking
5. Share, take turns, and play by the rules

Contrast this with the expectations for "desirable abilities" the very next year in first grade.

1. The ability to attend to a task for at least 10 minutes
2. The ability to express herself orally with teachers and peers
3. The ability to retell the plot and describe the main character after listening to a story

4. The ability to follow basic procedures for reading left to right, top to bottom
5. The ability to count objects and count aloud to 10
6. The ability to say the alphabet in order
7. The ability to see letter-to-sound relationships
8. The ability to identify beginning sounds
9. The ability to print her own name legibly (Tattershall & Creaghead, 1985, p. 32)

As children progress toward secondary school, language-based abilities such as the following become increasingly important.

- The ability to work independently
- Organizational skills
- Taking responsibility for work assignments
- Using the library
- Developing appropriate study habits
- Thinking and problem solving using language and mathematics
- Performing group problem solving
- The ability to discuss opinions
- Discriminating fact from opinion
- The ability to develop arguments for a number of issues

Many more changes in expectations occur, and students are expected to learn more sophisticated skills each year, sometimes with no direct explanation but just by inference based on teacher and peer behavior.

In the school environment, students must learn even different communication rules in addition to the rules of proper behavior (sit in your seat, don't talk to your neighbor, raise your hand). Question sequences are different from the typical routine experienced at home. For instance, many researchers (Sinclair & Coulthard, 1975; Mehan, 1978) report that school questions typically form a three-level sequence composed of the following parts.

1. The question ("What letter is at the beginning of the word *cat*?")
2. The answer ("*C.*")
3. The teacher's evaluation of the response ("That's right, David")

There are at least three differences between question routines existing at home and those at school. First, home questioning usually has a two-part sequence (typically the evaluation portion is not included, although it might be). Second, questions at home are most often asked to obtain "real" information from the child. Questions in the classroom are more to demonstrate knowledge that is already known to the teacher and most of the class. Finally, teachers spend significantly more time in questioning behavior than do parents.

Another difference in the classroom is the routine for turn allocation. Especially in the lower grades, the teacher usually chooses the speaker (child) and the child talks to the teacher (typically in an answering mode). The child rarely gets to address communications to other students unless he or she "sneaks" these communications during activities such as arts and crafts that are not designed for such interactions. Then, the teacher does not always reinforce the interactions. Thus, the speaker selection and interactions are not natural in the classroom.

Topic selection and maintenance also are different in the classroom setting. The teacher almost always chooses the topic of conversation, selects who will take turns, maintains the topic, and changes the topic when he or she sees fit. This is different from topic management in the natural environment, which is more arbitrary.

The purpose of this section is to show that the student entering school must learn a host of new routines, both verbal and nonverbal, and is faced with significantly different and more complex expectations than previously experienced at home. This requires a significant adjustment for the young child, and if a language disorder exists, the adjustment may be even more difficult or impossible. If the student with a language disorder has difficulty abstracting the rules for classroom participation, he or she may be faced with negative feedback. You can imagine how the routines can become even more complicated in the higher grades, where the student is confronted with several different teachers in the same day, all with different expectations and modifications of the basic school routine. For a student with a language disorder, this challenge may be insurmountable.

TEACHER TALK

Many studies have focused on the types of language teachers use in the classroom. Nelson (1984) summarizes data that were gathered on teacher language in first, third, and sixth grades. The major variables that Nelson examined were grammatical complexity of sentences, rate of speaking (speed), and fluency (pauses, hesitations). She found that the syntactic complexity increased with grade level, which made the language used in sixth grade more complex than that used in first grade. There was also more pausing and disfluency as the grade level increased. Finally, the rate of speech in syllables per second (sps) increased from first (4.5 sps), to third (5.4 sps), to sixth (5.3 sps) grade. Interestingly, in an earlier study, Nelson (1976) found that a rate of 5.0 syllables per second increased comprehension problems among normal children up to the age of 9 years.

Students with language disorders have difficulty with a number of aspects of linguistic material. For instance, more complex sentences are more difficult to understand for normal as well as students with language impairments. Many studies show that students with language learning disabilities have trouble with rapid auditory processing of information. The incorporation of teacher disfluencies, hesitations, and false starts serves only to add to the confusion as the grade level increases.

Wallach and Miller address another aspect of teacher talk: "Teachers make great use of rhetorical questioning in their teaching" (Wallach & Miller, 1988, p. 43). Teachers after approximately fourth grade make frequent use of nonliteral language such as idioms, analogies, similes, sarcasm, and indirect polite forms (Nelson, 1984; Stephens & Montgomery, 1985). Many children are able to handle some aspects of nonliteral language by age 8 years, but they do not acquire many nonliteral forms until as late as 13 years. Adolescents with language learning disabilities are especially vulnerable as language becomes more abstract.

Cuda and Nelson (1976) found that first-grade teachers use a high number of statements to direct attention and gain behavioral control of their classrooms. At the first grade level there is an emphasis on "how to do" reading, writing, and mathematics, using concrete materials with much assistance from the physical context of the classroom. By third grade, the teachers focus more on content subjects such as social studies, science, and geography than on the how-to aspects. Verbal instruction increases in importance as grade level rises, and by sixth grade, students are almost exclusively concentrating on content areas, using reading and writing as tools for learning. Therefore, after the first few grades in elementary school teachers assume that children have acquired the basic skills of reading, writing, and spoken language and that no review of these important requisites is needed. Sturm and Nelson state: "One of the many challenges in inclusive classrooms is monitoring and assisting the comprehension of lower functioning students without reducing the level of interaction for others" (Sturm & Nelson, 1997, p. 271).

CURRICULUM AND MATERIALS

A very important concept that many teachers are unaware of is called metalinguistics. This concept is critical to classroom teaching and the performance of students with normal language and language disorders. Although metalinguistics may be unfamiliar to many, it is probably the most important topic in this chapter. Because people often have difficulty grasping the notion of metalinguistics, we provide several examples here. Specifically, we describe the developmental unfolding in the child of this ability to focus on and think about language (i.e., what its parts are and how those parts relate to each other) (VanKleek, 1984).

Explicit language knowledge, sometimes defined under the general term *metalinguistics*, involves the ability to make conscious judgments about one's language. Adult language users are capable of making many metalinguistic judgments. They can decide whether sentences are grammatical, they can correct written language, and they can decide whether words have equivalent meanings. Children demonstrate metalinguistic ability when they can specify the first sound in the word *dog*, when they circle all the pictures that begin with the /k/ sound, and when they judge whether a sentence looks all right. The 3-year-old boy who says, "The zebra looks like a horse but he has funny stripes" would be unable to tell how many words are in the sentence or how many sounds are in the word *zebra* because the word and sound judgments require metalinguistic ability, which is a later acquisition. This demonstrates how a child can be capable of talking (as reflected in the zebra sentence) without being able to talk about talking (Wallach & Miller, 1988).

So, what does all this have to do with classroom teaching and students with language disorders? The first point that teachers need to realize is that much of their time in the early grades is spent teaching metalinguistic skills. For instance, Wallach and Miller state:

School activities . . . also require a great deal of metalinguistic ability. Even in the early grades, children are asked to compare sentences, to count the number of words in a sentence, to listen for the first sound in a word, to identify a rhyming word, and to decide which sentence is the "proper" way to say something. The discovery that the alphabet corresponds with particular sounds requires rudimentary metalinguistic ability. In addition standardized tests and intervention materials have a metalinguistic focus. . . . VanKleek (1984, p.187) writes, "It appears that verbal intelligence measures require that the child focus on and consciously manipulate language. Such tests often contain subtests in which children are asked to give definitions, rhyme, solve anagrams, check secret codes, complete verbal analogies, etc. Such an assessment tells us far more about a child's metalinguistic skills than how he or she functions using language in social interactions." (Wallach & Miller, 1988, p. 9)

Thus, you can easily see that elementary school teachers deal with metalinguistics on a daily basis. Teachers need to be aware of several important factors concerning metalinguistics. The first is that metalinguistic ability develops, as all language skills do, on a maturational timetable. That is, a child must have reached a particular level of linguistic maturity to perform and understand metalinguistic tasks. Note that many normal students do not acquire the ability to segment syllables into phonemes until they are about 6 years of age. Yet many students are involved in phonics programs either before or at the same time as these skills are developing. Also, figurative language and abstract language use may not be understood until well after age 8 years, yet authorities report that abstract and figurative language (analogies, dual word meanings) occurs in teacher utterances even at the first-grade level (Cuda & Nelson, 1976). If these skills are later developing ones for normal language students, then they are clearly going to cause extreme difficulty for youngsters with language impairments. In fact, many studies indicate that students with language learning disabilities have particular trouble with metalinguistic tasks (Hook & Johnson, 1978; Baker, 1982; Nippold & Fey, 1983; Simon, 1985). Nelson provides an example of the complexity of an actual teacher directive that relies heavily on metalinguistic ability:

What kind of animal do you see at the very top? And where is the rabbit? He's sitting on a radio. Did you ever see a real rabbit sit on a radio? What does rabbit begin with? "R", all right. And what about the thing he's sitting on? Say the word. Radio. Radio and rabbit both begin with the letter "r." OK, can you see how that letter is made? The capital "R" is how many spaces? Two spaces tall. And the small "r"? After your name is made at the space at the top, will you make a capital "R" and a small "r" on the lines that are shown right beside the rabbit? (Nelson, 1984, p. 165)

Note that in the preceding example the student must mentally shift from one metalinguistic task to another (location of sounds in words, uppercase versus lowercase letters, the correspondence between sounds and letters, the physical configurations that differentiate uppercase from lowercase letters). The teacher also asks the student to describe the picture, reflect on metalinguistic issues, and then to actually perform a writing task. Also note that the instructions for the writing task (the last sentence in the example) is a very complex sentence that reverses the order of events in time ("After your name is made in the space at the top, will you make . . ."). Finally, the instructions for the writing task are stated in the form of a question (polite form) rather than a directive. This type of indirect request is often very difficult for a student with a language impairment to understand.

Often, even the textbooks used by classroom teachers are infested with complex and sometimes incomprehensible instructions written by "experts" in the educational process (Lasky & Chapandy, 1976; Creaghead & Donnelly, 1982; Nelson, 1983). The classroom teacher often is encouraged by the textbook to read such directives verbatim to the students.

READING: A LANGUAGE-BASED SKILL

While we are discussing curriculum issues, it is pertinent to mention the teaching of reading, which is an important language skill. Teachers use a variety of approaches to teach reading. Reading, as a language skill, is particularly difficult to learn for children with language disorders. Catts and Kamhi state:

> The research reviewed in these studies clearly demonstrates that language deficits are closely associated with reading disabilities. In many cases, these language deficits precede and are causally linked to reading problems. Reading is a linguistic behavior, and, as such, it depends on adequate language development. Many children with reading disabilities have developmental language disorders that become manifested as reading problems upon entering school. (Catts & Kamhi, 2005, p. 115)

As in many academic realms and areas of professional practice, the popularity of certain teaching methods ebbs and flows according to the tenor of the times. Fifty years ago, the rule was phonics programs for reading instruction. Then, in the 1980s the whole-language movement affected reading instruction, and phonics training fell out of favor in many school systems. Now the pendulum has swung back toward an emphasis on phonological awareness. Some approaches use a highly metalinguistic approach (phonics) coupled with reading material that emphasizes decoding written words. This type of approach may be extremely difficult for a student with metalinguistic deficits, yet these skills may be the key to learning to read for such a child. Other approaches (e.g., whole language) emphasize meaning and comprehension of the written material and place less emphasis on phonemic awareness. They stress that language in any form (speaking, writing, reading, and listening) has real communicative value. This awareness provides an incentive for the various uses of language because all of the content areas in school depend on what language communicates, not on how effectively a speaker can "play with" sounds, letters, words, and sentences.

It is easy to see that children with language disorders may benefit greatly from a whole-language approach to reading instruction because it makes reading meaningful and relevant to their daily lives instead of focusing on phonetic aspects. However, even if the whole-language approach is used, children with language disorders still can benefit greatly from phonological awareness training to improve their reading ability (Kaderavek & Justice, 2004). The lesson here is that the teacher and SLP should work together to determine the most effective strategy for each student on the caseload, especially when that student is having difficulty with reading as well as oral communication. The teacher who is willing to consider a variety of approaches or a combination of methods in instruction is far more likely to succeed with students having communication impairments.

Much literature has suggested that reading difficulties may have a linguistic basis (Catts & Kamhi, 1986; Casby 1988; Catts & Kamhi, 2005). These same sources advocate that the SLP take on an increased role in working with students who have reading problems (see Chapter 6 for specific examples and references). It is important to identify students as early as possible who are at risk for reading and other literacy difficulties. Justice, Invernizzi, and Meier (2002) describe the design and implementation of an early literacy screening protocol for use in public school systems. The goal of the screening protocol is to examine early literacy skills and offer help to students before they fail at learning how to read. Justice et al. (2002) recommend that teachers and SLPs both participate in the literacy screening program as members of an educational team. The specific targets of literacy screening include written language awareness, phonological awareness, letter name knowledge, letter–sound correspondence, literacy motivation, and home literacy. Once a student has been identified as having difficulty with these important emerging literacy skills, a remediation program can be initiated. Recently, emergent literacy intervention programs have been developed for use in school environments that involve cooperation of teachers and SLPs (Kaderavek & Justice, 2004; Justice & Kaderavek, 2004). Kaderavek and Justice (2004) recommend an "embedded-explicit" approach to teaching emergent literacy. The classroom teacher conducts the embedded part of the approach in normal classroom routines that involve a print-rich environment, adult–child book sharing, and an emphasis on literacy in play. The SLP conducts the explicit part of the approach, which may involve direct service delivery, work with the entire class, or work in small groups where specific training on phonological awareness, print concepts, alphabet knowledge, and sound–letter correspondence is targeted. In another example of intervention, Fleming and Forester (1997) targeted work in the areas of metacognition, metalinguistics, phonology, and language use patterns in a collaborative (teacher and SLP) effort. They found that "integrating reading and language instruction proved to be mutually beneficial for both skill areas" (Fleming & Forester, 1997, p. 180). Payoffs for collaboration between the teacher and SLP can even be found in treatment of articulation/phonological disorders. Stewart, Gonzalez, and Page found that children with articulation disorders "learned to read sight words incidentally during articulation training and this learning generalized beyond printed words on cards to printed words on a list" (Stewart, Gonzalez, & Page, 1997, p. 115). Thus, SLPs and teachers need to begin to think in terms of multiple payoffs from their interactions with students. How can the SLP work with the student on communication and positively affect the student's academic performance and reading/writing abilities? How can the teacher enhance academic performance and at the same time facilitate better communication strategies? Answers to these questions will come from increased collaborative efforts and communication between teachers and speech-language pathologists.

Students with Voice Problems   A student in school with a disordered voice may be considered to have a handicap and qualify for SLP services. Recall that both PL 94-142 and the Individuals with Disabilities Education Act incorporate the broad definition of a handicapping condition as including academic, social, and emotional impacts on the student. A voice disorder, therefore, may qualify as an educationally handicapping condition and the student may qualify for speech-language services in the school. Imagine the difficulty a student has making friends in the classroom when he or she has a chronically hoarse and low-pitched voice or exhibits the facial scars from cleft lip and palate surgery along with a nasal-sounding voice, or if the student is a neck breather and hooked to equipment. In addition to daily issues surrounding the disorder and the social impact, teachers may express prejudice to these types of students and assume that they are less intelligent when that clearly is not the case.

Students Who Stutter   Students in elementary school who stutter can be the target of bullying. Adolescent students are in the throes of all sorts of social crises and stuttering when giving oral reports in class or trying to talk to someone of the opposite sex can be extremely traumatic. Panic over using the telephone, answering a teacher's question, asking for the correct movie ticket, and ordering in a restaurant also are common situations of fluency breakdown. Experiences with fluency failure build up over time and soon the person who stutters has full-blown situation and word fears that often evolve into avoidance behaviors and complete escapes, such as avoiding answering the phone, ordering a hamburger when a cheeseburger is really wanted, never asking for a date, and so forth. For decades, psychosocial attributes of stuttering have been investigated. Clearly, stuttering and the surrounding behavioral attributes of the disorder affect a person's quality of life on a daily basis.

COMMUNICATION DISORDERS AND QUALITY-OF-LIFE ISSUES: THE POSTSCHOOL YEARS

The previous section of this chapter discusses how communication disorders can affect the academic success of students. However, as described in other chapters, some communication disorders are either acquired during or continue on through the postschool years. In such cases, SLPs are not so much concerned with academic issues as they are with quality of life (QOL) issues. QOL refers to a person's ability to enjoy normal life activities. The enjoyment of normal life activities typically involves successful interpersonal relationships, occupational satisfaction, and pleasurable leisure activities. Certainly, communication disorders can affect an individual in all of these areas. In this section of the chapter, we identify effects communication disorders may have on QOL. SLPs, audiologists, and other professionals who deal with individuals with communication disorders must be aware of such potential effects because individuals are often hesitant to talk about such issues with professionals.

QUALITY-OF-LIFE ISSUES FOLLOWING GLOSSECTOMY

The person who has undergone a glossectomy may encounter many problems in addition to the speech and swallowing issues described in Chapter 4. Some of these additional problems may stem from communication and swallowing difficulties. For example, swallowing problems may cause a person to eat less and suffer from fatigue and other health problems related to poor nutrition. Embarrassment about eating and swallowing modifications resulting from surgery, along with difficulty being understood, may result in avoidance of social situations and contribute to depression on the part of the patient. Additionally, the reactions of a spouse or other family members, issues related to radiation and chemotherapy, fears about the recurrence of cancer, and emotional reactions to the experience all combine to affect the patient's quality of life.

QOL issues have become an increasingly important focus in the treatment of many medical conditions including oral cancer. SLPs and other health professionals who treat glossectomy patients on a continuing basis should be alert to QOL issues and take appropriate action or make referrals to address them. This is not always easy. Many patients may be hesitant to talk about problems of a personal nature, such as relationship issues with a spouse, family, or friends. Clinicians may not have the time to explore the patient's adjustment in sufficient detail. Myers (2005) suggests that clinicians treating patients with head and neck cancer should, at a minimum, screen for psychosocial distress, which commonly accompanies disorders of this nature. Several QOL screening procedures are available for use with cancer patients, and there is a growing literature on QOL issues. SLPs and other healthcare workers should be familiar with this area and select screening instruments that are most effective for their patients.

QUALITY-OF-LIFE ISSUES ASSOCIATED WITH HEARING LOSS

Mental and Physical Health Issues   Hearing loss can affect many parts of an individual's life including social, emotional, and occupational aspects (Chia et al., 2007). The effect that a hearing loss has on the quality of life of any individual varies according to many factors including, but certainly not limited to, age, age at onset of the hearing loss, the degree of hearing loss, family support, and general health. Two additional factors that appear to have a major impact on quality of life for people with hearing loss are amplification and, in the case of acquired loss, whether the onset was gradual or sudden.

With regard to amplification, it has been reported that patients who used some form of sensory aid demonstrated higher mood level, richer social relationships, and better performance in activities of daily living (Radcliff, 1998). People who experience a rapid onset of a severe or profound hearing loss face unique challenges. They and their family and friends have little or no time to adjust to the hearing loss. Many of these individuals experience misunderstanding from family and others who knew them prior to the hearing loss and therefore may suffer greater emotional distress as a result of the loss (Hallam, Ashton, Sherbourne, & Gailey, 2006). In addition to emotional health, significant degrees of hearing loss also appear to affect physical health (Crandell, 1998; Johnson, 2010). One cause of this influence on physical health may be that severe and profound hearing losses can interfere with effective communication between patients and physicians. Many healthcare providers may not be well prepared to communicate with patients who are deaf or hard-of-hearing (Witte & Kuzel, 2000).

Finally, recall that the inner ear has both hearing and balance functions. Some people with a sensorineural hearing loss may also have balance and dizziness issues. This can be especially difficult for older people for whom falls could result in serious, possibly life-threatening injuries. Healthcare professionals working with older persons with hearing loss must be aware of the possibility of balance problems.

Employment Issues   Among the factors that affect the quality of life of individuals with severe and profound hearing loss are employment issues. Ringdahl and Grimby (2000) report that individuals with a severe to profound hearing loss who had full-time employment scored better on a quality-of-life index than did those who had part-time or no employment. Until the latter part of the twentieth century, it was fairly common for deaf children to be educated in special schools for the deaf where they received vocational training, often in the area of printing and carpentry. Students with severe and profound hearing loss who desired a college education often felt that their choices were limited to the few universities that specialized in programs for the deaf such as Gallaudet University or the National Technical Institute for the Deaf (NTID) at the Rochester Institute of Technology. As Moores (1987) indicates, deafness itself precludes very few occupations. The primary issues affecting employment opportunities for individuals who are deaf are providing appropriate education and training and making reasonable accommodations in the workplace.

Because of public laws such as Section 504 of the Rehabilitation Act of 1973 and Americans with Disabilities Act of 1990, colleges and technical schools are now required to provide accommodations that allow deaf students to pursue a wide variety of professional and technical fields. As is true with all students, the selection of colleges by students with severe and profound hearing loss involves many individual variables. Regarding the choice of a postsecondary educational setting, Johnson (2010) suggests that students with hearing loss take the following steps.

- Investigate the quality of programs for students with disabilities.
- Determine the types of accommodations for those who are deaf and hard-of-hearing.
- Identify themselves as a student who will require accommodations and provide any required documentation.
- Communicate with the school well in advance of the first semester to allow it adequate time to provide appropriate accommodations.

Accommodations in the Workplace   The Job Accommodation Network (JAN) is a service provided by the U.S. Department of Labor's Office of Disability Employment Policy (ODEP). JAN's mission is to facilitate the employment and retention of workers with disabilities by providing employers, employment providers, people with disabilities, their family members, and other interested parties with information on job accommodations, entrepreneurship, and related subjects. With regard to individuals with hearing loss, JAN identifies the following questions to consider regarding the workplace.

1. What limitations is the employee with hearing loss experiencing?
2. How do these limitations affect the employee and the employee's job performance?
3. What specific job tasks are problematic as a result of these limitations?
4. What accommodations are available to reduce or eliminate these problems? Are all possible resources being used to determine possible accommodations?
5. Has the employee with hearing loss been consulted regarding possible accommodations?
6. Once accommodations are in place, would it be useful to meet with the employee with hearing loss to evaluate the effectiveness of the accommodations and to determine whether additional accommodations are needed?
7. Do supervisory personnel and employees need training regarding hearing loss?

Additionally, JAN lists more than 60 specific accommodations for employees with hearing loss, ranging from using written instructions for an employee with a hearing loss to hiring a sign language interpreter.

Deafness as a Cultural Difference   Many people who are deaf consider themselves part of a separate culture. Deaf culture is defined differently by some, but essentially it refers to people who are prelingually deaf, use sign language as their primary means of communication, and hold a set of beliefs about themselves and their connection to the larger society (Padden & Humphries, 1988). Many members of this culture resent what they view as attempts by hearing society to force them or their deaf children to communicate orally, and they resist such innovations as cochlear implants. Many Americans first became aware of the strength of feelings in the Deaf culture in 1988 when student protests over the appointment of a hearing person as president of Gallaudet University in Washington, DC (the world's only university in which all programs and services are specifically designed to accommodate deaf and hard-of-hearing students), forced the resignation of the university president and resulted in the appointment of the first deaf president in the school's history.

It is sometimes difficult for hearing individuals to understand the attitudes expressed by members of this Deaf culture, but differing views about the "best" way to do things are frequently at the heart of cultural differences, whether those cultures are religious, ethnic, or political in nature. Communication disorders professionals should attempt to understand and respect the various cultures they encounter in their work and keep in mind that ultimately the right to make decisions about rehabilitation and treatment belongs to the patient and his or her family.

QUALITY OF LIFE FOR PERSONS WITH VOICE DISORDERS

To underscore that contemporary health issues are the consequences of various disorders, the World Health Organization developed the International Classification of Impairment, Disability, and Handicaps (ICIDH). The updated ICIDH-2 emphasizes functioning as well as disability and health (World Health Organization [WHO], 2001). Recall from the discussion in Chapter 9 how the voice affects speakers and listeners. A voice deemed odd or not-normal-sounding may have negative consequences for the speaker in school, work, or society in general.

Adults may find negative consequences at work or in daily socialization. The woman with an atypical voice that is low pitched and gravelly sounding; the man with a high-pitched effeminate voice; the executive with a weak, soft, and breathy voice resulting from a paralyzed fold; and the salesperson who survived cancer by having a laryngectomy may all find that society is not tolerant. Will the person keep friends and colleagues, make the sale, convey authority, or even lose his or her job? Will the child at school be teased or bullied?

A voice disorder has both large and small impacts on daily life. The SLP may obtain patient impact ratings during a thorough voice assessment. For example, Jacobson and colleagues (1997) created the *Voice Handicap Index* to quantify the psychosocial consequences of a voice disorder. With this instrument, patients rate, on a 0–4 scale, issues and their handicapping impact along three domains. The physical domain asks for ratings on statements like, "I feel as though I have to strain to produce voice." The functional domain explores daily impacts of the voice through statements such as, "My voice makes it difficult for persons to hear me." In the emotional domain, the person rates emotional and psychological feelings that stem from the voice disorder. An example is to rate degree of agreement with statements such as, "My voice problem upsets me." The speech-language pathologist may also administer daily impact assessments before, during, and after treatment to help document improvement and functional impact of intervention. Two of these are mentioned below:

Ma and Yiu (2001) developed the *Voice Activity and Participation Profile*. As the name implies, this instrument evaluates the person's perception of the voice problems, the degree that daily activities are limited by the vocal issues, and the extent to which there are restrictions in daily life.

Bosley and Hartnick (2004) administered the *Pediatric Voice Outcomes Survey* to the parents of children pre- and post-surgery for different types of oral surgery and the impact on the child's speech and velopharyngeal competence.

QUALITY OF LIFE FOR PEOPLE WHO STUTTER

Recall that stuttering is a disorder of speech characterized by repetitions of sounds, syllables, and/or words but also by prolongation of speech sounds. These disrupt the normal forward flow of speech. In addition, there may be accompanied signs of struggling behavior, such as rapid eye blinks or tremors of the lips. Stuttering can make it difficult to communicate with others and it can be frustrating, even embarrassing. The intermittency of the disruptions—one minute speaking fine, and then suddenly stuck—adds further frustration. It is no wonder that stuttering often affects a person's quality of life.

Yaruss and Quesal (2002) write about the impact of stuttering on quality of life as discussed by the World Health Organization (WHO, 2001). He designed the *Overall Assessment of the Speaker's Experience of Stuttering (OASES–Adult)* that analyzes the quality of life and impacts of stuttering on a speaker's ability to pursue life goals in various domains, such as social interactions, economic independence, and so forth. Child and adolescent versions of this assessment tool have also been designed.

Craig, Blumgart, and Tran (2009) used a general measure of quality of life called the *Medical Outcomes Study Short Form-36* to assess the impact of stuttering on adults. Findings confirm that stuttering negatively affects the quality of life in the areas of vitality, social functioning, emotional functioning, and mental health status. Similarly, Robin and colleagues (2006) assessed the quality of life in adults who stutter.

Regardless of the particular quality-of-life scales used, the speech-language pathologist has a variety of reasons to use them. When administered pre- and post-treatment, these types of scales offer impact data on the success of intervention. Third-party payers (often insurance companies) appreciate quantitative information. The SLP may use quality-of-life scales to identify areas in a person's life that need focus in the treatment program. Examples might be the necessity to invest resources to address the emotional and psychological aspects of stuttering (Craig et al., 2009). Using quality-of-life techniques therefore may contribute to complete measurement protocols for the treatment of stuttering (Bramlett, Boothe, & Franic, 2006).

QUALITY OF LIFE FOR PERSONS WITH ADULT LANGUAGE DISORDERS

The quality of life after stroke or other brain-damaging episode has been used as an outcome measure following language treatment for aphasia (King, 1996). Because language is a key component of what makes someone human and allows him or her to socialize, it seems logical that adult language disorders negatively affect quality of life. Conversely, it seems logical that the degree of language recovery correlates with patient satisfaction, less frustration, and a more positive mood. Unclear is the extent to which type and severity of aphasia correlate with quality of life. Although it is generally true that the severity of aphasia, as measured by the *Western Aphasia Battery-Revised* (Kertsz, 2006) or the *Boston Diagnostic Aphasia Examination* (Goodglass, Kaplan, & Barresi, 2000), is a key determinant of patient quality of life, individual circumstances may alter this broad statement. Individual factors that matter, for example, include the provision of social interactions and lack of a monotonous routine. Residing at home versus in a residential facility matters less than the quality of care and interaction provided to adults with language disorders.

King (1996) investigated older adults one to three years after they had a stroke. Both satisfaction and importance of items were ranked within four domains: health and functioning, socioeconomic, family, and psychological-spiritual. Overall, the poststroke adults highly rated their quality of living. The family domain received the highest ratings, and the health and functioning domain was lowest rated. Noteworthy was that 30 percent of the adults scored in the depressed range, suggesting that depression is a long-term outcome of stroke.

In recent years, a language-focused outcome measure has been used. The *Aphasia Quality of Life Scale-36* is an assessment instrument that has been shown to be valid and reliable and so is commonly used in assessing the quality of life in adults with language impairments (Hilari, Byng, Lamping, & Smith, 2003).

QUALITY OF LIFE FOR PERSONS WITH SWALLOWING DISORDERS

Swallowing disorders, whether in children or adults, present clear challenges to a person's quality of life. Recall that dysphagia is a chronic health condition. If you consider quality of life from the point of view of daily satisfaction and well-being, certainly eating and swallowing impairments have a negative impact each and every day. Imagine the student who cannot participate in classroom birthday parties and who feels humiliated daily at lunchtime for eating unusual foods and requiring the assistance of a teacher or school nurse. Think about the adult who survived cancer through head and neck surgery or radiation but cannot find joy at mealtimes with coworkers and friends because of an altered swallowing mechanism and special diet. Consider the grandparent who had a stroke and who is being treated for aphasia and is learning safe swallowing strategies while receiving muscle electrical stimulation to strengthen swallowing muscles. All these types of patients, and many more, share an emotion: the constant fear of choking. Dysphagia indeed affects the physical, social, and psychological quality of life.

The entire healthcare team is important in treating the medical situation that causes dysphagia and in rehabilitating a safe swallow (or finding other avenues of nutrition), and the team can affect, positively or negatively, the patient's reaction to the swallowing challenges. Providing education about changes in swallowing resulting from a disease process or its treatment can improve the person's degree of confidence in the modified situation and swallowing. Feeling understood and accepted, and having confidence can boost the patient's emotional state of health. Eating is a social activity, and having the confidence to swallow safely and not feel embarrassment for eating differently (maybe eating slowly, perhaps with a head tilt, or eating foods of different consistencies and textures) can help the person's outlook on life. Persons with dysphagia need to establish this social reconnection to friends. Also, diet changes or restrictions may decrease the satisfaction of eating.

Tibbling and Gustafsson (1991) report the impact of dysphagia on quality of life. Based on a mailed questionnaire survey with a low return rate, only 8 percent of adults older than age 59 years reported symptoms of dysphagia. Reported symptoms tended to be either esophageal or pharyngeal. But importantly, half of these individuals reported anxiety at meals. Some stated that their degree of anxiety made them want to eat alone. Often there were reports of gastrointestinal symptoms such as chest pain, heartburn, and regurgitation.

Ekberg et al. (2002) interviewed adults living in long-term care facilities. Their questionnaire covered background, eating habits, personal feelings and importance, seeking help, and medical status. Results indicate that dysphagia created social and psychological consequences and was not well recognized, diagnosed, or managed. Many residents reported avoiding eating with others and felt panicked or anxious at mealtimes. Less than half the adults interviewed reported that eating was enjoyable and more than half indicated that they were eating less and remained hungry.

To improve swallowing and hence improve the quality of life for patients, speech-language pathologists often apply neuromuscular electrical stimulation to muscles in the neck and surrounding area. Clark et al. (2009) did an evidence-based systematic review of this literature. Dysphagia affects the quality of life in numerous ways: physically, emotionally, socially, and nutritionally.

No matter which type of communication disorder a person experiences, there are real-world consequences. The effects of a speech, language, hearing, or swallowing impairment can be far-reaching and present significant academic, social, psychological, vocational, and general quality-of-life issues. This is why SLPs work so hard to identify, assess, and treat children and adults who have difficulty with communication. Professional treatment can have a tremendous impact on individuals' quality of life, and perhaps that is why communications professions, education, and allied health specialties are fields so gratifying to work in.

Term to Know

Phonological awareness

Study Questions

1. Discuss how a speech-language pathologist and a reading specialist can work together to identify and remediate children who are at risk for reading problems.
2. Identify some problems that a person with a significant hearing loss may encounter in the workplace. Then, identify some accommodations that would overcome those problems.
3. Describe how a hearing loss might affect an individual's physical and mental health.

Bibliography

Adams, M. (1990). *Beginning to read: Thinking and learning about print*. Cambridge, MA: MIT Press.

Allen, T. E. (1986). Patterns of academic achievement among hearing impaired students: 1974 and 1983. In A. N. Schildroth & M. A. Karchmer (Eds.), *Deaf children in America*. Boston, MA: Little, Brown.

Apel, K., Masterson, J. J., & Hart, P. (2004). Integration of language components in spelling: Instruction that maximizes students' learning. In E. R. Silliman & L. C. Wilkinson (Eds.), *Language and literacy learning in schools*. New York, NY: Guilford Press.

Aram, D., & Nation, J. (1980). Preschool language disorders and subsequent language and academic difficulties. *Journal of Communication Disorders, 13*, 159–170.

Baker, L. (1982). An evaluation of the role of metacognitive deficits in learning disabilities. *Topics in Learning and Learning Disabilities, 2*, 27–35.

Ball, E., & Blachman, B. (1991). Does phoneme awareness training in kindergarten make a difference in early word recognition and developmental spelling? *Reading Research Quarterly, 26*, 49–66.

Baron, B., Baron, C., & MacDonald, B. (1983). *What did you learn in school today?* New York: Warner Books.

Bashir, A., Kuban, K., Kleinman, S., & Scavuzzo, A. (1983). Issues in language disorders: Considerations of cause, maintenance, and change. In J. Miller, D. Yoder, & R. Shiefelbusch (Eds.), *Contemporary Issues in Language Intervention*, ASHA Reports 12, The American Speech-Language-Hearing Association: Rockville, MD.

Berg, F. S. (1986). Characteristics of the target population. In F. S. Berg, J. L. Blait, S. H. Viehweg, & A. Wilson-Vlotman (Eds.), *Educational audiology for the hard of hearing child*. Orlando, FL: Grune and Stratton.

Bird, J., Bishop, D., & Freeman, N. (1995). Perception and awareness of phonemes in phonologically impaired children. *European Journal of Disorders of Communication, 27*, 289–311.

Blachman, B. (1991). Early intervention for children's reading problems: Clinical applications of the research in phonological awareness. *Topics in Language Disorders, 12*, 51–65.

Blachman, B., Ball, E., Black, R., & Tangel, D. (2000). *Road to the code: A phonological awareness program for young children*. Baltimore, MD: Paul H. Brookes.

Boseley, M. E., & Hartnick, C. J. (2004). Assessing the outcome of surgery to correct velopharyngeal insufficiency with pediatric outcomes surgery. *International Journal of Pediatric Otorhinolaryngology, 68*(11), 1429–1433.

Brackett, D., & Maxon, A. B. (1986). Service delivery alternatives for the mainstreamed hearing-impaired child. *Language Speech and Hearing Services in Schools, 17*, 115–125.

Catts, H. W. (1991). Early identification of reading disabilities. *Topics in Language Disorders, 12*, 1–16.

Catts, H. W., & Kamhi, A. G. (2005). *Language and reading disabilities* (2nd ed.). Boston, MA: Allyn & Bacon.

Chia, E., Wang, J., Rochtchina, E., Cumming, R., Newall, P., & Mitchell, P. (2007). Hearing impairment and health-related quality of life: The blue mountains hearing study. *Ear and Hearing, 28,* 187–195.

Clark, H., Lazarus, C., Arvedson, J., & Schooling, T. (2009). Evidence-based systematic review: Effects of neuromuscular electrical stimulation on swallowing and neuro activation. *American Journal of Speech-Language Pathology, 18,* 361–375.

Clarke-Klein, S. (1994). Expressive phonological deficiencies: Impact on spelling and development. *Topics in Language Disorders, 14,* 40–45.

Cowan, W., & Moran, M. (1997). Phonological awareness skills in children with articulation disorders in kindergarten to third grade. *Journal of Children's Communication Development, 8,* 31–38.

Craig, A., Blumgart, E., & Tran, Y. (2009). The impact of stuttering on the quality of life in adults who stutter. *Journal of Fluency Disorders, 34*(2), 61–71.

Crandell, C. (1998). Hearing aids: Their effects on functional health status. *Hearing Journal, 51,* 22–30.

Creaghead, N., & Donnelly, K. (1982). Comprehension of superordinate and subordinate information by good and poor readers. *Language, Speech, and Hearing Services in Schools, 13,* 177–186.

Creaghead, N., & Tattershall, S. (1985). Observation and assessment of classroom pragmatic skills. In C. Simon (Ed.) *Communication skills and classroom success: Assessment of language-learning disabled students.* San Diego, CA: College-Hill.

Cuda, R., & Nelson, N. (1976). Analysis of teacher speaking rate, syntactic complexity, and hesitation phenomena as a function of grade level. Presented at the annual meeting of the American Speech-Language-Hearing Association, Houston, TX.

Davis, J. (1974). Performance of young hearing-impaired children on a test of basic concepts. *Journal of Speech and Hearing Research, 17,* 342–351.

Davis, J., & Blasdell, R. (1975). Perceptual strategies employed by normal-hearing and hearing-impaired children in the comprehension of sentences containing relative clauses. *Journal of Speech and Hearing Research, 18,* 281–295.

Dobie, R. A., & Berlin, C. I. (1979). Influence of otitis media on hearing and development. *Annals of Otology, Rhinology, and Laryngology, 88*(suppl. 60), 48–53.

Ehri, L. C., Nunes, S. R., Willows, D. M., Schuster, B. V., Yaghoub-Zadeh, Z., & Shanahan, T. (2001). Phonemic awareness instruction helps children learn to read: Evidence from the National Reading Panel's meta-analysis. *Reading Research Quarterly, 36,* 250–287.

Ekberg, O., Hamby, S., Woisard, V., Wuttge-Hannig, A., & Ortega, P. (2002). Social and psychological burden of dysphagia: Its impact on diagnosis and treatment. *Dysphagia, 17,* 39–146.

Everhart, R. (1953). The relationship between articulation and other developmental factors in children. *Journal of Speech and Hearing Disorders, 18,* 332–338.

FitzSimons, R. (1958). Developmental, psychosocial, and educational factors in children with nonorganic articulation problems. *Child Development, 29,* 481–489.

Fleming, J., & Gorester, B. (1997). Infusing language enhancement into the reading curriculum for disadvantaged adolescents. *Language, Speech and Hearing Services in Schools, 28*(2), 177–180.

Flynn, P., & Byrne, M. (1970). Relationship between reading and selected auditory abilities of third-grade children. *Journal of Speech and Hearing Research, 13*, 731–740.

Goldsworthy, C. L. (1998). *Sourcebook of phonological awareness activities.* San Diego, CA: Singular.

Goodglass, H., Kaplan, E., & Barresi, N. (2000). *The assessment of aphasia and related disorders.* Hagerstown, MD: Lippincott Williams & Wilkins.

Hall, M. (1938). Auditory factors in functional articulatory speech defects. *Journal of Experimental Education, 7*, 110–132.

Hall, P., & Tomblin, J. (1978). A follow-up study of children with articulation and language disorders. *Journal of Speech and Hearing Disorders, 43*, 227–241.

Hall, S. L., & Moats, L. C. (2002). *Parenting a struggling reader: A guide to diagnosing and finding help for your child's reading difficulties.* New York, NY: Broadway Books.

Hallam, R., Ashton, P., Sherbourne, K., & Gailey, L. (2006). Acquired profound hearing loss: Mental health and other characteristics of a large sample. *International Journal of Audiology, 45*, 715–723.

Ham, R. (1958). Relationship between misspelling and misarticulation. *Journal of Speech and Hearing Disorders, 23*, 294–297.

Hilari, K., Byng, S., Lamping, D., & Smith, S. (2003). *Stroke and Aphasia Quality of Life Scale-39 (SAQOL-39)*: Evidence of acceptability, reliability, and validity. *Stroke, 34*, 1944–1950.

Hill, S. & Haynes, W. (1992). Language performance in low achieving elementary school students. *Language, Speech and Hearing Services in Schools, 23*, 169–175.

Holm, V. A., & Kunze, L. H. (1969). Effect of chronic otitis media on language and speech development. *Pediatrics, 43*, 833–839.

Hook, P., & Johnson, D. (1978). Metalinguistic awareness and reading strategies. *Bulletin of the Orton Society, 28*, 62–78.

Jacobson, B., Johnson, A., Grywalski, C., Silbergleit, A., Jacobsen, B., & Benninger, S. (1997). The *Voice Handicap Index (VHI)*: Development and validation. *American Journal of Speech-Language Pathology, 6*(3), 66–70.

Jensema, C. J. (1975). *The relationship between academic achievement and demographic characteristics of hearing-impaired children and youth.* Series R, No. 2. Washington, DC: Office of Demographic Studies, Gallaudet College.

Johnson, C. (2010). *Aural rehabilitation: A contemporary issues approach.* Boston, MA: Pearson.

Justice, L., Invernizzi, M. & Meier, J. (2002). Designing and implementing an early literacy screening protocol: Suggestions for the speech-language pathologist. *Language, Speech and Hearing Services in Schools, 33*, 84–101.

Justice, L. & Kaderavek, J. (2004). Embedded-explicit emergent literacy intervention I: Background and description of approach. *Language, Speech and Hearing Services in Schools, 35*, 201–211.

Kaderavek, J., & Justice, L. (2004). Embedded-explicit emergent literacy II: Goal selection and implementation in the early childhood classroom. *Language, Speech, and Hearing Services in Schools, 35*, 212–228.

Kertesz, A. (2006). *Western Aphasia Battery—Revised.* New York, NY: Psychological Corporation.

King. R., Jones, C., & Lasky, E. (1982). In retrospect: A fifteen year follow-up report of speech-language disorders in children. *Language, Speech, and Hearing Services in Schools, 13*, 24–32.

King, R. B. (1996). Quality of life after stroke. *Stroke, 27*, 1467–1472.

Kodman, F. (1963). Education status of the hard-of-hearing child in the classroom. *Journal of Speech and Hearing Research, 28*, 297–299.

Lahey, M. (1988). *Language disorders and language development.* New York, NY: Macmillan.

Lindamood, C., & Lindamood, P. (1998). *The Lindamood phoneme sequencing program for reading, spelling and speech* (3rd. ed.). Austin, TX: Pro-Ed.

Lombardino, L., Bedford, T., Fortier, C., Carter, J., & Brandi, J. (1997). Invented spelling: Developmental patterns in kindergarten children and guidelines for early literacy intervention. *Language Speech and Hearing Services in Schools, 28*, 333–343.

Ma, E., & Yiu, E. (2001). Voice activity and participation profile assessing the impact of voice disorders on daily activities. *Journal of Speech, Language, and Hearing Research, 44*, 511–524.

Magnusson, E. (1991). Metalinguistic awareness in phonologically disordered children. In Y. Mehmet (Ed.), *Phonological disorders in children* (pp. 87–120). New York, NY: Routledge.

Magnusson, E., & Naucler, K. (1990). Reading and spelling in language-disordered children—Linguistic and metalinguistic prerequisites: Report on a longitudinal study. *Clinical Linguistics and Phonetics, 4*, 49–61.

Marschark, M., Lang, H., & Albertini, J. (2002). *Educating deaf students: From research to practice.* New York, NY: Oxford University Press.

Maxwell, S. & Wallach, G. (1984). The language-learning disabilities connection: Symptoms of early language disability change over time. In G. Wallach, & K. Butler (Eds.) *Language Learning Disabilities in School-Age Children.* Baltimore: Williams & Wilkins.

Mehan, H. (1978). Structuring school structure. *Harvard Educational Review, 48*, 32–64.

Moores, D. (1987). *Educating the deaf: Psychology, principles and practices.* Dallas, TX: Houghton Mifflin.

Muter, V., Hulme, C., Snowling, M., & Stevenson, J. (2004). Phonemes, rimes, vocabulary, and grammatical skills as foundations of early reading development: Evidence from a longitudinal study. *Developmental Psychology, 40*, 665–681.

Myers, C. (2005). Quality of life and head and neck cancer. In P. Doyle & R. Keith (Eds.). *Contemporary considerations in the treatment and rehabilitation of head and neck cancer: voice, speech and language.* Austin, TX: Pro Ed.

Nelson, N. (1976). Comprehension of spoken language by normal children as a function of speaking rate, sentence difficulty and listener age and sex. *Child Development, 47*, 299–303.

Nelson, N. (1984). Beyond information processing: The language of teachers and text-books. In G. Wallach, & K. Butler (Eds.) *Language learning disabilities in school-age children*. Baltimore: Williams & Wilkins.

Nippold, M., & Fey, M. (1983). Metaphoric understanding in pre-adolescents having a history of language acquisition difficulties. *Language, Speech and Hearing Services in Schools, 14*, 171–180.

Olson, R., & Byrne, B. (2005). Genetic and environmental influences on reading and language abilities and disabilities. In H. Catts & A. Kamhi (Eds.). *The connections between language and reading disability*. Mahwah, NJ: Lawrence Earlbaum Associates.

Padden, C., & Humphries, T. (1988). *Deaf in America: Voices from a culture*. Cambridge, MA: Harvard University Press.

Paul, P. V., & Quigley, S. P. (1987). Some effects of early hearing impairment on English language development. In F. N. Martin (Ed.), *Hearing disorders in children*. Austin, TX: Pro-Ed.

Pressnell, L. (1973). Hearing-impaired children's comprehension and production of syntax in oral language. *Journal of Speech and Hearing Research, 16*, 12–21.

Preston, J., & Edwards, M. L. (2009). *Speech sound disorders: Red flags for literacy problems*. A paper presented at the annual meeting of the American Speech-Language-Hearing Association. New Orleans, LA.

Quigley, S., & Thomure, R. (1968). *Some effects of hearing impairment on school performance*. Urbana, IL: University of Illinois, Institute for Research on Exceptional Children.

Quigley, S., Wilbur, R., Power, D., Montanelli, D., & Steinkamp, M. (1976). *Syntactic structures in the language of deaf children*. Urbana, IL: University of Illinois, Final Report Project No. 232175, U.S. Department of Health, Education and Welfare, National Institute of Education.

Radcliffe, D. (1998). The high cost of hearing lost: What our publics need to know. *The Hearing Journal, 51*, 21–30.

Ringdahl, A., & Grimby, A. (2000). Severe profound hearing impairment and health-related quality of life amongst post-lingual deafened Swedish adults. *Scandinavian Audiology, 29*, 266–275.

Robin, E., Bramlett, R., Bothe, A., & Duska, F. (2006). Using preference-based measures to assess quality of life in stuttering. *Journal of Speech, Language, and Hearing Research, 49*, 381–394.

Shriberg, L. (1982). Programming for the language component in developmental phonological disorders. *Seminars in Speech, Language and Hearing, 3*, 115–126.

Shriberg, L. D., & Austin, D. (1998). Co-morbidity of speech-language disorder: Implications for a phenotype marker of speech delay. In R. Paul (Ed.), *The speech-language connection* (p. 73-117). Baltimore, MD: Paul H. Brookes.

Shriberg, L. D., & Kwiatkowski, J. (1994). Developmental phonological disorders I: A clinical profile. *Journal of Speech and Hearing Research, 37*, 1100–1126.

Simon, C. (1985). The language-learning disabled student: Description and assessment implications. In C. Simon (Ed.) *Communication skills and classroom success: Assessment of language-learning disabled students.* San Diego, CA: College-Hill.

Sinclair, J. & Coulthard, R. (1975). *Towards an analysis of discourse: The English used by teachers and pupils.* Oxford, UK: Oxford University Press.

Stackhouse, J. (1982). An investigation of reading and spelling performance in speech disordered children. *British Journal of Disorders of Communication, 17,* 53–60.

Stackhouse, J. (1997). Phonological awareness. In B. W. Hodson & M. L. Edwards (Eds.), *Perspectives in applied phonology.* Gaithersburg, MD: Aspen.

Stephens, M. & Montgomery, A. (1985). A critique of recent relevant standardized tests. *Topics in Language Disorders, 5,* 21–45.

Stewart, S., Gonzalez, L. & Page, J. (1997). Incidental learning of sight words during articulation training. *Language, Speech, and Hearing Services in Schools, 28(2),* 115–126.

Stoel-Gammon, C., & Dunn, C. (1985). *Normal and disordered phonology in children.* Austin, TX: Pro-Ed.

Strominger, A. & Bashir, A. (1977). A nine year follow-up of language delayed children. Presented at the annual convention of the American Speech-Language-Hearing Association, Chicago, IL.

Sturm, J. & Nelson, N. (1997). Formal classroom lessons: New perspectives on a familiar discourse event. *Language, Speech, and Hearing Services in Schools, 28(3),* 255–273.

Tangel, D., & Blachman, B. (1992). Effect of phoneme awareness instruction on kindergarten children's invented spelling. *Journal of Reading Behavior, 24,* 223–258.

Tattershall, S. & Creaghead, N. (1985). A comparison of communication at home and school. In D. Ripich & F. Spinelli (Eds.) *School discourse problems.* San Diego, CA: College-Hill.

Tibbling, L., & Gustafsson, B. (1991). Dysphagia and its consequences in the elderly. *Dysphagia, 6,* 200–202.

Tye-Murray, N. (1998). *Foundations of aural rehabilitation: Children, adults, and their family members.* San Diego, CA: Singular.

Tyler, A. & Watterson, K. (1991). Effects of phonological versus language intervention in preschoolers with both phonological and language impairment. *Child Language Teaching and Therapy, 7,* 141–160.

U.S. Department of Labor. Office of Disability Employment Policy. (n.d.). Job Accommodation Network Website. Retrieved June 17, 2010, from http://www.jan.wvu.edu.

VanKleek, A. (1984). Metalinguistic skills: Cutting across spoken and written language and problem-solving abilities. In G. Wallach, & K. Butler (Eds.) *Language learning disabilities in school-age children.* Baltimore: Williams & Wilkins.

Wallach, G. & Butler, K. (Eds.) (1994). *Language learning disabilities in school-age children and adolescents.* New York: Merrill.

Wallach, G. & Miller, L. (1988*). Language intervention and academic success.* San Diego, CA: College-Hill.

Webster, P., & Plante, A. (1992). Effects of phonological impairment on word, syllable, and phoneme segmentation and reading. *Language, Speech, and Hearing Services in Schools, 23*, 176–182.

Wiig, E. & Semel, E. (1976). *Language disabilities in children and adolescents.* Columbus, OH: Merrill.

Wilcox, J., & Tobin, H. (1974). Linguistic performance of hard-of-hearing and normal hearing children. *Journal of Speech and Hearing Research, 17*, 286–293.

Winitz, H. (1969). *Articulatory acquisition and behavior.* New York, NY: Appleton-Century-Crofts.

Witte, T., & Kuzel, A. (2000). Elderly deaf patients' health care experiences. *Journal of the American Board of Family Practice, 13*, 17–22.

World Health Organization. (2001). *International Classification of Functioning, Disability, and Health (ICIDH-2).* Geneva, Switzerland.

Yaruss, S., & Quesal, R. (2002). *Overall assessment of the speaker's experience of stuttering—adult.* Upper Saddle River, NJ: Pearson.

GLOSSARY

A

abducted: Taken away from home or midline position: vocal folds in an open position.

acute care hospital: A clinical facility in which patients are initially seen after a traumatic event (e.g., stroke, head injury) and are discharged after they are physiologically stable.

adducted: Moved to the home or midline position: vocal folds in a closed position.

affricate: A consonant sound that is produced by stopping the flow of air, and then releasing the air through a narrow opening, creating friction noise. In English, the <u>ch</u> as in *church* and the <u>dg</u> as in *fudge* are affricates.

African American English (AAE): A dialect.

air conduction test: A hearing assessment in which test tones are sent via the air into the outer ear. This is usually done using headphones.

Alternative/Augmentative Communication (AAC): A term encompassing all forms of communication used to assist in expression of thoughts, needs, wants, and ideas; may include use of gestures, symbols, pictures, and writing and may employ various delivery methods, with or without technology.

alveolar ridge: The ridges that contain the sockets of the lower and upper teeth. More commonly, the area just behind the upper incisors that serves as the place of articulation for <u>t</u>, <u>d</u>, <u>s</u>, <u>z</u>, <u>l</u>, and <u>n</u>.

ambient noise: Noise in the surrounding environment.

American Academy of Audiology (AAA): A professional organization that provides advocacy, leadership, education, public awareness, and research in the areas of hearing and balance disorders.

American Sign Language (ASL): The predominant system of manual communication used in the United States and Canada by individuals who are deaf. Also known as Ameslan or ASL.

American Speech-Language-Hearing Association (ASHA): The professional organization of speech-language pathologists and audiologists that provides guidelines for training of professionals and conduct of clinical practice in communication disorders.

Americans with Disabilities Act (ADA): Enacted in 1990, this act provides comprehensive civil rights protection for qualified individuals with disabilities.

Ameslan: American sign language.

ankyloglossia: A condition in which the lingual frenulum is short limiting the movement of the tongue.

aphasia: Language impairment after language acquisition, typically in adults, and often attributed to stroke, tumor, other disease, or trauma. Receptive and/or expressive impairments vary in severity and type, and rarely is there complete loss such that *dysphagia* is a more accurate term.

apraxia of speech: A type of motor speech disorder affecting a person's ability to translate the brain's intended speech plans into the actual motor plan, disrupting volitional movement patterns rather than automatic movements or movement weakness (such as dysarthria).

articulation: The process of physically producing speech sounds.

articulator: A structure used to produce a speech sound. Moveable articulators include the lips, tongue, soft palate, and mandible. Immovable articulators include the alveolar ridge, hard palate, and teeth.

artificial larynx: A device (e.g., electronic, pneumatic) that acts as a substitute glottis or vibratory sound source for a person without a larynx so that the person can produce articulated speech.

ASHA position on social dialects: The American Speech-Language-Hearing Association takes the position that social dialects are legitimate forms of communication and not disorders of speech or language.

assimilation: The modification of a speech sound resulting from the influence of another sound in close proximity. This usually results in a speech sound substitution error as opposed to more minor differences resulting from coarticulation.

ataxia: Inability to coordinate voluntary muscular movements, such as gait, and attributed to damage or disease of the cerebellum.

athetosis: Slow, recurrent, involuntary wormlike movements of various parts of the body associated with damage to the brain (particularly in the basal ganglia).

atresia: A deformity of the outer ear that may narrow or occlude the ear canal and can result in a conductive hearing loss.

Attention Deficit Hyperactivity Disorder (ADHD): A syndrome, usually diagnosed in childhood, characterized by a persistent pattern of impulsiveness, short attention span, and often hyperactivity that interferes with cognition and language so that it affects academic, occupational, and social performance.

audiogram: A graphic representation of a subject's performance on a hearing test.

audiologist: A communication disorders professional who specializes in assessing and treating hearing problems and other conditions related to the ear. Currently, certification as an audiologist in the United States requires a doctoral degree (typically an AuD or PhD).

audiology: The profession which involves the study, assessment, and treatment of hearing and balance disorders.

audiometer: An instrument used to assess hearing sensitivity.

audition: Processing sensory information through the auditory system (hearing).

auditory: Pertaining to hearing.

auditory processing disorder (APD): A problem recognizing or interpreting sounds in the environment although hearing acuity is normal. Skills such as sound discrimination, recognition, and recognition in noise may be affected.

auditory stimulation: A technique used in treating speech sound disorders in which the clinician provides a spoken model of the target sound.

auditory training unit (ATU): An amplification device in which the microphone is worn by the speaker (often a teacher) and the receiver is worn by the listener (often a student in a classroom).

auditory-verbal therapy: A therapy approach designed to teach children with hearing loss to make maximum use of *the hearing* provided by a hearing aid or a cochlear implant for *understanding speech* and *learning to talk*.

Augmentative/Alternative Communication (AAC): Communication for those with impairments or restrictions on the production or comprehension of spoken or written language; there are low-tech or high-tech (computerized) options.

aural rehabilitation: Training individuals with hearing problems to improve their communication skills.

auricle: Also called the pinna. The visible external portion of the ear.

avoidance behaviors: Tricks or crutches that persons who stutter may use in an attempt to circumvent disfluency, for example, substitution of certain words for words that start with difficult sounds.

B

babbling: The stage of pre-language development in which children produce strings of consonant-vowel syllables. Begins at about 6 months of age.

BACIS: The foundations of communicative development. Biological, access to language model, cognitive, intent to communicate, and social interaction.

back vowel: Vowels produced with the tongue placed toward the back of the oral cavity. Back vowels include <u>oo</u> as in "too," <u>o</u> as in "no," and <u>a</u> as in "father."

behind-the-ear aid: Hearing aid in which most of the components are contained in a unit worn behind the pinna of the outer ear.

bidialectalism: Having proficiency in two dialects. Also, a teaching method in which several dialects are used in educational materials.

bilabial: Consonants produced by the articulation of both lips. The consonants <u>p</u>, <u>b</u>, <u>m</u>, and <u>w</u> are bilabial.

bilingualism: Speaking two languages, one a first language and the other a second language.

bone conduction test: A hearing assessment in which test tones are sent directly to the inner ear by vibration of skull bones. A bone conduction test bypasses the outer and middle ear.

bound morphemes: A unit of language that is meaningful only when it is attached to another unit. Plural markers such as "s" and past tense markers such as "ed" are bound morphemes.

Broca's aphasia: A type of language impairment characterized by damage to Broca's area in the frontal lobe with nonfluent expressive speech, disrupted syntax, and relatively intact auditory comprehension.

C

canal aids: Tiny hearing aids which fit entirely into the auditory canal.

CCC: A credential called the Certificate of Clinical Competence in either audiology or speech-language pathology granted by ASHA.

central lisp: The substitution of a "th" like sound for "s" and "sh."

central nervous system (CNS): The portion of the nervous system encased in a bony covering including the brain and spinal cord.

cerebral cortex: The outermost layer of the cerebrum. It consists of about six layers of neurons. Considered gray matter as opposed to the nerve fibers, or white matter, below.

cerebral palsy: A group of nonprogressive disorders of movement and posture caused by abnormal development of, or damage to, motor control centers of the brain before, during, or after birth.

cerebration: The role of the nervous system in regulation of speech.

Certificate of Clinical Competence (CCC): A credential issued by the American Speech-Language-Hearing Association after completion of prescribed coursework, practicum experience, passing of a national examination, and completion of the Clinical Fellowship Year.

cerumen: Ear wax.

child find: A program conducted in the community that is designed to identify children with developmental delays in motor, cognitive, communicative, or social domains. The goal is to facilitate early identification and intervention.

circumlocutions: A type of avoidance behavior where a difficult word or phrase is described rather than said; talking around the concept.

cleft lip: A separation in the upper lip and in some cases the alveolar ridge. The separation may occur on one or both sides. The condition is congenital, resulting from the failure of the structures forming the lip to meet and fuse properly during embryonic development.

cleft palate: A separation in the soft or soft and hard palates. The condition is congenital, resulting from the failure of the structures forming the palate to meet and fuse properly during embryonic development.

Clinical Fellowship Year (CFY): A mentorship typically occurring during the first year of working professionally as an audiologist or speech-language pathologist and one component of qualifying for the CCC.

closed head injury (CHI): A type of traumatic brain injury (TBI) in which the scalp and membranes remain unbroken though deeper damage to the brain and brainstem may be significant.

cluttering: A type of fluency disorder that often is part of a more pervasive language, reading, or cognitive disturbance; excessive speech rate and part-word repetitions are part of the milieu.

coarticulation: The influence of one speech sound on the production of another speech sound in the same utterance.

cochlea: The snail-shaped portion of the inner ear related to hearing function.

cochlear implant: A surgically implanted device that directly stimulates the auditory nerve.

cognates: Sounds that are the same in manner and place of articulation but that differ in voicing.

communication: Transmission of information from sender to receiver that does not necessarily use speech and language. This can include gestures, facial expressions, or vocal productions.

communicative intent: People communicate for a reason. The two major communicative intents are *imperative* (communicating to influence another's actions) and *declarative* (communicating to influence another's attention).

community clinic: A clinical facility that provides services for speech, hearing, and language disorders that is sponsored by some community agency (e.g., Sertoma International).

compensatory articulation: An alternate production of a speech sound to offset physical or structural barriers preventing the typical production of that sound.

conductive hearing loss: A hearing loss caused by a problem in the outer or middle ear.

confabulation: Language output that contains untruths, often told with elaborate false details not connected with reality.

congenital hearing loss: A hearing loss present at birth.

context generalization: The transfer of correct production of a target sound to other phonetic environments.

contextual tests: Speech sound production tests in which a target sound is assessed in several different phonetic environments.

conversational repair strategies: Mechanisms used to maintain a conversation when the conversation breaks down such as "you went where?"

cranial nerves: Part of the peripheral nervous system. Twelve pairs of nerves which emerge from the brain and brainstem and innervate, among other structures, the speech and hearing mechanism.

cued speech: A system of communication used by individuals with hearing loss. Speech reading is paired with manual cues to help the listener distinguish among sounds which look similar when spoken.

D

deaf: A term used to describe individuals whose hearing loss is so great as to preclude the understanding of speech through the ear alone.

decibels (dB): The unit used to measure sound intensity.

decoding: Taking meaning from a coded message. An essential skill in receptive language.

dementias: A group of disorders of varying etiologies (causes) characterized by declines in cognition, intellect, language, memory, and other skills of daily living.

developmental apraxia of speech (DAS): A motor speech disorder seen in children characterized by difficulty planning and executing the sequence of motor movements required for speech.

dialect: A rule-governed variation of a language spoken by a definable group of people characterized by their culture, ethnicity, or geographical region.

dialect importation: When two dialects are spoken in close geographic proximity, they borrow from one another and incorporate features from the other dialect.

dialectal continuum: Dialects differ from Standard English by a maximum number of linguistic features. Speakers can incorporate many or few of these differences along a continuum of use.

diaphragm: The dome-shaped muscle that separates the thoracic and abdominal cavities.

differential diagnosis: Sorting one type of disorder from another, as in determining among different forms of aphasia, motor speech disorders, fluency disorders, and the like.

diphthong: A vowel sound which is produced by gliding from one vowel sound to another. The vowel sounds in "eye," "boy," and "cow" are diphthongs.

diplophonia: A condition in which the voice simultaneously produces two sounds of different pitch.

direct treatment: Intervention that directly works with the client as opposed to indirectly modifying speech and language through significant others (e.g., parent, teacher, spouse).

disfluent: Speech that is unsmooth or disrupted by any number of events such as hesitations, repetitions, prolongations, and the like.

disorders of resonance: A branch of voice disorders attributed to articulatory and vocal tract transmission issues rather than issues at the level of the glottis.

distortion: A speech sound production error in which the speaker attempts the appropriate phoneme but fails to produce it with complete acoustic accuracy.

due process: A guarantee under the law that parents have status as a full member of the rehabilitation team and can ask questions about goals, procedures, and how they are implemented. The parent also has the right to object to procedures and have the child's program reviewed by an impartial judge.

dysarthria: A group of motor disorders characterized by muscular weakness rather than deficits of cortical planning (as in apraxia); various types of motor-speech impairment exist that may affect aspects of respiration, phonation, articulation, and resonance.

dysphagia: Disorders of swallowing.

E

ear mold: The portion of a hearing aid which fits into the ear canal.

ear training: A stage in traditional treatment for speech sound problems in which the child is taught to identify and discriminate the target sound through hearing.

early multiword communication: A period in language development when a child speaks in two- to four-word utterances (e.g., "mommy eat," "daddy drive car," "doggie eat big bone").

edema: A condition of abnormally large fluid volume in the circulatory system or in tissues; fluid retention and swelling in the vocal folds affect voice production and quality.

encoding: Placing information into a coded message. An essential skill for expressive language.

esophageal speech: A technique for speaking after total laryngectomy that involves swallowing or injecting a small ball of air and its subsequent expulsion to produce vibrated noise in the upper esophageal segment that is shaped into audible speech using articulators.

establishment: The process of teaching a client to perform a communicative behavior that was previously absent from his or her repertoire. For example, teaching a child or adult to produce a new grammatical, phonetic, or vocabulary form.

ethnocentric: The tendency for a person to view other cultures and make value judgments from the perspective of his or her own culture.

eustachian tube: A passage connecting the middle ear cavity with the pharynx.

evaluation: Assessment and diagnosis of a communication disorder through standardized and nonstandardized testing.

expressive language: The use of a coded system to communicate ideas to others.

external auditory meatus: A portion of the outer ear. The passageway running from the aurical or pinna to the tympanic membrane. Also known as the auditory canal.

F

Fetal Alcohol Syndrome (FAS): A birth defect resulting from excessive alcohol intake by the mother during pregnancy.

final position: The position of the last sound in a word.

fluency disorder: Pathology of speech characterized by frequent or marked lack of smoothness in connected speech; several types of fluency disorders exist such as developmental stuttering, neurogenic stuttering, and cluttering.

fluent: Speech that is smooth flowing and void of interruptions (or has only slight but normal interruptions); a communicative aspect that merits consideration in a variety of patients including voice, adult language, motor speech, and stuttering evaluations.

fluent aphasia: Expressive language output that retains smoothness and continuity, even when nonsensical.

fluent verbal output: Spoken language that retains characteristics of being fluent, that is smooth and forward flowing without hesitations and undue effort; often used to describe some forms of aphasia output.

formal testing: Use of standardized testing in assessment of communication.

frequency: The number of cycles per second of a sound wave. The number of vibrations per second of a sound source such as the vocal folds.

fricative: A consonant sound produced by forcing air through a narrow opening. The sounds f, v, th, s, z, sh, zh (as in *vision*), and h are fricatives.

front vowel: Vowels made with the tongue toward the front of the mouth. The vowel sounds in "bee," "bit," "may," "red," and "fat" are front vowels.

functional voice disorders: A disorder with no known structural, physiological, or neurologic cause. A group of voice disorders that have no underlying medical cause and that may, in the early stages, show little or no laryngeal tissue changes.

fundamental frequency: The rate of vibration of the vocal folds based on age, sex, and body stature that is perceived as the pitch of the voice.

G

generalization: The ability of communication goals to transfer to environments (e.g., classroom, home) outside the treatment setting.

generative: Use of a finite set of rules to create an infinite number of utterances as in the rules of syntax.

glossectomy: The surgical removal of all or part of the tongue.

glottal: Referring to the level of the larynx.

H

habitual pitch level: A controversial concept that refers to the average pitch of a person's voice that is typically used.

hair cells: Specialized cells in the cochlea that change pressure waves associated with sound to neural impulses.

hard-of-hearing: A term used to describe individuals whose hearing loss makes difficult, but does not preclude, the understanding of speech through the ear alone.

hearing impairment: Below normal hearing ability.

hearing threshold: The lowest loudness level at which a sound can be heard 50 percent of the time.

hemiplegia: Paralysis affecting only one side of the body.

hertz (Hz): The unit used to measure the frequency of a sound.

high vowel: Vowels made with the tongue elevated above the resting position. Vowels in the words "bee," "hit," "no," and "took" are high vowels.

HIPAA: Health Information Portability and Accountability Act of 1996. This act establishes measures that ensure the security and privacy of healthcare information maintained by healthcare providers, both public and private.

Hispanic English (HE): A dialect of English spoken by people who have Spanish as a first language.

hypernasality: The presence of excessive or inappropriate nasal resonance accompanying speech.

I

identification: The process of locating persons with communication impairments with the aim of further assessing them and providing appropriate treatment.

incidence: A quantified description of how many persons have or have had a particular disorder; for example, the 4–5 percent incidence figure for stuttering includes those in the population who stutter or used to stutter.

incus: One of the three bones in the middle ear.

indirect treatment: A form of therapy in which teachers, parents, or medical professionals accomplish communication treatment goals in the natural environment instead of direct intervention by the SLP.

Individualized Education Program (IEP): A formal statement of assessment information and treatment objectives for children between the ages of 3 and 21 years in public school settings. The IEP must be reviewed and updated annually.

Individualized Family Service Plan (IFSP): Children between birth and 3 years of age must be evaluated with the help of parents or caregivers. The professionals and parents jointly develop an assessment and treatment plan that is evaluated and updated every six months.

Individuals with Disabilities Education Act (IDEA): A federal law mandating procedures for providing assessment and treatment services to students with disabilities in the public school system.

industrial audiologist: An audiologist who specializes in noise abatement, monitoring of hearing health in industrial settings, and prescription of hearing protection for workers to prevent hearing loss.

informal evaluation: Nonstandardized testing of a client. For example, use of a conversational speech sample instead of administration of a standardized test.

initial position: The position of the first sound in a word.

inner ear: That part of the ear consisting of the cochlear and vestibular portions.

intensity: The strength of a sound.

interdisciplinary: Professionals from multiple disciplines (e.g., education, psychology, communication disorders) focusing on a client for evaluation and/or treatment. This model has more communication/cooperation among the disciplines than does multidisciplinary models and less than transdisciplinary models.

intervocalic: Occupying a position between two vowels. For example, the l̲ in "yellow."

in-the-ear aids: Hearing aids in which all components fit into the ear.

J

jargon: Nonsensical speech-language output; a feature of some types of aphasia, particularly Wernicke's.

joint referencing: When a caregiver and a child focus on the same object or event in the communicative context. For example, a parent and a child might be looking at a book together. Joint referencing provides an opportunity to stimulate language by exposing a child to appropriate linguistic models.

L

labiodentals: Consonant sounds formed by the lips and teeth. The sounds f̲ and v̲ are labiodentals.

lack of affect: Not displaying emotion, whether in facial expression, vocal tone, or verbal output.

language: A system of rules and symbols that allows information to be transmitted from sender to receiver. The system includes semantics, syntax, morphology, phonology, and pragmatics.

language deficit: The view that deviations from Standard English represent disorders of communication (this is not currently believed by linguists).

language difference: Dialects are viewed as simply different forms of linguistic communication and not disorders of communication.

language stimulation/modeling: Language stimulation/modeling takes place when a parent or clinician demonstrates the correct use of language in a natural situation. Types of language stimulation are self-talk, parallel talk, imitation, and expansion.

laryngectomy: The partial or complete surgical removal of the larynx as may be necessary in cases of laryngeal cancer.

laryngologist: A physician who specializes in the diagnosis and treatment of laryngeal disorders.

larynx: The tubular structure consisting of cartilages and muscles housing the vocal folds. It is located above the trachea and below the hyoid bone.

lateral lisp: A speech sound error affecting s, sh, and their voiced cognates. Air escapes around the sides of the tongue rather than being channeled down the middle resulting in a "slushy" sound.

least restrictive environment: This is basic to the notion that children with special needs receive services in an environment that does not impose undue limitations or isolation on them. For example, a child with a language disorder must be served to whatever extent possible in the typical classroom and be allowed to interact on a regular basis with normally developing students.

limited language: A period in which children are communicating nonverbally (using gestures), in single words, or in short multiword utterances.

lingua-alveolar: Consonant sounds formed by the tongue and the alveolar ridge. The sounds t, d, s, z, l, and n are lingua-alveolar.

lingua-dental: Consonant sounds formed by placing the tongue between the teeth. The th sounds (voiced and voiceless) are lingua-dental.

lingua-palatal: Consonant sounds formed by the tongue and hard palate. The initial sounds in "show," "choose," and "jump" are lingua-palatal as is the medial sound in "vision."

lingua-velar: Consonant sound formed by the tongue and the soft palate. The sounds k, g, and ng are lingua-velar.

linguistic unit generalization: Transferring the correct production of a target sound from one level of linguistic unit to another. Typically the progression is from syllables, to word, to sentences, to connected speech.

lipreading: Observing the lip, mouth, and facial movements of a speaker in order to interpret the spoken message.

lisp: An articulation error involving sibilant sounds (s, z, sh, zh, ch, and dg). Lisps are typically frontal, in which the tongue is too far forward, or lateral in which air escapes around the sides of the tongue.

long-term care facility: A medical facility that provides ongoing care to patients who are not able to live at home; often called a nursing home.

loudness: The subjective perception of the intensity of sound.

low vowel: Vowels made with the tongue positioned below the resting position. The vowels in the words "fat," "fall," and "law" are low vowels.

M

macroglossia: A condition in which the tongue is abnormally large.

maintenance: A stage of traditional treatment for speech sound disorders in which the frequency of contact between the client and clinician is reduced.

malleus: One of the three bones of the middle ear.

malocclusion: A condition in which the upper and lower teeth are not properly aligned.

manner of articulation: The way in which the articulators shape a sound.

manual methods: The use of sign language for communication.

mean length of utterance (MLU): A length measurement involving computation of the average number of morphemes produced in utterances gathered in a language sample. Morphemes can be free (e.g., *car, dog*) or bound (e.g., *-ed, -ing*) and are still counted in the computation. The calculation is the total number of morphemes produced in a language sample divided by the number of utterances.

medial position: The position occupied by sounds that are neither the first nor last sounds in a word.

medically fragile children: Children with chronic illnesses who require long-term intensive and specialized medical treatment.

metathetic errors: A speech sound error in which the sounds in a word are produced in the wrong order. For example, "pasghetti" for "spaghetti."

microglossia: A condition in which the tongue is abnormally small.

microtia: *See* atresia.

middle ear: The portion of the ear from the tympanic membrane to the cochlea.

mild hearing impairment: A hearing loss between 26 and 40 dB.

mild-to-moderate hearing impairment: A hearing loss between 41 and 55 dB.

minimal pair: Two words differing by a single sound or feature (e.g., *pat* and *bat*).

mixed cerebral palsy: A type of cerebral palsy that occurs in about 10 percent of children with cerebral palsy; the combination may involve two or more types such as having the tight muscle tone of spastic CP and the involuntary movements of athetosis CP as a result of different areas of nervous system involvement.

mixed hearing loss: A hearing loss with both conductive and sensorineural components.

moderate hearing impairment: A hearing loss between 56 and 70 dB.

monotone: A voice characterized by lack of frequency fluctuations; a flattened range of tonality.

morpheme: The smallest meaningful unit of language. Unbound morphemes have meaning when standing alone (e.g., the word *boy*). Bound morphemes have meaning only when attached to unbound morphemes (e.g., plural markers such as the *-s* in *boys* or tense markers such as the *-ed* in *batted*).

morphology: The linguistic rules for the use of morphemes in language. For example, word endings such as *-ed*, *-ing*, and the plural *-s*.

motor speech disorder: A general term that includes apraxia and dysarthria as types of speech disorders resulting from neurologic damage that affects the motor programming and/or control of speech muscles.

multidisciplinary: Professionals from multiple disciplines (e.g., education, psychology, communication disorders) focusing on a client for evaluation and/or treatment. This model has the least amount of interdisciplinary communication/cooperation.

muscular dystrophy: A group of inherited disorders in which strength and muscle bulk gradually decline; nine types of muscular dystrophy are generally recognized.

N

nasal emission: Air escaping from the nose during the production of speech.

nasals: Consonant sounds produced with the nasal cavity coupled to the oral cavity. The sounds m, n, and ng are nasals.

naturalistic treatment: Providing therapy for communication disorders using natural activities such as play or conversation in the client's normal environment such as home or school.

negative practice: Intentionally practicing an incorrect response in order to sharpen the distinction between a correct and incorrect response.

neologism: Literally means "new word" that, though nonsensical, is embedded within an utterance when a person with aphasia speaks.

neoplastic voice disorders: A collection of disorders affecting the laryngeal mechanism in which there is an abnormal new growth of tissue; a mass that when biopsied may prove benign or malignant.

neurogenic stuttering: A type of fluency disorder that is acquired following neurologic damage (e.g., stroke, traumatic injury) or disease; often of adult onset as opposed to developmental stuttering in children.

neurogenic voice disorders: A collection of voice disorders that originate from a neurologic issue.

neurologist: Physician who specializes in conditions of the nervous system.

neuromuscular problems: A family of motor-based, neurologic issues.

neurotic stuttering: A type of fluency disorder that typically has a sudden onset following psychological trauma and that presents with severe, struggled forms of disfluency.

nonfluent aphasia: Expressive language output that lacks smoothness and continuity, often with disfluency types such as hesitations, reduced utterance length, lack of small parts of speech, and word retrieval impairment.

nonverbal communication: The use of gestures in communication such as reaching, pointing, showing, and giving.

O

omission: A speech sound production error in which a sound is deleted.

open head wound: A type of traumatic brain injury (TBI) in which the scalp and membrane is penetrated, for example, a gunshot wound.

oral methods: Communication techniques taught to deaf and hard-of-hearing persons which employ speech as the primary method of communication.

organ of Corti: The structure within the cochlea housing the hair cells.

organic disorder: An anomaly having a structural, physiological, or neurologic cause.

ossicles: The three bones of the middle ear: the malleus, incus, and stapes.

ossicular chain: *See* ossicles.

other disfluencies (ODs): Types of disfluency that are characteristic of persons who do not stutter (as contrasted to stuttering-like disfluencies, or SLDs).

otitis media: An inflammation of the middle ear.

otolaryngologist: A physician who specializes in diseases of the ear, nose, and throat.

otologists: A physician specializing in disorders of the ear.

otosclerosis: A conductive hearing problem that results from a bony growth around the stapes.

ototoxic: Damaging to the hearing mechanism.

outer ear: The portion of the ear consisting of the pinna and the external auditory meatus.

oval window: The portion of the cochlea which contacts the stapes.

P

papilloma: Benign epithelial tumor, such as a wart or wartlike cluster, that is thought to be viral in nature; may occur throughout the body including on or around the vocal folds.

paraphasia: Incorrect but real words used in utterances that often bear some resemblance (phonetic or semantic) to the intended words.

paraplegia: Complete paralysis of the lower half of the body including both legs, usually caused by damage to the spinal cord.

paraprofessionals: Personnel trained to do highly specific tasks under the supervision of a teacher or speech-language pathologist to provide support for the program. In the case of teachers, this includes teacher's aides and in speech-language pathology involves speech-language pathology assistants.

paresis: Condition of muscular weakness, but not paralysis, often attributed to some sort of neurologic damage.

pattern analyses: A speech sound analysis technique which identifies patterns such as phonological processes which underlie sound errors.

peripheral nervous system (PNS): The peripheral nervous system. The portion of the nervous system that exits the bony covering and carries nerve signals to muscles and end organs. Consists primarily of the cranial and spinal nerves.

pharynx: The tubular structure that begins above the larynx and continues upward behind the oral and nasal cavities.

phonation: The production of voice in the larynx.

phonatory disorders: Disorders of voice that are laryngeal in nature as opposed to vocal tract resonance issues.

phoneme: The smallest unit of sound capable of making a difference in meaning. A family of sounds considered to be the same for purposes of changing the meaning of a word.

phonetic context: The sounds which surround a target phoneme.

phonetic environment: *See* "phonetic context."

phonetic placement: A treatment technique for speech sound errors in which the child is given instructions on where to place the articulators to correctly produce the target sound.

phonological awareness: The understanding that words are made up of smaller units (syllables, phonemes) and the ability to manipulate those units.

phonological disorder: A problem related to the cognitive-linguistic aspects of speech sound production.

phonological process: A simplification of adult forms of words typically used by children in their phonological development between 2 and 4 years of age. These simplifications may include alterations of syllabic structure and substitution of easier sounds for more difficult sounds or sound sequences.

phonology: The study of the rules that govern the use and organization of speech sounds in a language.

phonotrauma: Any abuse or misuse of the vocal folds that may lead to various lesions, such as polyps or nodules; the accumulated stress from voicing.

pinna: The portion of the outer ear that is visible on the side of the head. It is also known as the auricle.

pitch: The subjective perception of the frequency of a sound.

pitch breaks: Sudden, often fleeting, pitch changes in the voice when speaking; breaks may pitch higher or lower.

PL 99-457: A federal law specifying guidelines for providing services to children between birth and 3 years of age.

place of articulation: The location in the vocal tract where a sound is produced.

position generalization: The transfer of correct production of a target sound from one word position (initial, medial, final) to another.

postlingual hearing loss: A hearing loss acquired after language was developed.

postponement devices: A type of avoidance behavior that may be used to delay an utterance attempt until it can be more fluent.

postvocalic: Following a vowel.

pragmatics: The use of language in a communicative context taking into account such variables as communication intent, listener perspective, and social status.

prelingual hearing loss: A hearing loss which occurred prior to the development of language.

presbycusis: Age-related hearing loss.

prevalence: A quantified description of how many persons have a particular disorder at any given point in time; for example, the prevalence of stuttering is less than 1 percent of the population in any given year.

prevention: A program carried out by audiologists and speech-language pathologists to reduce the occurrence of communication disorders.

prevocalic: Preceding a vowel.

primary stuttering: A term once used to describe the early stage of developmental stuttering in which a child has easy repetitions and little awareness of disfluencies, as contrasted with the secondary stage.

private practice: A clinical practice in which a professional audiologist or speech-language pathologist provides services to clients from a private office setting.

profound hearing impairment: A hearing loss of 90 dB or greater.

psychogenic voice disorders: A group of voice disorders that have their origin in psychological issues of voice usage.

pure tone audiometer: An instrument for testing hearing which produces tones at various frequencies and intensities.

Q

quadriplegia: Complete paralysis of the body from the neck down.

quality: A perceptual attribute of the voice that may be attributed to glottal issues or even supraglottal resonance; the spectral characteristics of the voice yield perceptual terms such as *breathy, harsh, hoarse,* and a host of others.

R

receptive language: The ability to understand spoken or written messages.

referrals: A method of identifying persons with communication disorders by relying on professionals and parents to refer an individual for assessment.

regional dialect: A dialect that is commonly seen in particular geographic areas (e.g., Southern English).

rehabilitation hospital: A clinical facility to which patients are transferred for rehabilitation services (e.g., physical, occupational, speech therapy) after being discharged from an acute care hospital.

representative language sample: An assessment task for language in which a conversational or play sample is gathered in an attempt to re-create the client's typical communication style. This is contrasted with standardized testing in which clients name pictures or perform tasks that do not represent "real" communication.

resonance: The effects of the size and shape of a cavity on the sound passing through it.

respiration: The inhalation and exhalation of air; breathing.

reverberation: Echoes caused by sound bouncing off walls, ceilings, and floors.

rigidity: A form of cerebral palsy or adult dysarthria characterized by muscles being nonflexible.

rule based: Linguistic productions are part of a rule-based system that governs all areas of language such as semantics, syntax, morphology, phonology, and pragmatics.

S

school register: A type of style shifting in which children speaking AAE use a unique form of their dialect when speaking to adult authority figures such as teachers. This dialect is usually more elaborate in that words and morphemes are included instead of reduced.

screening: The process of briefly assessing communication abilities to determine whether a person should undergo a more intensive assessment. Screenings typically take less than five minutes.

screening test: A test designed to identify those members of a large group who are most likely to have a particular trait or disorder.

secondary stuttering: A term once used to describe the later-developed stage of stuttering in which the speaker has noticeable, nonrhythmic disfluencies and/or avoidance behaviors, as contrasted with the primary stage.

Section 504 of the Rehabilitation Act: A law passed in 1973 that precludes discrimination in terms of access to or benefits from any institution receiving federal financial support. This assumes that such institutions will provide appropriate accommodations for students with disabilities so that they can participate in all reasonable activities.

semantics: The linguistic rules governing word meaning and the selection of vocabulary words for utterances.

semivowel: Speech sounds that are produced when the degree of occlusion in the vocal tract is greater than for vowels but less than that for most consonants. In English, w̲, y̲ (as in *young*), l̲, and r̲ are semivowels.

sensorineural hearing loss: A hearing loss resulting from problems in the inner ear or the nerve pathway leading to the brain.

severity: The degree of something; the extent of involvement, as in the severity of stuttering, aphasia, or other communication disorder, to which a rating might be applied (mild, moderate, severe, or percentage data).

sibilant sound: A consonant sound produced with a hissing sound such as s̲, s̲h̲, and c̲h̲.

Signing Exact English (SEE): A manual communication system that accurately reflects the vocabulary and syntax of spoken English.

single-word communication: A period in language development when a child speaks in one-word utterances (e.g., "ball," "mommy," "doggie").

site of lesion: This refers to the place or location of brain damage.

situation generalization: The transfer of correct production of a target sound from one circumstance to another. For example, from a treatment room to a playground.

slight hearing impairment: A hearing loss between 16 and 25 dB.

sound and feature generalization: Transferring the correct production of a sound or a feature such as voicing to a similar sound or another sound containing the target feature.

spasticity: A form of cerebral palsy or adult dysarthria characterized by muscles being overactive or resistive to stretch.

specifically language impaired (SLI): A term referring to children who have impairments in language but who are age appropriate in cognition, motor ability, and social-emotional ability.

speech: The oral production of language using the human vocal tract.

speech appliance: A device used to assist an individual with the production of speech sounds. Palatal lifts and speech bulbs are considered speech appliances.

speech community: A definable group that uses a particular social dialect (e.g., Hispanic English).

speech-language pathologist: The communication disorders professional who deals with the assessment and treatment of speech, language, and swallowing disorders.

speech notebook: A method for a speech-language pathologist to communicate with parents and teachers. It may contain assignments, rewards, progress reports, or any other information the SLP wishes to convey.

speechreading: *See* lipreading.

spontaneous recovery (aphasia): Improvement of function following brain damage resulting from innate healing and neural plasticity; the time period when treatment may generate optimal improvements.

spontaneous remission (fluency): Also called spontaneous recovery; an unexpected improvement or cure from developmental stuttering that may occur without treatment; outgrowing stuttering.

Standard American English (SAE): A controversial term that refers to the language used by the group in society with power and wealth and the mainstream media. In the United States, SAE is often said to be similar to Midwestern English.

stapes: One of the three bones of the middle ear.

starter device: A word, sound, or action used by a speaker to aid in initiation speech, as may be employed by a person who stutters.

stoma: A hole or "mouth" that can be surgically created; in the field of communication disorders, stoma is short for *tracheostoma*, which is an opening through the neck and into the trachea.

stop consonant: A consonant sound produced by completely occluding the vocal tract, and then in most but not all cases suddenly releasing the built-up air. These sounds are sometimes called plosive or stop-plosive sounds. In English, the stop consonants are p̲, b̲, t̲, d̲, k̲, and g.

street register: A type of style shifting in which children speaking AAE use a unique form of their dialect when speaking to peers. This dialect is usually more restricted in that words and morphemes are reduced or eliminated.

structured treatment: Providing therapy for communication disorders using structured activities usually involving drillwork. This treatment is usually provided in a therapy room and not in the patient's natural environment.

stuttering (developmental stuttering): One of several types of fluency disorders; it first appears in childhood and in the absence of pervasive neurologic symptoms (as might be seen in cluttering or in neurogenic stuttering).

stuttering-like disfluencies (SLDs): Types of disfluent speech behaviors that are typical of persons who stutter, as contrasted to other disfluencies (ODs) that typify the speech of persons who do not stutter.

style shifting: The tendency of a dialect speaker to change speech and language depending on the communicative situation and type of listener with whom they are interacting. For instance, an AAE speaker may use more dialectal features with friends than with Standard English speakers.

subglottic pressure: Exhaled air pressure that builds beneath closed vocal folds and, when sufficient, can blow open the vocal folds to initiate phonation.

submucous cleft palate: A condition in which the mucosal surface of the soft palate is intact but there is a separation in the underlying muscles.

substitution: A speech sound error in which one sound is produced in place of another. Words or phrases that a speaker uses to replace more difficult ones in an attempt to avoid stuttering.

successive approximation: A technique used in treating speech sound errors in which a client is taught to move from a sound that can be produced correctly to the target sound in steps.

syndrome: Multiple anomalies present in a single individual that all have one primary cause.

syntax: The linguistic rules governing word order or grammar in sentences.

T

TE speech: A form of verbal communication that is possible in persons with a total laryngectomy when the surgeon creates a hole or fistula in the trachea–esophagus wall such that exhaled pulmonary air can vibrate the upper esophageal segment for articulated speech.

threshold: With regard to hearing, the loudness at which a sound is just noticeable. The lowest intensity required for a person to hear a sound 50 percent of the time.

threshold test: A hearing test with the purpose of identifying the lowest intensity level at which a person can hear specific frequencies 50 percent of the time.

tongue thrust: An infantile swallowing pattern in which the tongue moves forward during the swallow.

TORCH infections: A group of infections that, when they occur in a pregnant woman, may affect her unborn fetus and result in a number of congenital disabilities including hearing loss. TORCH is an acronym for *t*oxoplasmosis, *o*ther diseases such as syphilis and hepatitis, *r*ubella, *c*ytomegalovirus, and *h*erpes simplex viruses.

total communication: A system of communication for individuals who are deaf that combines spoken and manual language aspects.

trach tube: There are many types of tracheostomy tubes that maintain a surgical opening between the trachea (windpipe) and the neck; an abbreviated term for the apparatus placed in this neck opening is trach tube.

tracheostomy: A hole or opening that can be surgically created in the neck and into the trachea for ease of breathing in some medical conditions or when the larynx has been removed surgically in a laryngectomy; can be shortened to *stoma.*

transdisciplinary: Professionals from multiple disciplines (e.g., education, psychology, communication disorders) focusing on a client for evaluation and/or treatment. This model has the most interdisciplinary communication/cooperation compared to other approaches.

transitional forms: Utterances used by some children at about 12 months of age which are used consistently to refer to objects or people, but are not based on the adult form of any word.

traumatic brain injury (TBI): A generic term encompassing both open head wounds and closed head injuries; surviving patients present with a host of issues including cognitive, communicative, attentional, perceptual, and emotional.

treatment: Direct and indirect; therapy for a communication disorder. This can be done directly in group or individual sessions or indirectly through a consultative model using teachers or parents in service delivery.

tremor: An involuntary, rhythmic alternating movement that may affect muscles of any part of the body; linked to rapid contraction and relaxation of muscles and a common symptom of nervous system disorders.

tympanic membrane: Also known as the eardrum. It is the membrane that separates the external ear canal from the middle ear space.

tympanometer: An instrument used to assess middle ear function.

U

unbound or free morphemes: A unit of language that is meaningful when it occurs alone and which cannot be divided into smaller meaningful units. A word such as "boy" is an unbound morpheme.

university-based clinic: A clinical facility that is part of a university training program in communication disorders in which students gain clinical practicum experience.

V
___

Velocardiofacial Syndrome (VCFS): A condition which includes cleft palate, heart anomalies, and atypical facial characteristics resulting from the deletion of a portion of the long arm of chromosome 22.

Velopharyngeal Inadequacy (VPI): A condition in which the velum (soft palate) and pharynx do not completely separate the nasal cavity from the oral cavity during speech. When the cause is a short palate, the term *velopharyngeal insufficiency* may be used. When the cause is a paralyzed or weak palate, the term *velopharyngeal incompetence* may be used.

velum: The soft palate.

ventilating tubes: Small tubes surgically placed in the eardrum to help drain fluid from the middle ear.

vernacular: A variety of a dialect that is typically used by lower socioeconomic classes in a culture. The vernacular is usually more restricted in terms of function words or word endings than is the version of the dialect spoken by the middle class.

vestibular: Relating to the portion of the inner ear which has to do with balance.

vocabulary spurt: A period in language development, typically around 18 months of age, when the child experiences a marked increase in the size of his or her vocabulary.

vocal folds: Two folds of muscle and their epithelial cover in the larynx. When the vocal folds are set into vibration by air from the lungs, voice is produced.

vocal hygiene approach: A focus on care of the voice through education and reduction of phonotraumas rather than direct clinical manipulation of vocal parameters.

vocal mutation: Rapid growth changes associated with puberty affect the larynx and can cause dramatic changes in the voice; this period is termed vocal mutation and may last 18 months; see also *voice mutation*.

vocal nodules: Nodules (and polyps, though nodules are firmer) are noncancerous growths on the vocal folds that affect manner and quality of voice production; can be unilateral or bilateral and occur in a characteristic location suggesting phonotrauma as a contributing cause.

vocal tract: The area from the larynx to the lips and nostrils. Includes the pharynx, oral cavity, and nasal cavity.

vocalic: Vowel-like.

voice: The sound produced by the vibration of the vocal folds in the larynx.

voice quality: One of the main attributes perceived in the human voice is the tonal quality which may be expressed by adjectives such as smooth, rough, harsh, hoarse, and so forth.

voice treatment: Professional intervention that may focus modifying vocal production along any number of parameters as needed by the circumstance.

voicing: Producing a sound with phonation.

W

Wernicke's aphasia: A type of language impairment associated with damage to Wernicke's area in the temporal lobe of the brain and characterized by fluent expressive (even jumbled) speech and auditory comprehension.

whole-class language experience: A language activity in which an entire classroom participates.

INDEX

A

AAA. *See* American Academy of Audiology
AAC. *See* alternative/augmentative communication
AAE. *See* African American English
abducted vocal folds, 42, 248
ABR. *See* auditory brainstem response
abuse. *See* vocal abuse
academic organization. *See* school system
academic success
   communication disorders and, 391–398
   defining, 389
   with hearing loss, 396–397
academically at risk students, 398
activities of daily living (ADLs), 390
acute care hospitals, 2
ADA. *See* Americans with Disabilities Act
ADD. *See* Attention Deficit Disorder
Adderall, 381, 385
adducted vocal folds, 42, 248
ADHD. *See* Attention Deficit Hyperactivity Disorder
ADLs. *See* activities of daily living
adolescents. *See* puberty, vocal mutation
      during; students
adult language disorders
   aphasias, 341–345
   assessment of, 347–350
   case history information for, 348
   dementias, 347, 350
   educational setting tips for, 352

healthcare professionals tips for, 352–353
language of confusion, 346–347, 350
language of generalized intellectual
      deterioration, 347
QOL issues for, 411–412
right hemisphere impairment, 346, 349–350
treatment principles for, 350–351
adults
   apraxia of speech in, 365
   communication disorders and QOL issues for
      post-school, 406–413
   dysarthria in, 364–366
   neurologic impairments in, 364–368
   stuttering, assessment of, 238–239
   stuttering, treatment of, 239
   swallowing disorders in, 367–368
   voice disorders in, 255–256, 263–264
advocacy, 5–7
affricates, 46–47
African American English (AAE), 194
   individuality/differences within, 200–201
   roots of, 196
   SAE, switching between, 208
   SAE compared to, 201–204
   semantics in, 204
   street register compare to school register in, 200
   style shifting in, 200
   syntax in, 204